SMART BANDAGE TECHNOLOGIES

DESIGN AND APPLICATION

To Mícheál and Caibridh

SMART BANDAGE TECHNOLOGIES

DESIGN AND APPLICATION

JAMES DAVIS

School of Engineering, Ulster University, Jordanstown, Northern Ireland, United Kingdom

ANNA McLISTER

School of Engineering, Ulster University, Jordanstown, Northern Ireland, United Kingdom

JILL CUNDELL

School Health Sciences, Ulster University/Belfast Health and Social Care Trust, Northern Ireland, United Kingdom

DEWAR FINLAY

School of Engineering, Ulster University, Jordanstown, Northern Ireland, United Kingdom

ELSEVIER

AMSTERDAM • BOSTON • HEIDELBERG • LONDON
NEW YORK • OXFORD • PARIS • SAN DIEGO
SAN FRANCISCO • SINGAPORE • SYDNEY • TOKYO

Academic Press is an imprint of Elsevier

Academic Press is an imprint of Elsevier
125 London Wall, London EC2Y 5AS, United Kingdom
525 B Street, Suite 1800, San Diego, CA 92101-4495, United States
50 Hampshire Street, 5th Floor, Cambridge, MA 02139, United States
The Boulevard, Langford Lane, Kidlington, Oxford OX5 1GB, United Kingdom

British Library Cataloguing-in-Publication Data
A catalogue record for this book is available from the British Library

Library of Congress Cataloging-in-Publication Data
A catalog record for this book is available from the Library of Congress

ISBN: 978-0-12-803762-1

For information on all Academic Press publications
visit our website at https://www.elsevier.com/

Publisher: Joe Hayton
Acquisition Editor: Fiona Geraghty
Editorial Project Manager: Maria Convey
Production Project Manager: Lisa Jones
Designer: Matthew Limbert

Typeset by Thomson Digital

CONTENTS

ABOUT THE AUTHORS

James Davis is Professor of Biomedical Sensors at Ulster University. He is a member of the Royal Society of Chemistry and is a Chartered Chemist. His principal interests lie in the design and development of electrochemical sensors for a range of biomedical applications such as wound monitoring, catheter diagnostics, and ostomy management. His research has been supported by the Engineering and Physical Sciences Research Council, Wellcome Trust, Heart Research, United Kingdom; National Institutes of Health, United States, Ireland; Juvenile Diabetes Research Foundation as well as numerous industrial and commercial sponsors. The team members have been involved in wound diagnostics and the design of smart dressings over the past decade and are presently designing systems for the early identification of infection.

Anna McLister completed her undergraduate studies in Biomedical Engineering and is presently completing her PhD within Prof Davis' group. She is engaged in the development of new diagnostic devices for monitoring wound healing. The main focus of her research has been on the design of electrochemical sensors for the decentralized/outpatient monitoring of chronic wounds associated with diabetic foot disease. Her work has involved the design of disposable screen printed sensors modified to confer selectivity toward monitoring wound pH.

Jill Cundell is a Lecturer Practitioner at Ulster University and Belfast Health and Social Care Trust. She has extensive clinical experience in the management of the High Risk Foot, working clinically in Belfast Health and Social Care Trust. She has an MSc in Wound Healing and Tissue Repair (2005) from Cardiff University and is currently undertaking a PhD—Evaluation of the characteristics of leucocyte-rich platelet-rich plasma from participants with diabetes at Ulster University. She received a SOCAP Distinguished Member Award in 2007 and is also an FCPod Med (2011) FFPM RCPS (Glasg) (2012) and a Chartered Scientist.

Dewar Finlay is Reader in Electronic Engineering at Ulster University. He holds a BEng degree in Electronic Systems and a PhD in Computing. He currently teaches courses on digital signal processing and engineering computing to students undertaking both undergraduate and postgraduate studies in Electronic and Biomedical Engineering. His research is focused on the application of technology in healthcare with particular emphasis on connected health and diagnostic algorithms relating to cardiology. He currently serves as a member of the Board of Directors of Computing in Cardiology and is a member of the Editorial Board for the Journal of Electrocardiology.

PREFACE

The development of new materials for use in wound dressing has captured the attention of scientists and engineers for decades and there have been many advances in the design and processing of new systems that can aid healing. In many cases, this pursuit and reporting of new polymer systems has been largely an iterative process, but, in recent years, the quest for dressings that can interact with the wound has brought about a step change in thinking. The advent of "smart" systems has been a rather fashionable label with a vague definition, but it does capture the essence of a move away from passive dressings to those that can respond in a specific manner to the prevailing wound conditions. This can offer an opportunity to facilitate and enhance the wound-healing processes, but it can also provide important diagnostic information about the condition of the wound and the biochemical processes at play. This book aims to cast a spotlight on both the material aspects of the so-called "interactive" dressings and those that aim to provide clinicians with insights into the wound dynamics.

It must be said that this book provides only a glimpse of the research that is being conducted into wound diagnostics and is by no means an attempt to encompass the whole topic. There is an inevitable bias toward electrochemical techniques as this reflects the specialism of the authors, but these are viewed in a hyper critical light and there is, nevertheless, a determined effort to provide some balance through the incorporation of alternative methodologies. Many of these competing approaches are, in fact, ahead of the electrochemical approaches in terms of their progress toward market and there is a healthy competition which, we believe, comes through in the discussion. In some respects, the book aims to serve as a scientific travelogue in the pursuit of a smart dressing that meets the core criteria necessary for implementation within the clinic or home. It charts the current wound management landscape and highlights the different routes that have been taken in the past and how they continue to inform present and future designs. The content reflects a holistic approach and determinedly attempts to avoid providing a treatise on one particular niche. Each chapter is extensively referenced and the authors are satisfied that the reader can easily go "off piste" to follow whichever technique/technology lies at the heart of their search.

A browse through any bioanalytical or materials journal will reveal a large selection of manuscripts purporting to have designed a new type of sensor for the supremely sensitive detection of some target biomarker or other. In many cases, the authors will have characterized the fundamentals of the system and the materials involved but the transfer of the technology to a real application is often overlooked or is simply incorporated as a minor component in an effort to assuage the editorial requirement for real-world demonstrations. It could be anticipated that a large selection of these materials (or sensors) could, in principle, be adapted for use in wound management, but there are severe hurdles to be overcome before any such system could be considered for further development. This book aims to contextualize the many challenges that lie ahead in the translation of what can be a lab bench based material or device to a format intended for use either on or by a patient (or healthcare provider). The various chapters, we hope, provide a rounded view—highlighting the nature of wounds, the factors involved in their healing, and the options available for their management. It brings together existing approaches and outlines the design issues being addressed in the development of new systems. The authors hope that in providing such a broad remit that the reader is given a detailed overview of the main issues and will be able to examine the emergence of new "smart" bandage systems in a critical light.

JD, AMcL, JC, DF, 2016

ACKNOWLEDGMENTS

The material discussed within this book has been the result of many years of research at the sharp end of electrochemistry and materials science with numerous forays into the world of clinical translation. An army of students, undergraduate, masters, and postgraduates have contributed many of the results documented and discussed in the various chapters. The authors express their gratitude to the many whose contribution has given them inspiration and encouragement to pursue the development of new systems for wound diagnostics and the production of this book. We would also like to specifically thank Maria Convey for her extreme patience and encouragement in enabling us to bring the various chapters together.

LIST OF ABBREVIATIONS

ABTS	2,2-Azinobis-(3-ethylbenzothiazoline-6-disulfonic acid)
ADC	Analogue-to-digital converter
ADP	Adenosine diphosphate
AHLs	Acyl-homoserine lactones
AI	Autoinducers
AIP	Autoinducing peptides
ATP	Adenosine triphosphate
BAN	Body Area Network
BED	Bioelectric dressings
bTEFAP	Bacterial tag encoded FLX amplicon pyrosequencing
CatG	Cathepsin G
CCD	Charge-coupled device
CEA	Cultured epithelial autografts
CMC	Carboxymethyl chitosan
CRP	C-reactive protein
CTGF	Connective tissue growth factor
CV	Cyclic voltammetry
CVI	Chronic venous insufficiency
DFU	Diabetic foot ulcer
DGGE	Denaturing gradient gel electrophoresis
DSP	Digital signal processing
ECM	Extra cellular matrix
EGF	Epithelial growth factors
EPS	Extracellular polymeric substances
FGF	Fibroblast growth factors
GM-CSF	Granulocyte macrophage colony stimulating factor
GUV	Giant unilamellar vesicles
HA	Hyaluronic acid
HNE	human neutrophil elastase
IDSA	The Infectious Disease Society of America
IGF	Insulin-like growth factor
IL	Interleukin
IPN	Interpenetrating network
KGF	Keratinocyte growth factor
LED	Light-emitting diode

MALDI-TOF	Matrix-assisted laser desorption ionization time-of-flight mass spectrometry
MMP	Matrix metalloproteases
MPO	Myeloperoxidase
NPWT	Negative pressure wound therapy
PAN	Personal area networks
PDGF	Platelet-derived growth factor
PEG	Poly(ethylene glycol)
PEO	Poly(ethylene oxide)
PG	Peptidoglycans
PGA	Polyglycolic acid
PHEMA	Poly (hydroxyethylmethacrylate)
PLA	Polylactide
PLGA	Poly(lactic-co-glycolic acid)
pNA	p-Nitroanilide
POCT	Point of care testing
PS	Polyurethanes
PUSH	Pressure Ulcer Scale of Healing
PVA	Poly(vinyl alcohol)
PVD	Peripheral vascular disease
PVdC	Poly(vinylidenechloride)
PVP	Poly(vinyl pyrrolidone)
QS	Quorum sensing
RBB	Remazol Brilliant Blue
RFID	Radiofrequency identification
rhPDGF	Recombinant human platelet-derived growth factor
ROS	Reactive oxygen species
SAM	S-adenosylmethionine
SPE	Screen-printed electrode
SQW	Square wave voltammetry
TGF	Transforming growth factor
TGF-β	Transforming growth factor beta
TNF	Tumor necrosis factor
UT	University of Texas ulcer classification
VAC	Vacuum-assisted closure
VEGF	Vascular endothelial growth factors
VLU	Venous leg ulcer
XO	Xanthine oxidase
XPS	X-ray photoelectrospectroscopy

CHAPTER ONE

Introduction to Wound Management

J. Davis, A. McLister
School of Engineering, Ulster University, Jordanstown, Northern Ireland, United Kingdom

1.1 INTRODUCTION

Small cuts and scratches are part and parcel of everyday life and most people, providing the trauma to the skin is relatively minor, will cede responsibility for repair of the wound to the myriad of biochemical processes that govern wound healing. In effect, beyond the simple cleansing of the wound, the body will be expected to act to reestablish the integrity of the skin barrier on its own accord with only the briefest oversight from the patient. This is not however always the case and the healing processes that would normally regulate tissue regeneration can become slowed or stalled [1–4]. The latter can arise as a consequence of numerous factors such as infection, compromised nutritional status, and poor circulatory supply. More often than not, however, a slow healing wound arises as a consequence of a comorbid condition (typically diabetes, spinal surgery, etc.) and, as a result, the true impact of their management is often hidden behind the cloak of these other conditions [1]. Slow healing wounds, typically termed chronic wounds, have been widely regarded as a "silent epidemic" that affects a significant proportion of the world's population but, it is only in recent years that they have been regarded by funding agencies as a major issue that has significant impact in socioeconomic terms [1,4].

Considering the impact on the patient themselves and their families dealing with the consequences of the daily management of a chronic wound, it quickly becomes clear that the total cost is simply immeasurable [1,4]. Chronic wounds are invariably long-term conditions which are painful, debilitating, and compromise the quality of life for sufferers [1–4]. Current approaches to the management of the wound often require that those afflicted take sick leave from their work until their wounds are healed [4]. Sadly, the situation can all too readily progress to the point at which, for many patients living with nonhealing wounds, amputation of an affected limb may be required [4,5]. This can dictate a change in the nature of employment and can, in severe cases, render the sufferer permanently disabled and unable to work [4,6,7]. There is a pressing need for a greater understanding of the processes involved in wound healing and the production of a new generation of dressing that can actively encourage wound closure.

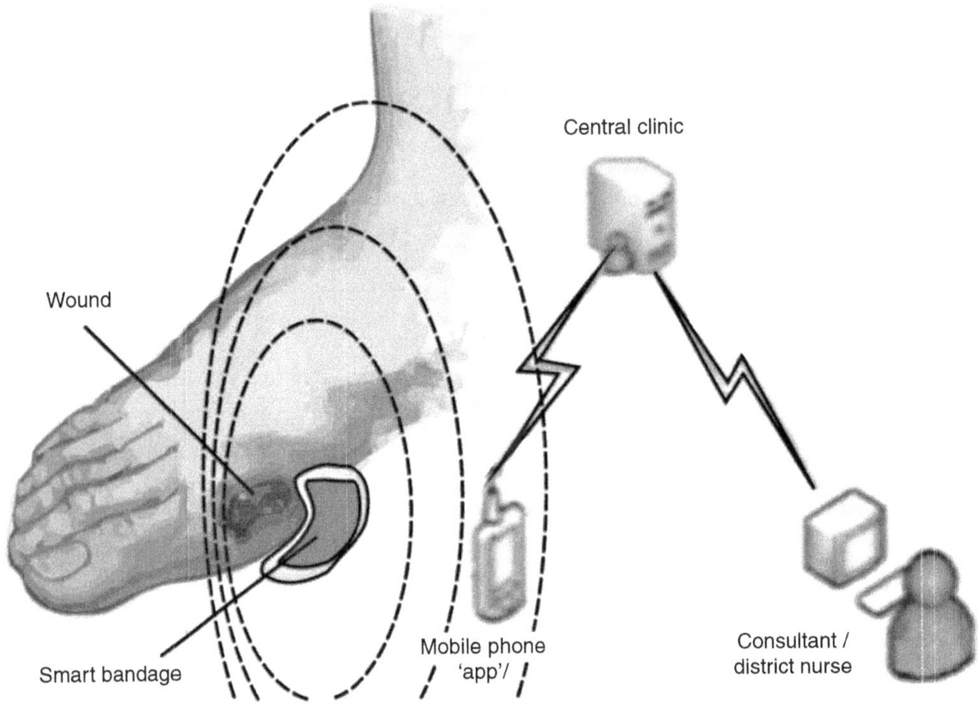

Figure 1.1 ***Connected health approaches to chronic wound monitoring [8].***

The aim of this book has been to provide an overview of the different approaches that have been taken in the development of bandages and wound dressings, and to provide some insights into the emergence of new technologies that could revolutionize the way wounds are treated in the future. New materials capable of being translated into innovative, interactive dressings abound within the literature, but there is also a need to ensure that the material is clinically effective and economically viable given the current pressures on healthcare budgets. One aim is for the development of intelligent, decentralized, wound care technologies that can monitor the condition of the wound—reporting directly to the patient and/or healthcare practitioner such that more informed decisions can be taken in regard to treatment (Fig. 1.1) [8,9]. Ultimately, it would be hoped that these systems could act autonomously to facilitate the healing processes or minimize complications such as inflammation or infection [8–10].

It can be envisaged that the development of new technologies that can reduce treatment times and minimize complications will have major impact, vastly improving patient outcome and delivering substantial cost benefits. One of the key findings in the

World Union of Wound Healing Societies' report: "Diagnostics and Wounds: A Consensus Document" was that "diagnostic tools need to be moved into the clinic or the patient's home to ensure optimal care is provided for patients with wounds" [11]. At present, there are few commercially available technologies to address this recommendation. The realization of such smart systems that promote healing but which could also provide feedback or telemetry on the healing dynamics are however now beginning to appear with increasing regularity within the literature [8,9,12,13].

It can be envisaged that the remote/periodic electronic measurements of physical and chemical markers within the wound would have a significant impact on current wound management practices through providing the care team with a robust picture of the cellular and biochemical health of the wound. Such technologies could be pivotal in reducing costs through increasing the efficiency of the treatment regime. In particular, bandage pressure, dressing moisture, wound pH, and temperature are key factors in the decision processes that direct intervention. A system that can alert a patient that a dressing needs replaced or inspected due to an "irregularity" within the wound could easily rationalize nursing effort and markedly cut costs through a combination of greater efficiency and the saving due to complications being minimized [8,9].

There is now a need to consider the principles that underpin these systems to identify their key characteristics and the impact they can have on the wound. The design of such smart systems requires an interdisciplinary approach and the involvement of a network of expertise. There are four broad areas which are central to the development of interactive or "smart" bandages and dressings: monitoring healing, understanding the dynamics of healing and the material interactions, treatment interventions, and the electronics for facilitating the intelligence needed for establishing control over the other three [14]. An indication of the specialisms which play a pivotal role in the development, application, and validation processes is highlighted in Fig. 1.2 along with their tentative initial alignment. The latter represents the traditional discipline-specific aggregations but such boundaries and distinctions are becoming increasingly blurred.

This book does not seek to provide low-level details of the underpinning physiology, chemistry, physics, and electronics that are increasingly applied to wound dressings but rather seeks to train a spotlight on the different strategies and to inform the reader, at a relatively high level, of the major properties of the materials and their exploitation and clinical application. There is a bias toward the management of diabetic foot ulcers (DFU) within the book as it reflects the direct research interests of the authors but, it must be noted, the materials and methodologies will, almost invariably, have application across the spectrum of chronic wound management. Before considering the nature of the material developments, it is necessary to identify the significance of wound care and to map the healthcare landscape in which new dressings will be employed.

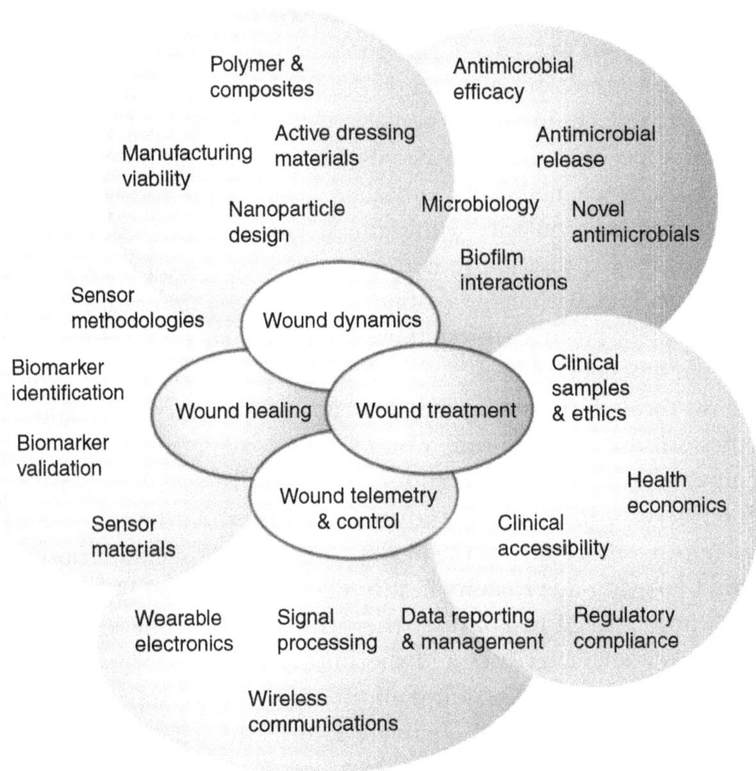

Figure 1.2 ***Multidisciplinary input necessary for smart bandage development [14].***

1.2 WOUNDS: ACUTE AND CHRONIC

It is inevitable that everyone will suffer from a wound of some sort during their lifetime but, in the vast majority of cases, it will heal in a relatively short period of time. The latter are generally classed as acute wounds and can vary tremendously in nature from superficial abrasions to the much more dramatic, such as surgical incisions [15]. Despite the nature and circumstances of the injury, the only significant complication to arise in the normal healing cycle is likely to be infection but, otherwise the wound would be expected to heal in a relatively short period of time. Wounds can be placed into various categories depending on nature and extent of the injury and some of the more common are highlighted in Fig. 1.3.

Dowsett et al. [16] acquired considerable insights into the present state of wound care in the United Kingdom through a combination of surveys targeted at wound care practitioners. Their report uncovered that 74% of wounds needing clinical attention are being managed within the community [16]. This is of particular significance as are

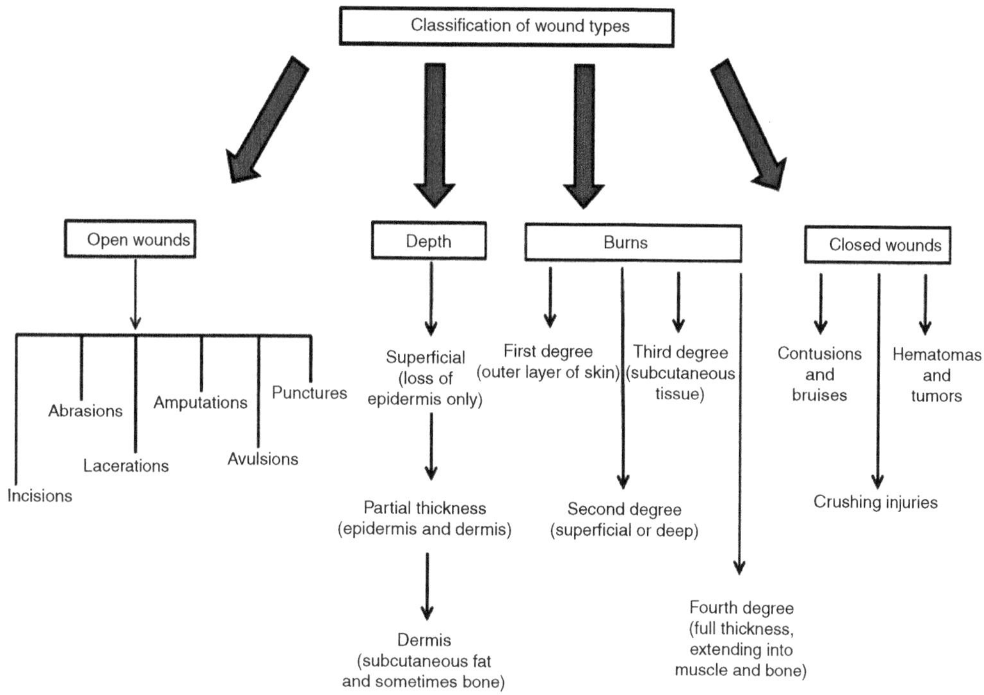

Figure 1.3 ***Acute wound categorization [15].***

the types of wound which are regularly treated by community nurses. A breakdown of the more prevalent wound type is detailed in Fig. 1.4.

As mentioned previously, the healing process can come to a halt with the result that the patient is left in limbo with no clear sign of improvement. At this stage there is a need for more targeted clinical interventions to restart the process. While the normal, acute wound, inflammatory phase will typically cease after a period of several weeks [15–17], in the case of chronic wounds it can persist for months and potentially for years [16–18]. The results of the Dowsett survey indicated that some 40% of wounds can take more than 3 months to heal [16] as indicated in Fig. 1.5. At this stage the wound would begin to fall into the chronic classification category.

Chronic wounds fail to heal through either repeated trauma or as a consequence of an underlying physiological condition such as diabetes [18]. This results in a disruption to the normal sequence of events that leads to successful healing [19–21]. The condition is exacerbated by additional complications that can affect the bones, joints, and nerves, and where there is an excessive production of exudate, maceration of the tissue can also occur. These factors can significantly impede normal healing processes [22] and the aim of the dressing is to enable remedial action to be taken such that the conditions for stimulating/reactivating the processes necessary for healing and wound closure are

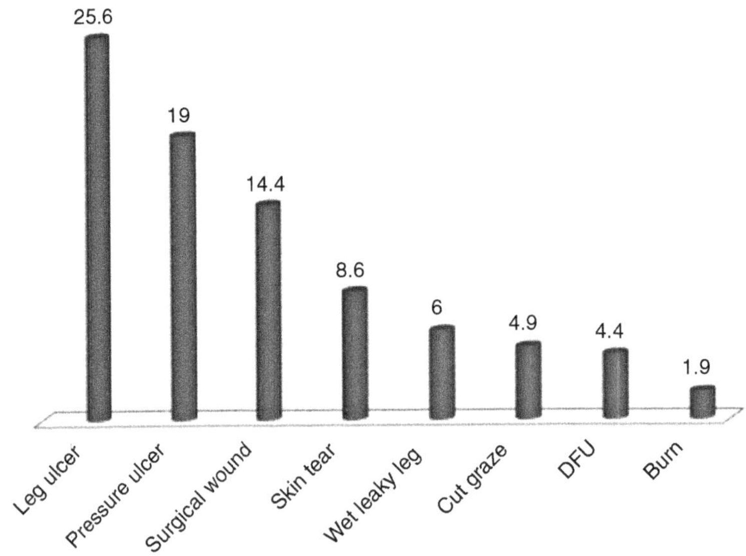

Figure 1.4 ***Prevalence of various wound types in the United Kingdom.*** *(Adapted from Dowsett et al. [16]).*

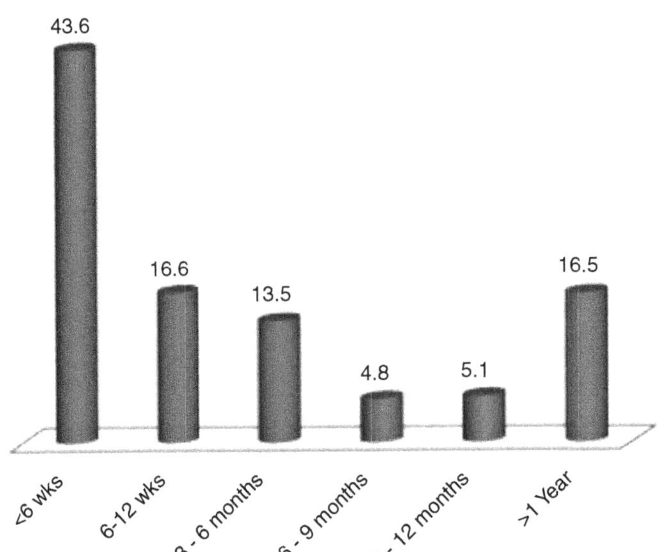

Figure 1.5 ***Wound healing time.*** *(Adapted from Dowsett et al. [16]).*

promoted. Given the data detailed in Fig. 1.4, the candidates most likely to exhibit slow healing/chronic wound characteristics are venous leg ulcers, pressure ulcers, and diabetic foot ulcers and these form the majority of the wounds taking over 1 year to heal [16].

1.2.1 Pressure Ulcers

Pressure ulcers result from pressure being applied to the skin which leads to a breakdown in the underlying tissue and are commonly known as "bedsores" or "pressure sores." The formal definition of a pressure ulcer is: "localized injury to the skin and/or underlying tissue usually over a bony prominence, as a result of pressure, or pressure in combination with shear and/or friction" [23]. The severity of the condition is typically graded in terms of: superficially discolored/bruised skin (Grade 1), broken/damage skin (Grade 2), open wound (Grade 3), which if left untreated can progress to the point where the underlying muscle or bone becomes exposed, damaged, or infected (Grade 4). These are illustrated in Fig. 1.6 along with the more common sites of ulceration. The additional pressure at the wound site causes the blood flow to the skin to slow or cease such that the affected skin becomes starved of oxygen and nutrients. This compromises the affected tissue leading to the onset of ulceration [23]. The critical considerations are: how much pressure and for how long? The common assumption is that they occur in patients who are immobile but this is not always the case. While even small degrees of pressure on the skin over a lengthy time period can lead to ulceration, ulceration can also occur over relatively short durations where the pressure has become excessive.

The majority (72%) of those afflicted with pressure ulcers are over 65-year old and are liable to have some comorbid condition (diabetes, dementia, stroke). A worrying trend is that the prevalence of pressure ulcers tends to be high in critical care units and

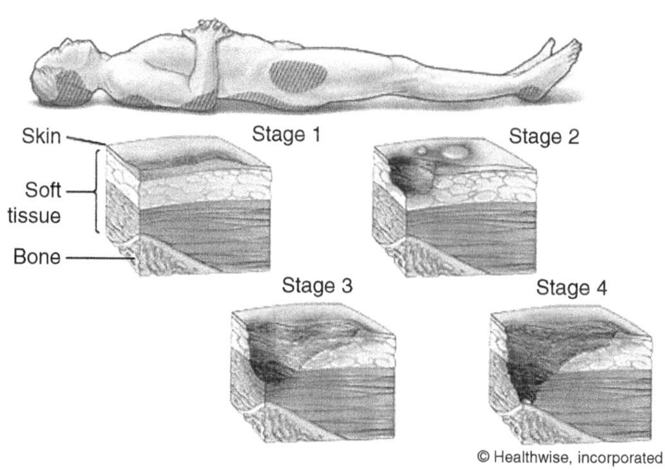

Figure 1.6 ***Sites vulnerable to pressure ulcers and injury categorization.***

figures for both the United States and Europe suggests that it stands at over 20% of admissions [23,24]. One-third of those were estimated to be at a severe grade (3 or 4) and, rather startlingly, 58% were hospital acquired. The importance of reducing the number suffering from pressure ulcers has long been recognized and, in recent years, there has been a raft of studies attempting to promote and assess new strategies. The core intention has been to reduce the number of category 3 and 4 wounds. A particularly successful approach has been the SSKIN system which involves surface, skin, keep moving, incontinence, and nutrition [16]. The key is diligence in monitoring the patients for skin damage. This is an ideal concept but, in the real world, where there are pressures on the care setting to cut costs and staff time, the vigilance of staff can be compromised to the detriment of the patient. It has been estimated that up to 29% of those suffering from a pressure ulcer reside with a long-term care facility [25,26] and the failure to prevent pressure ulcers within such settings has resulted in increasing litigation. Thus far, the judicial processes have favored the claimants in up to 87% of cases [26,27].

Residential care homes are not however the only concern as the number of hospital patients who develop pressure ulcers has seen increases of 63% over the past decade [28] and, it has been reported that in 2007, there were more than a quarter million preventable cases [29]. It is little surprise to find that there has been an ever-increasing range of technological solutions to aid prevention and treatment and they can go some way to addressing these concerns—the application of polymer gels is one example where their application has been reported to be effective in reducing hospital acquired pressure sores with a reduction of some 70% [16].

1.2.2 Venous Leg Ulcers

Venous leg ulcers tend to develop when there is a problem with the circulation of blood in the leg veins causing an increase in pressure which gradually damages the blood vessels within the skin. As a result, the skin becomes fragile and can be prone to ulceration and the development of an open wound. The pathophysiology of the condition is complex but is largely attributed to chronic venous insufficiency (CVI) and is caused by the failure of the calf muscle pump (Fig. 1.7), which is responsible for venous blood flow. An added complication is abnormal flow—typically backflow or reflux and in most cases, the complications arise through dilated veins and or faulty valves [30].

It is known that CVI leads to the development of venous hypertension which results in distension of the capillary walls and transfer of the blood constituents into the surrounding tissues. The leakage of fibrinogen is particularly problematic as it is converted into fibrin which subsequently forms deposits that, it has been postulated, act as a barrier to the passage of oxygen and nutrients to the tissues. The result is hypoxia and the onset of ulceration [31,32], though whether the fibrin "cuffs" are wholly responsible remains a matter of debate [33]. It has been also been suggested that the fibrin effectively traps growth factors, thereby preventing their action and hence prolonging the process of healing [34].

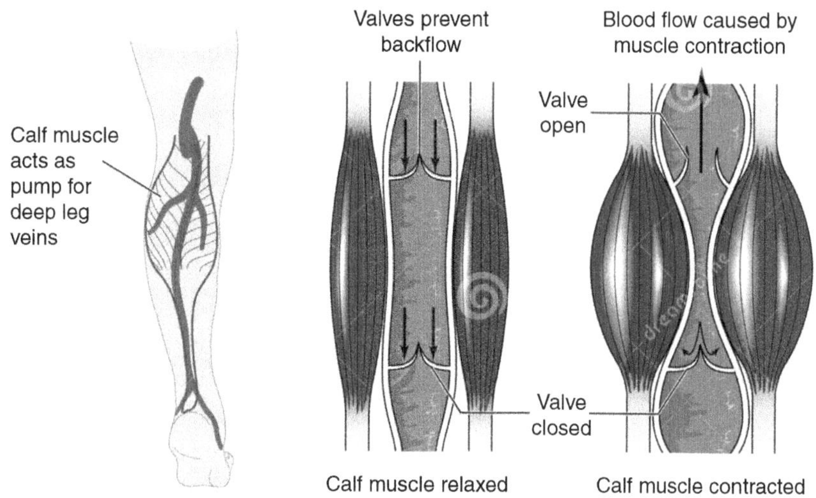

Figure 1.7 ***Action of the calf pump.***

It has been suggested that venous insufficiency may also induce an accumulation of white blood cells (leukocytes) in the small blood vessels, releasing a host of inflammatory factors (proteolytic enzymes, cytokines, and reactive oxygen species) [35,36]. These will invariably contribute to ulceration and, if prolonged, will further increase the vascular damage and promote chronic wound formation [35,36]. It is also possible that this cellular build-up within the confines of the small vessels could result in blockage which will exacerbate the ischaemia. The ulcer can arise anywhere on the leg or foot and it has been estimated that there are some 600,000 patients at any one time in the United States [37,38]. The global prevalence is estimated to lie in the 1–3% region [38].

1.2.3 Diabetic Foot Ulceration

The pathophysiology of Diabetic Foot Ulcers is considered in depth in Chapter 2 and used as a model example for the clinical approach to the assessment, treatment, and management of chronic wounds. In summary, however, diabetes presents numerous complications with sensory, motor, and autonomic neuropathies being among those of direct significance to the onset of DFUs [5,39]. The critical issue in considering DFUs is that sensory neuropathy can greatly reduce awareness of pressure, heat, or injury which would otherwise warn the patient through the normal expression of pain or discomfort. As a consequence, it is all too easy for mechanical trauma to occur through simply being unaware of the events/incidents that is causing it. Repetitive damage inevitably leads to ulceration [39]. Motor neuropathy leads to issues with joints and muscle within which inevitably impairs the foot biomechanics, changes the patient's normal gait, and results in pressure on the foot being unevenly distributed. Where the latter is focused on bony prominences, the stress arising from ambulation will damage the underlying skin and an ulcer will arise [40]. Autonomic neuropathy principally affects the skin whereby increases risk of crack and fissures as a consequence of dry areas and leaves the patient susceptible to infection and ulceration [41].

1.3 WOUND HEALING

Once a wound has formed, an organized series of processes will normally proceed until the wound has been bridged by scar tissue [42]. These stages in healing are discussed in detail within Chapter 2 in the context of DFU treatment but, it is useful to survey the range of processes and the protagonists involved here such that the options that exist in the treatment plan can be more fully understood. The process of healing involves a complex interplay of many biochemical and cellular species such as parenchymal cells, blood cells, and a huge array of soluble mediators. The latter can be important in providing some diagnostic information on the condition of the wound and will be discussed in greater depth in Chapter 6. There are three overlapping phases which dominate the healing process and are classified as the inflammatory, proliferative, and tissue remodeling phases [42]. A summary of their temporal relationship in acute and chronic wounds is highlighted in Fig. 1.8.

1.3.1 Inflammation

The inflammatory phase is the immediate response to the trauma and sets about preparing the groundwork for the remaining two phases. The wound swells and there is the inevitable bleeding which is a primary mechanism through which debris and

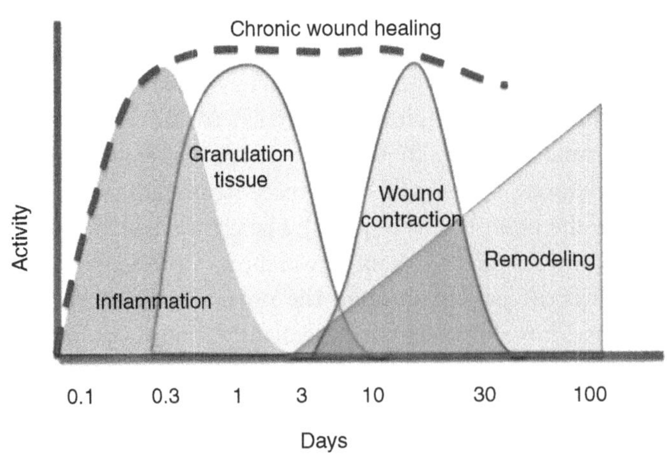

Figure 1.8 ***The various stages of healing in acute and chronic wounds.***

toxins can be removed. Coagulation is needed for wound protection and hemostasis. Soon after an injury, inflammatory cells are sent to the site of the wound and a fibrin plug is formed. This consists of platelets embedded into polymerized fibrinogen, fibronectin, vitronectin, and thrombospondin. It immediately fends of any bacteria as well as providing temporary coverage. While converging within the plug, platelets aggregate and release growth factors such as platelet-derived growth factor (PDGF) and transforming growth factor (TGF). Inflammatory cells such as neutrophils and macrophages aid in wound debridement whereby dead cells are removed. They both produce key growth factors as well as mediators that help fuel the repair process. Over the following 2–3 days, dermal and inflammatory cells at the wound site produce a powerful arrangement of growth factors and cytokines. From previous granulation, the presence of macrophages, fibroblasts, and endothelial cells initiates the process of wound contraction [42,43].

1.3.2 Proliferation

As the inflammatory phase begins to simmer down, the migration of cells within the wound bed occurs and epidermal cells at the wound margins begin to increase in number in a prelude to wound contraction. It has been estimated that during this phase cells may travel 3 cm or more which when considered the scale is an incredible journey. The presence of extra cellular matrix (ECM) proteins, angiogenesis, contraction, and keratinocyte migration are essential components in this phase. Matrix proteins provide substrates for cell movement, which facilitates the change in cell behavior and provides structures to reestablish the integrity and function of the tissue. Granulation tissue begins to appear and is composed of new connective tissue and tiny blood vessels and is due to the fibroblast and macrophage activity, which provides a source of growth factors that maintains angiogenesis and fibroplasias [43,44]. This culminates in the production of collagen and new capillaries which aids contraction of the wound edges.

1.3.3 Tissue Remodeling

The previous stages generally take a few days to several weeks to complete depending on the nature and size of the injury and assuming that there are no underlying conditions that impede the dynamics of the various conditions. The final stage usually commences thereafter but in the case of chronic wounds which have become stalled in the previous stages (as indicated in Fig. 1.9), there can be a significant delay of months and, in the worst cases, years after the initial injury. This phase is typified by the remodeling of the dermal tissue whereby fibroblasts continue to stimulate collagen synthesis. Collagen is released in the ECM where it attains its characteristic triple helix form and begins to form more significant structures through intra and intermolecular interactions. The end result is a highly stable and strong collagen mesh [45,46].

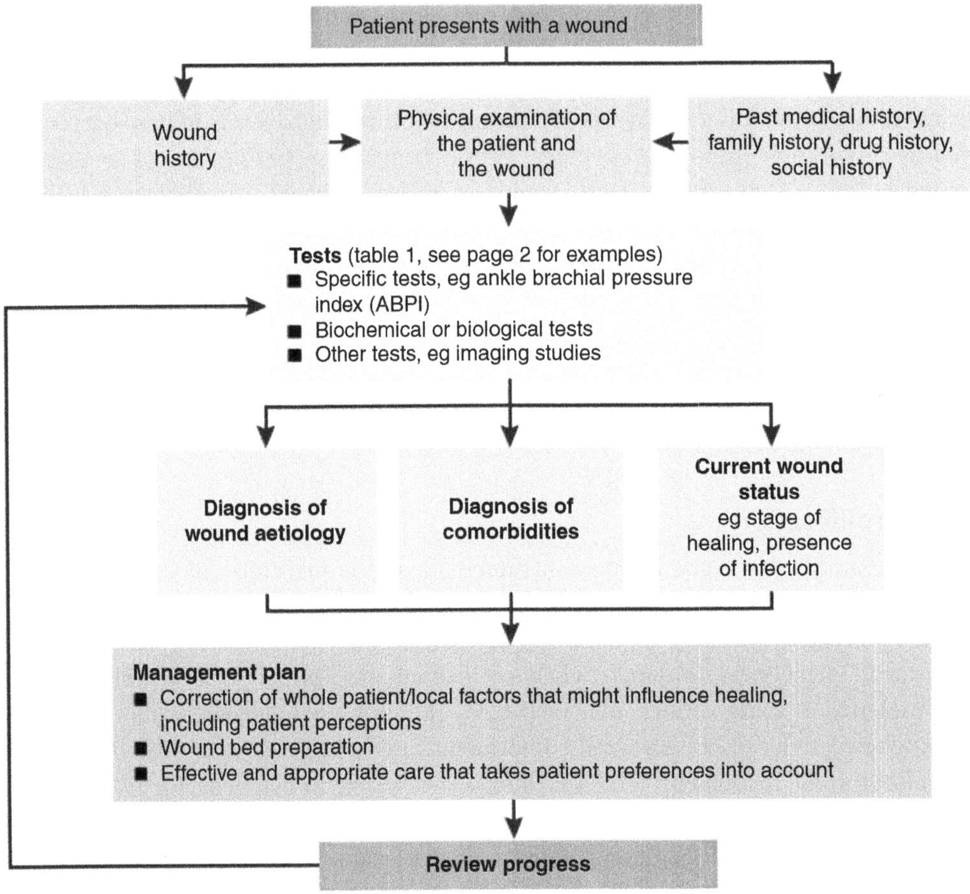

Figure 1.9 ***Generalized wound management plan [11].***

1.4 WOUND MANAGEMENT STRATEGIES

Examination of chronic wounds relies principally on the classical approaches to clinical assessment involving consideration of the patient's medical history combined with a preliminary physical examination. The latter typically involves consideration of wound location, exudates, pain, oedema, lipodermosclerosis, and hyperpigmentation and will almost inevitably be followed by a number of tests through which to determine the wound aetiology, comorbidities and to gauge the current status of the wound. The basic approach, as advocated by Harding and colleagues [11] in their "Diagnostics and wounds – A consensus document," is summarized in Fig. 1.9 [11]. The over-riding aim is to develop an appropriate management plan through which the wound can be regularly monitored and appropriate interventions employed to promote healing progression.

1.4.1 Scoring Systems

A series of tests, essentially prognostic tools, are generally employed at the time of consultation to aid the assessment process outlined in Fig. 1.9. Wound classification based on the application of a scoring system is normally used at the outset and is a rapid profiling method that can be linked to the development of strategies for clinical management and prediction of outcome and typically involves the physical assessment of the wound characteristics. Chronic wounds are highly variable with different causes and prognoses and, therefore, it follows that there is a clear requirement for an unambiguous system of classification with a common language that is readily translated from one care setting to another [5,47]. Taking Diabetic Foot Ulcers as an example, a variety of scoring systems have been proposed (Fig. 1.10) but as yet none has been universally accepted and the absence of a definitive classification system can be attributed to the diversity of wounds encountered in clinical practice. A large number of factors can contribute to the healing progression or indeed the failure to heal and, there can be considerable difficulty in determining which of the many aetiological factors predominate in a particular wound. This is compounded by the absence of simple and robust methods to determine the extent or severity of those factors (particularly ischaemia, neuropathy, and infection) [5,47]. It is also possible that there may be multiple ulcers and different lesions—all of which will possess their own distinct characteristics and it is clear that the outcome of one may be influenced by the outcome of the others.

Ideally, the classification system needs to be simple enough to be remembered and thus employed but, must retain enough precision to be useful. The latter is dependent on the clarity of the terms used to categorize the wound (ie, distinguishing between exudate and slough) and thus ensure that ulcers and lesions will be classified similarly across different care settings [5,47,48]. This is vital to ensure continuity given the mobility of both patients and the clinical staff. This all assumes that the classification system

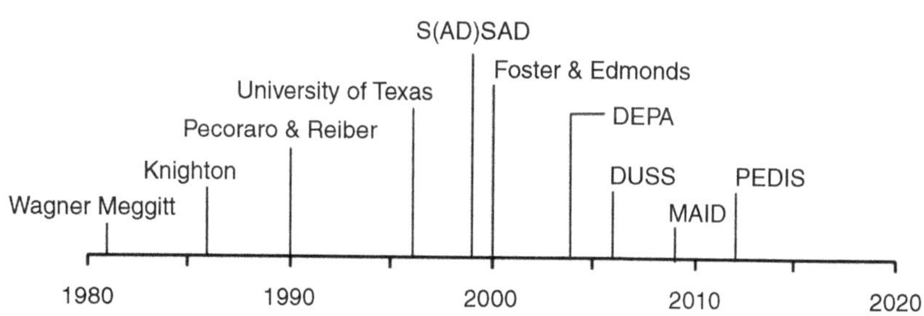

Figure 1.10 ***Evolution of DFU scoring systems.***

Table 1.1 Wagner Meggitt classification scale

Grade	Description
0	Intact skin (only foot symptoms like pain exist)
1	Superficial ulcer
2	Deep ulcer to tendon, bone or joint
3	Deep ulcer with abscess or osteomyelitis
4	Forefoot gangrene
5	Whole foot gangrene

will be universally adopted. As no definitive classification system exists, there has been a gradual evolution in the design of scoring systems as the shortcoming of one is typically addressed in more recent adaptations (Fig. 1.10) [48]. The intended use of the classification system must also be carefully weighed, as a system designed purely for clinical care can be relatively descriptive while one used for audit purposes associated with research studies will generally possess a far greater degree of structure to aid comparison across large population data sets [5,48]. There are extensive literature resources comparing and contrasting their respective merits and limitations [47,48], and a detailed examination of each is beyond the scope of this book but, a summary, highlighting the commonalities and differences in classifying foot ulcers, is considered.

The Wagner–Meggitt system was one of the earliest forms and is used to classify DFUs into six categories based on wound depth and the extent of gangrene [49–51] and is highlighted in Table 1.1 and Fig. 1.11. The system only deals explicitly with infections (deep wound abscess, joint sepsis, or osteomyelitis) in Grade 3 and there is essentially no differentiation between the different types.

The University of Texas (UT) ulcer classification (Table 1.2), in contrast, utilizes a 4×4 matrix in which the depth of the wound and presence (or absence) of infection or

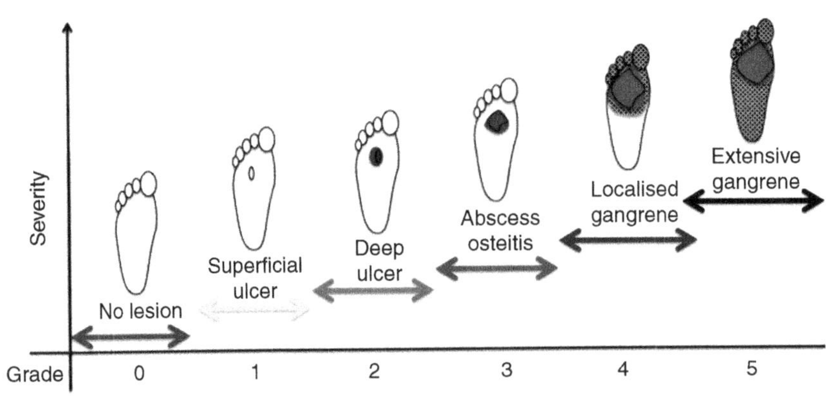

Figure 1.11 ***Graphical representation of the Wagner–Meggitt scoring system.***

Table 1.2 University of Texas (UT) classification scale

Grade	Description
0	Preulcerative site, or healed ulcer.
1	Ulcer through the epidermis ± dermis, but not to tendon, capsule or bone 1A—without infection or ischaemia 1B—with infection but no ischaemia 1C—with ischaemia 1D—with ischaemia and infection
2	Ulcer to capsule or tendon 2A—without infection or ischaemia 2B—with infection but no ischaemia 2C—with ischaemia 2D—with ischaemia and infection
3	Ulcer to bone or joint 3A—without infection or ischaemia 3B—with infection but no ischaemia 3C—with ischaemia 3D—with ischaemia and infection

ischemia are related [52,53]. This is a more comprehensive scale and includes risk stratification and expresses tissue breakdown, infection, and gangrene separately. The system has been found to successfully predict the likelihood of complications in a number of studies [52,53].

1.4.2 TIME Framework and Wound Bed Preparation

There are many factors that are vital to the delivery of effective wound management and, although the peculiarities of a given injury will set up different assessment criteria, the TIME approach has been shown to be useful. The TIME concept has been recognized for many years and aims to provide a simple though logical procedural framework for wound management. The basic format (highlighted in Table 1.3) is based on clinical observation of four key factors and from those a series of actions can be enacted [15,54–56].

The TIME framework is a useful, albeit simple, tool through which to identify the key barriers to healing and it offers the primary foundation for a plan of care to overcome these and reinitiate healing. The core tenet of the system is effective wound bed preparation, but it must be noted that if a wound is stalled, there will be a mixture of factors involved and it is vital to consider the wider context of the condition and the patient [53]. The TIME approach therefore is merely a framework that has been integrated within much more elaborate care systems. A detailed patient assessment will uncover the underlying aetiology and other factors that may be instrumental in delaying or prolonging healing (ie, poor nutrition) [54]. There are numerous examples of where the TIME

Table 1.3 Time framework for wound bed preparation

Observation	Pathophysiology	Action
Tissue nonviable or deficient	Dead cells and debris impede migration of cells and healing and serves a breeding ground for bacteria	Debridement
Infection or inflammation	Uncontrolled inflammation process or infection may perpetuate a cycle of repeated injury and prevent cellular migration and wound bed reconstruction	Introduce: antimicrobials, protease inhibitors, antiinflammatories
Moisture balance	Deficient moisture will impede cellular migration and transport of growth factors. Excess moisture can induce maceration of periwound tissue	Apply moisture balancing dressings Apply absorbant dressings or negative pressure therapy for exudate removal
Edge of wound	A migrating epithelial edge is a visible indicator that healing is taking place.	Reconsider assessment Debridement Skin grafts Adjunctive therapies

Source: Adapted from Dowsett and Newton [54].

ethos can be applied—one example that is the "Care Cycle" which revolves around the wound preparation is detailed in Fig. 1.12 [54].

The "Care Cycle" is but one of many approaches to the management of wounds and while different categories of injury (ie, PU, venous leg ucler (VLU), DFU) will have evolved their own particular approach, most will still have the TIME ethos, or elements thereof, contained within.

1.4.3 Wound Diagnostics

There is little doubt that the classification systems are useful from an auditing perspective, but it must be noted that they are the first step in informing the follow-up procedures—this will invariably necessitate the scheduling of further wound imaging or laboratory tests. A wide range of tests are available to the clinician to aid wound diagnosis and the subsequent management of the wound. The types of test can be broken down into three distinct categories: nonspecific, diagnostic, and theranostic [10]. These reflect the degree to which they indicate an appropriate intervention as indicated in Fig. 1.13. General tests, such as checking for the presence of systemic inflammatory markers (ie, C-reactive protein), temperature or blood pressure, may not be specific to the wound and therefore although they help to inform the clinician, they do not, by themselves, indicate a particular diagnosis [10]. Diagnostic tests are more specific and require little in the way of interpretation and provide unambiguous answers relating to a specific physiological or

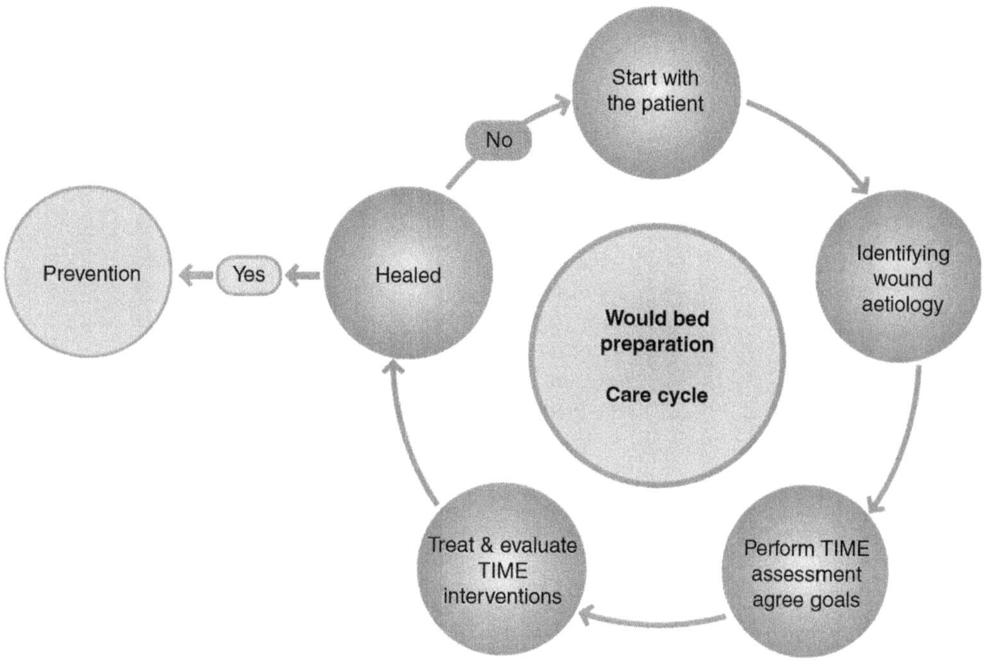

Figure 1.12 ***Wound bed preparation "Care Cycle" [54].***

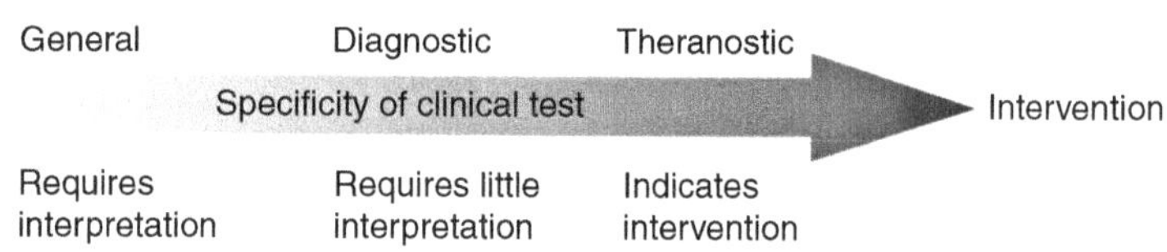

Figure 1.13 ***Diagnostic tests and their impact.*** *(Adapted from World Union of Wound Healing Societies 2008) [11].*

biochemical condition and can be used directly to influence subsequent interventions. Theranostic tests, in contrast to the other two, do not directly lead to a diagnosis but are confirmatory in regards to the need for a specific intervention. The identification of a haemolytic streptoccoi within the wound fluid would be an example of a theranostic, whereby the outcome points toward the prescribing of a specific antibiotic [11].

The development of theranostics is an ever-increasing area as the potential to accurately direct treatments promises more favorable outcomes and, importantly, has knock-on effects in terms of health economics. Personalized healthcare and stratified medicine are key areas of research at present and likely to become critical in future clinical practice [11].

Table 1.4 General diagnostic tests

Type	Description	
Wound specific	Dimensions	C
	Odema	C
	Erythema/heat	C
	Wound bed condition	C
	Wound margin	C
	Location	C
	Exudate color, odor, quantity	C
	Pain	C
General tests	Temperature	C
	Pressure	C
	Reflexes and sensation	C
	Arterial pulses	C
	Monofilament sensitivity	C
Biological tests	Microbial culture	L
	Wound histology	L
	White cell count	L
	Erythrocyte sedimentation	L
Biochemical tests	Glucose	C/L
	Hemoglobin	L
	Plasma albumin	L
	Lipids	L
	Urea and electrolytes	L
	HbA1C	L
	Rheumatoid factor	L
	CRP	L
Miscellaneous	Oxygen	C
	Ankle brachial pressure index	C
	High frequency ultrasound	C

Source: Adapted from World Union of Wound Healing Societies [11].

It is unlikely that a test for one specific marker will be considered a suitable tool for the diagnosis of all chronic wounds and therefore, it is much more realistic to expect that a number of tests will be employed. Typical examples of the type of test that would be considered in the assessment of a chronic wound are highlighted in Table 1.4 [11]. The majority of these can be done directly within the clinic at the time of consultation (C), but the biological and biochemical analysis will almost invariably require the dispatch of wound/blood samples to a central clinical laboratory (L). As such, there will be inevitable delays in processing and reporting which can compromise the treatment plan. It must be noted that the tests highlighted in Table 1.4 have changed little in recent decades but, there is a pressing need for new diagnostics which can be employed during the clinic assessment or, as indicated in the later sections, by the development of smart technologies that perform the analysis automatically within the actual dressing.

1.5 WOUND TREATMENT TECHNOLOGIES

The principal aim of wound management is to heal the wound as quickly as possible, restoring function without causing the patient undue pain. Historically, the main approach would have been to cleanse the wound and then simply protect it from exogenous contaminants. The evolution of wound treatment practices is discussed in Chapter 3, but suffice to say that informed intervention in the healing processes is a relatively recent advance given the long history of human injury. Advances in science and engineering have provided key insights into the relationships that exist between the cellular and molecular players within the wound and how they can be perturbed for the benefit of the patient. It is only in the past 50 years that maintaining a moist wound environment has been recognized as being advantageous for encouraging the wound healing processes [57]. The apparent randomness of early medical approaches has largely given way to new functional materials designed to specifically interact with the wound [15,58,59]. At one point, the primary wound dressing available to the clinician would have been cotton gauze/cotton wool pad, while now it is possible to cover pharmacy shelves with a multitude of different products, each possessing a variety of materials, additives, functions, and forms [59]. The core remit of this book is to explore the material aspects of these dressings and to examine new approaches to their design and application, but it must be noted that dressings are only one part of the story of wound management technologies and there have been significant advances in procedures and instruments. The range of wound management technologies that are presently available to the clinician are summarized in Table 1.5. It is important to note that there have been tremendous advances in skin graft techniques and tissue engineering and, there is a wide spectrum of commercial grafts and scaffolds available which have been shown to be a versatile addition to the clinician's tool box [59,60]. A detailed discussion of these approaches is beyond the scope of this book, but an overview is provided here to illustrate the key points and benefits of the approach. Similarly, the uses of negative pressure and hyperbaric oxygen are two approaches that have been found to be particularly useful for the treatment of chronic wounds and these are briefly described and considered in the following subsections. It must be noted that each of these complementary aids to wound healing will still be dependent on the application of an appropriate dressing to maintain the healing process through to closure.

The skin is capable of remarkable feats of bioengineering without prompting but, when the injury is sufficiently severe, wound aids (be they dressing or tissue scaffold) will be necessary. Is such a diversity of dressings necessary? This can be answered to some

Table 1.5 Wound technologies and healing aids

Negative pressure wound therapy
Hyperbaric oxygen therapy
Topical oxygen therapy
Electrical stimulation, diathermy, pulsed electromagnetic fields
Pulsed radiofrequency energy
Low-frequency noncontact ultrasound—MIST
Extracorporeal shock wave therapy—DermaPACE
Growth factors
Acellular matrix tissues
Xenograft dermis
Xenograft acellular matrices
Human dermis
Human pericardium
Placental tissues
Bioengineered allogeneic cellular therapies
Stem cell therapies

Source: Adapted from Frykberg and Banks [60].

extent by an appreciation of the equally great diversity of wound type and the peculiarities presented by individual patients. Almost all of the dressings which are commercially available will conform to the core criteria of an idealized dressing but selecting the appropriate aid for a given patient to accelerate healing is a considerable challenge and there is certainly no universal bandage or dressing to accomplish this [15,58–60].

Different wounds require different treatments and thus, the wide variety of dressing ensures that there will be a system which can be tailored to a particular wound. The dressing can also be employed to modify the wound environment through the physicochemical properties of the materials contained within the dressing. This aspect is discussed at length in Chapter 4, but as eluded to in Table 1.4, dressings can be used to control moisture. In fact, dressings can be employed to influence all four factors in the TIME philosophy and many more besides.

1.5.1 Skin Grafts and Engineered Tissues

Dressing technology is a vital part of wound management but there are occasions where despite their intricate design, physicochemical properties, and bioactive functionalities, they are unable to advance the healing. These situations typically occur where a substantial amount of damage has been inflicted and epidermal and dermal skins layers have been lost. Such situations represent an overwhelming challenge and would normally involve the use of autografts—sections of tissue harvested from a donor site identified on the same patient [61,62]. There are issues with such procedures: scarring, pain, infection, and a limited source of material [63,64]. In addition, it has been noted that the proliferation potential of cells in the excised graft is inversely proportional to the patient age [65,66]. The latter clearly poses an issue as significant proportion of those with chronic wounds will be elderly [16].

Autologous grafts have been promoted as a much more effective and clinically (and patient) acceptable approach to autografting. Cultured epithelial autografts (CEAs) were first demonstrated by O'Connor and coworkers and involved harvesting cells through punch biopsy and subsequently grown in vitro [67,68] where it is possible to obtain a 1,000-fold expansion within a month [69]. Sheets of epithelia can be grown and easily grafted onto the wound bed to encourage healing [70,71]. It must be remembered that the grafts are incredibly fragile and their transfer to the wound exposes the cells to a much harsher environment where there are a multitude of enzymes that can easily disrupt their structure and reduce viability [71,72]. It is little surprise therefore that a critical determinant in the successful transfer and "take" of the graft is the degree to which it attaches to the wound bed. The latter is crucial for the protection, proliferation, and differentiation of the cells [73,74]. The effectiveness of the approach has been studied in a number of chronic wounds with a range of success. Work conducted by Hefton and coworkers is among the more promising with complete healing observed within 28 days of the graft compared with wounds that had previously, over a 2-month period, shown no response to conventional treatment [70].

The main disadvantage to the CEA approach relates principally to the time required to grow the sheets and, as noted previously, the proliferation rate can be greatly reduced in the case of elderly patients [63]. The delay is critical in terms of burn patients in whom there is need for speedy treatment but even in chronic wound scenarios, a 4-week wait can render the patient susceptible to infection which will further compromise the ability of the graft to adhere to the wound bed.

1.5.2 Negative Pressure Wound Therapy

The application of a vacuum dressing—a specially designed foam sealed by an occlusive dressing—enables the efficient removal of exudate and reduces the build-up of metalloproteinases, bacteria, and other toxins which impede wound repair [75]. The removal of the excess fluid minimizes the risk of edema, but there is much more to this technique. A key advantage is the ability to stimulate blood flow to the underlying tissues, whereby it has been shown to stimulate angiogenesis, the formation granulation tissue and to aid the contraction of the wound edges [76,77]. It has become a standard technique within hospital settings for the treatment of both acute and chronic wounds and has found application in the management of skin grafts [78–83]. There is an abundance of evidence to support the efficacy of the approach toward chronic (venous leg and diabetic foot) wounds [75,84,85]. The systems have advanced considerably since their introduction in the 1990s and have been adapted in a multitude of ways to suit different applications and wound types. One important addition has been the option to include antimicrobial agents within the foam dressing [86–89]. The main drawback, however, has been the relative bulk of the equipment but there has been substantial progress in minimizing the device footprint. Mechanically powered and eminently portable negative pressure wound therapy systems have now begun to appear and could easily be applied within a community treatment plan [90,91]. In recent studies, these portable devices have shown to offer considerable benefits for DFU patients [92,93].

1.5.3 Oxygen Therapies

Hyperbaric oxygen therapy is more commonly associated with the treatment of decompression sickness in divers and its use as a wound healing therapy may seem a little odd, but it has been advocated as a very versatile addition to the wound management armoury when dealing with chronic ulcers. As with deep sea divers, the patient is placed in a sealed vessel containing 100% pressurized oxygen (typically 1.5–3 atm) for an hour or more, whereby the hyperbaric environment results in the plasma within the tissues becoming hyperoxygenated [94,95].

The role of oxygen in chronic wound management cannot be understated as it serves as a feedstock for the cellular processes that drive healing and is a vital weapon in infection control [94,95]. Clearly, impaired oxygenation and perfusion will compromise the healing effort [96,97]. As with negative pressure wound therapy, oxygen therapies have been proffered as a treatment for diabetic ulcers where there is a compromised circulation that effectively restricts the transfer of oxygen to the cells within the wound bed. It has been postulated that, through increasing tissue oxygenation, higher rates of wound healing could be induced and could significantly reduce the risk of major amputation [94,97–99]. There are, however, many conflicting reports on the performance of hyperbaric techniques and while there have been many studies on its application within the treatment regimes of DFU and VLU patients, there are significant variations in the trial outcomes [60,94–96].

The need for a hyperbaric chamber is a clear drawback to the technique but topical administration of oxygen to an ischemic wound has arisen as an alternative and much more accessible approach. Rather than have the patient confined with a high-pressure vessel, pure oxygen is injected into an inflatable bag which effectively surrounds the wound area. There are many advantages to this approach (cost, lower risk of oxygen toxicity, portability) but, as with the chamber approach, the efficacy of the approach can be contentious [60].

An alternative spin on the topical administration of oxygen has emerged in recent years where advanced dressings have been designed to deliver oxygen directly to the cells. In principle, it addresses the same clinical issues as the previous approaches but in a more readily accessible format and, through promoting more rapid healing, promises better cost-benefits. There are many different approaches to the design of oxygen delivery devices. One of the more simple approaches involves the use a composite film possessing an occlusive film and a semipermeable lower film. The latter is typically in the form of a foam dressing containing oxygen microbubbles that are released when the dressing becomes moistened with wound fluid [100]. This enables the dressing to effectively supersaturate the wound fluid with oxygen for several days. There are many other approaches of varying complexity and which can be applied and controlled by the patient. The mechanism through which they act and the purported efficacies of these "active oxygen" dressings are considered in more detail within Chapter 4.

1.5.4 Electrostimulatory Techniques

The use of electrical stimulation for the treatment of chronic wounds is well established and there are numerous studies to suggest that there is a distinct healing benefit to the patient [101–103]. The skin normally possesses an electropotential of around 30–100 mV between the stratum corneum and the underlying dermis but, upon injury, the loss of the epithelial cells essentially removes the potential difference [104]. The body actually uses electrical energy (galvanotaxis or electrotaxis) to aid the recruitment of cells necessary to repair the damage and it has been demonstrated that human keratinocytes can alter their behavior accordingly [104–106]. It has been suggested that the application of an electromagnetic field induces the upregulation of nitric oxide production resulting in greater angiogenesis and improved healing time [103]. Many different approaches have been employed and there are extensive reviews on the techniques [105,106], but one example is of considerable interest: bioelectric dressings [106]. These are important hybrid systems that bring the main benefits and characteristics of a wound dressing but also enables electrical gradients to be established which can be used in concert to stimulate wound healing. These dressings and the materials used in their construction are considered in Chapter 4.

1.5.5 Ultrasound Technologies

The use of ultrasound is not restricted to diagnostic applications but has been used as a tool to aid debridement of the wound [107]. Ultrasound is known to give rise to a number of physical effects (thermal and nonthermal) which depend on the frequency and intensity of the source [108]. The application of high-frequency, high-intensity ultrasound tends to generate thermal effects, whereas low-frequency systems (the most commonly utilized) induce mechanical effects—principally cavitation and acoustic streaming. Depending on the relative position of the transducer at the wound site, low ultrasound can be either low or high intensity (in direct contact with the wound). Debridement is usually facilitated by high-intensity application where the generation and subsequent collapse of cavitational bubbles within the tissue reduces the structural integrity of the devitalized tissue and aids its removal [109]. It is suggested that low-intensity applications create acoustic streaming which has an impact on a variety of biochemical processes within the wound (protein synthesis, growth factor production, fibrinolysis) [110–114]. The debriding effect has been shown to be beneficial when dealing with thick fibrinous slough and necrosis but, while the technique can aid the physical cleanup of the wound bed, its overall influence on the rate of wound healing is far from clear [107,115,116].

1.6 WOUND INFECTION

A key issue with the development of a chronic wound is the susceptibility of the patient toward infection [5,11]. The longer a wound remains unhealed, the greater the opportunity and probability of infection. Bacteria contaminate most open wounds and, in many cases, exert little influence on the healing dynamics and do not unduly impede wound closure. Some bacterial strains are more than problematic and can be life threatening. Staphylococcus aureus, Pseudomonas, aeruginosa, Streptococcus pyogenes, and some Proteus, Clostridium, and Coliform species are among the more common culprits of infection [117,118]. These are largely adventitious species and their colonization of the wound can often be attributed to inadequate control measures. The onset of infection does not simply impede the healing process but leads to cellulitis and, if not treated, bacteremia and septicemia. In general, there are several stages toward which a clinician assessing a wound looks: contamination, colonization, critical colonization, and infection [11]. The relative differences between each stage are summarized in Fig. 1.14.

Contamination is the least troublesome of the stages and elicits no response from the patient's immune system. Colonization, similarly, exerts little influence on the healing process as the populations are still sufficiently low. Critical colonization, however, is the point at which the microbes begin to aggressively proliferate and will begin to impact on the healing process. Infection occurs where the microbes induce the immune response—typified by the classic signs of redness, pain, swelling, raised temperature, and fever. If left untreated, the infection will transform into a systemic issue which could be life threatening. Local infection gives rise to cellulitis and the destruction of the soft tissue and will be

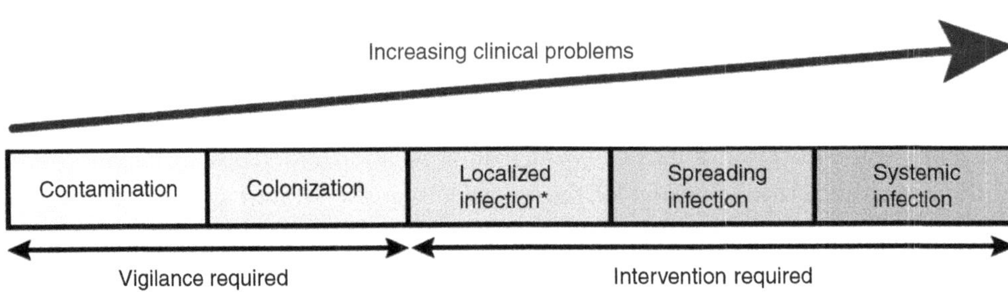

Figure 1.14 ***Effect of bacterial growth on wound healing.*** *(Adapted from World Union of Wound Healing Societies 2008) [11].*

a major setback to the tissue reconstruction which has occurred prior to microbial growth [119,120]. One major issue with microbial growth is the deposition of biofilms and it is widely accepted that the latter is a key mediator in chronic wounds [119–121].

The main approaches to treating wound infection are based on the topical and/or systemic administration of antimicrobial compounds to reduce the bioburden. As part of the assessment processes, it is likely that any suspicion of infection will have meant that a swab of the wound will have been sent for microbiological testing to identify possible candidates and therefore enable selection of an appropriate antimicrobial. The wound will also be debrided to remove compromised tissue and biofilm that would harbor the microbes and which could serve as a barrier to the antimicrobials [122,123]. The introduction of antimicrobial dressings has increased dramatically in recent years and their composition and application are discussed in depth in Chapter 7. Silver-impregnated dressings, however, will be fresh in the mind of most readers and are available in most pharmacies. A quick examination of the number of reports using silver within wound dressing over the past few decades is highlighted in Fig. 1.15. It would appear that silver is major new discovery but its use in combating infection is far from recent and has been used for several millennia [124].

The use of silver can be quite contentious and, while there are studies to indicate some cytotoxicity, there is a substantial body of evidence to indicate that it does improve

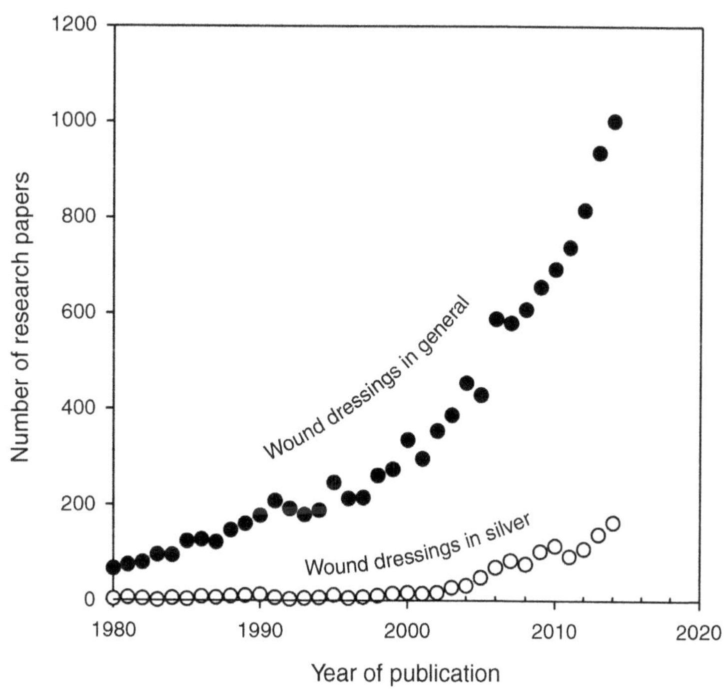

Figure 1.15 ***Research growth in wound dressings.***

the healing process [124,125]. The increasing prevalence of resistant bacteria is an obvious worry for healthcare providers and there is a continuing search for new approaches and these are discussed in later sections of the book.

1.7 HEALTH COSTS

The economic burden on the healthcare provider alone for treating chronic wounds is liable to be greatly exacerbated through an austere financial climate, increasing health care costs, an aging population, and sharp increases in the incidence of diabetes and obesity. There are wildly varying estimates of the cost of treatment associated with wounds but, in most cases, these equate to multibillion figures irrespective of country. In the United Kingdom, it has been estimated that some 650,000 patients suffer from some form of wound that requires clinical intervention with published reports suggesting that the combined cost to the NHS for their treatment reaches approximately £3 billion per year [1]. Costs within the United States are estimated at a more hefty $25 billion—a consequence of the greater population but also partly associated with an atypical medical care system [4].

The need for sustained clinical attention in the management of chronic wounds is clearly of fiscal concern and thus, the speedy reinstatement of normal wound healing is, without question, the desired outcome from the perspectives of the patient, the clinician, and the medical administrator. At present, chronic wounds require a high staff overhead associated with the nurse/consultant time and this is liable to remain so for the foreseeable future. Chronic wounds can arise from a number of conditions but, a momentary focus on those arising principally as a consequence of diabetes can be illuminating. The global figure for diabetes worldwide is expected to rise from 370 million at present, to some 552 million people by 2030 [126,127]. It is widely recognized that some 5–7% of diabetic patients in the UK have had, or presently manage, a foot ulcer [128,129] but, more worrying, are the predictions that the lifetime probability of a diabetic developing a chronic foot ulcer lies in the region of 10–25% [130]. The economic cost can be staggering when considering that the cost of treating a single DFU incident in the United States equated to $28,000 over a 2-year period [131] with the inpatient costs for major amputations in the realm of $31,000 [132,133].

Diabetic ulcers are only one example of a wound type that presently places a significant burden on health care resources. VLUs are another critical player and affect 1–3% of the adult population [134] and, as with DFUs, they can recur with alarming frequency—12-month recurrence rates range between 18% and 28% [135]. This cycle causes an immeasurable toll on the patient whose wound, despite receiving regular clinical treatment, fails to progress [134–137]. In the majority of cases, the healing processes are stalled with a state of prolonged inflammation and, as with DFU, there is a continual risk of early localized infection which can quickly escalate to life-threatening events [138,139].

Table 1.6 Patient costs for the treatment of a venous leg ulcer

		Euro	Frequency
Bandage costs	Lower leg	93	/6 months
	Upper leg	118	/6 months
	Pelvis	150	/6 months
Outpatient costs	Physiotherapist	33	/month
	Therapist of Lymphatology	43	/month
	Nurse	14	/dressing
	Consultant	45	/3 months
	Specialized Outpatient clinic	21	/month
Hospital costs	Arterial surgery	6,733	
	Vein surgery	2,972	
	Meshgraft	7,611	
	Hospitalization	5,139	
	Conservative Therapy and VAC	3,457	

Source: Adapted from Augustin et al. [140].

Augustin and coworkers conducted a cross sectional study of 147 institutions in Germany involved in the care of VLUs and found that the annual treatment costs were just short of 10,000 Euros per patient per year [140]. Indications of the material and staff overheads involved in the treatment and management of a venous leg ulcer are highlighted in Table 1.6. These figures have been adapted and abridged from the work by Augustin and coworkers [140] and are presented primarily to emphasize material and procedural nature of the management plan.

It has been speculated that, in general, only some 5% of the cost is actually attributed to the actual materials required for dressing and treatment with the vast majority—estimated to be around 80%—being largely staff-related [1]. This is dependent to a large extent on the severity of the condition and the mobility of the patient. Elderly patients who are frail or immobile will be unable to attend clinics and, will invariably have a high reliance on district/community nursing to maintain the wound. Likewise, those whose condition has deteriorated will inevitably become hospitalized. In either case, the material costs are trivial to the time spent dealing with the patient [1,140].

Chronic wounds are a pernicious poison from a psychological perspective, it is a disability and, the recognition of this and the limitations imposed on the patient, has an impact on the wound outcomes. It is easy to see how a vicious circle can ensue and, it is inevitable that patients will encounter difficulties in maintaining a commitment to their employer whilst striving to manage their health [141–143]. In an austere financial climate, pressures on employers to cut cost are usually translated to staff reductions which removes much of the flexibility necessary to accommodate an employee with a demanding medical illness. This can mean that many are denied employment as a consequence [144]. There have been endless surveys targeted at examining the quality of life and the impact such conditions have but, few really convey the anguish that can arise. Irrespective of age, a chronic wound will mean lost working hours, potential job loss and financial insecurity. Philips et al. conducted an extensive survey on patient suffering from leg ulceration and found 68% of respondents found the managing their condition had a negative effect on their daily routine and, not unsurprisingly, there was a strong correlation between the amount of time consumed by the management needs and emotions of anger, isolation and resentment. These inevitably lead to depression which will do little to aid recuperation [145–148].

It has been estimated that in the United States alone, the annual bill for working days lost as a consequence of a skin disorder is around US$39 billion [4]. Examining the individual components, venous leg ulcers are reported to lead to 2 million work days lost to the condition (irrespective of whether it relates to illness or attending clinics to receive treatment) with and overall bill of $2 billion [4,146,147]. It is easy to appreciate from the data in Table 1.6, the degree of inconvenience that must be endured in the treatment of a venous leg ulcer but, it is impossible to fully understand the psychological cost. It can be suggested that prompt assessment and treatment are essential in the management of a chronic wound along with suitable follow up to ensure that healing is progressing [145–149]. As Dowsett and coworkers have discovered, some 74% of patients are treated in the community [16] and with pressures on resources, it cannot always be assumed that that such criteria are presently being met or can be in the future.

1.8 FUTURE STRATEGIES AND TECHNOLOGICAL SOLUTIONS

The cost of treating chronic wounds is, and will be, a tremendous burden to health care services irrespective of geographical location as they affect large swathes of the global population. The figures highlighted in Section 1.6 will inevitably be subject to error and are likely to substantially underestimate the true costs as they take no real account of the impact on the patient and their families. It is clear from the work of Dowsett and coworkers [16], that the majority of wounds are treated in the community and this creates additional problems over resources at a time where budgets are decreasing but chronic wounds are ever expanding [1,4,5]. The term "silent epidemic" is often used and it represents a fair assessment of the issue facing healthcare administrators and clinical staff who are on the front line. Aging populations combined with an increased prevalence of obesity and diabetes has led to extremely pessimistic predictions suggesting substantial increases in pressure, venous and foot ulcers in the near future [1,4]. As chronic wounds take longer to heal, infection is an ever-present hazard and one that is further complicated by the increasing threat of antimicrobial resistance.

At present, there are continuing motions within most healthcare providers to rationalize resources and seek better efficiencies. It is of course a matter of speculation as to what impact this may have on patient care but, when faced with a wave whose crest keeps increasing, it is clear that there needs to be alternative solutions. The best solution is undoubtedly prevention and, as Dowsett's study indicates, gains are certainly been made in terms of educating care staff toward reducing the incidence of preventable pressure ulcers [16]. This can only go so far, but the situation is not all doom and gloom. The second approach is to heal the wound faster. Tremendous efforts are being made in the development of new dressings designed to improve healing as highlighted in Fig. 1.15, moreover, these figures take no account of the extensive work conducted by commercial dressing manufacturers.

As the processes involved in healing have become better understood, interactive dressings have appeared and these have offered better opportunities to stimulate particular processes or remove factors that might otherwise impede healing. The term "smart" has been applied to various biomedical devices in recent years and, in some respects, the term can appear as a trendy jargon label added to a manuscript to encourage publication while there is little evidence of any inherent intelligence to the device. It does, however, reflect an ongoing pursuit of dressings that can respond to the prevailing conditions within the wound without the need for intervention by the clinician. This is a critical factor for, if the majority of wounds are to be treated in the community, regular/routine access to a nurse may be limited. There is no implication that such technologies will replace the oversight provided by a dedicated care team, rather, they will complement the management plan. A critical issue, particularly in relation to infection, is the delay in seeking assistance. The deployment of a smart system that can proactively deal with critical colonization—offering either autonomous treatment or alerting the patient would overcome many of the delays encountered in conventional medical practice. Dressings that can accomplish such tasks are already passing the conceptual stage as indicated in Fig. 1.16.

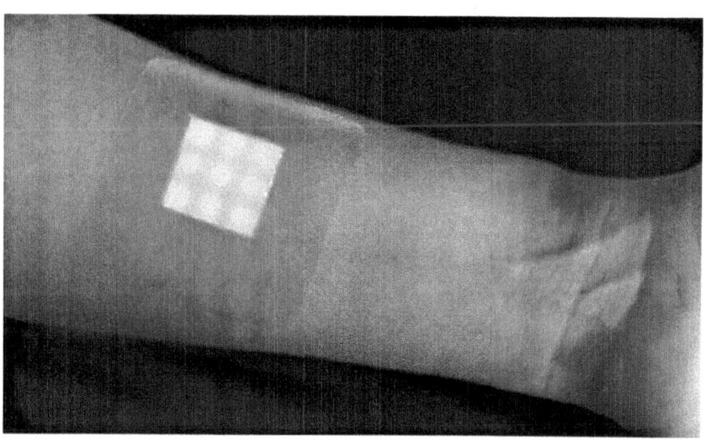

Figure 1.16 ***"Smart" dressing designed to alert the patient to an infected wound.*** *(Reproduced with permission University of Bath).*

There is no doubt that infection is a critical issue in chronic wounds but deciding how to re-stimulate healing processes in a wound that has been in a chronic phase for many months or years requires a knowledge of the cellular and molecular interactions and the nature of the inhibition. There is a need for "smart" systems that can provide detailed information of the wound and how the various protagonists change over time such that the dressing selection can be judiciously managed. The design of dressing to enhance healing are described in Chapter 4, those that can provide diagnostic information are introduced in Chapter 5 and those designed to combat infection are discussed in Chapter 6. There is also a need to discuss the electronic infrastructure necessary to bring the components together and this is covered in Chapter 7.

REFERENCES

[1] Posnett J, Franks PJ. The burden of chronic wounds in the UK. Nursing Times 2008;104(3):44–5.
[2] de la Torre JI, Chambers JA, Chronic Wounds, Medscape.com. Available at: http://emedicine.medscape.com/article/1298452-overview#showall; 2015.
[3] Dreifke MB, Jayasuriy AA, Jayasuriya AC. Current wound healing procedures and potential care. Mater Sci Eng C 2015;48:651–62.
[4] Sen CK, Gordillo GM, Roy S, Kirsner R, Lambert L, Hunt TK, Gottrup F, Gurtner GC, Longaker MT. Human skin wounds: a major and snowballing threat to public health and the economy. Wound Rep Reg 2009;17:763–71.
[5] Wounds International. International best practice guidelines: wound management in diabetic foot ulcers. Available at: <http://www. woundsinternational.com/>; 2013.
[6] Waters N, Holloway S. Personal perceptions of the impact of diabetic foot disease on employment. Diabetic Foot Canada 2013;1:32–40.
[7] Price P, Krasner DL. Health-related quality of life and chronic wounds: evidence and implications for practice. In: Krasner DL, Rodeheaver GT, Sibbald RG, Woo KY, editors. Chronic wound care, a clinical source book for healthcare professionals. 5th ed. Malvern: HMP Communications; 2012. p. 77–84.
[8] McLister A, Phair J, Cundell J, Davis J. Electrochemical approaches to the development of smart bandages: a mini-review. Electrochem Commun 2014;40:96–9.
[9] Dargaville TR, Farrugia BL, Broadbent JA, Pace S, Upton Z, Voelcker NH. Sensors and imaging for wound healing: a review. Biosens Bioelectron 2013;41:30–42.
[10] Zhou J, Tun TN, Hong SH, Mercer-Chalmers JD, Laabei M, Young AER, Jenkins ATA. Development of a prototype wound dressing technology which can detect and report colonization by pathogenic bacteria. Biosensors Bioelectron 2011;30:67–72.
[11] World Union of Wound Healing Societies (WUWHS). Principles of best practice: wound infection in clinical practice. An international consensus. London, UK: MEP Ltd. Available at: <http://www.mepltd.co.uk/>; 2008.
[12] Mehmood N, Hariz A, Fitridge R, Voelcker NH. Applications of modern sensors and wireless technology in effective wound management. J Biomed Mats Res B Appl Biomats 2014;102B:885–95.
[13] Ochoa M, Rahimi R, Ziaie B. Flexible sensors for chronic wound management. IEEE Rev Biomed Eng 2014;7:73–86.
[14] McLister A, Phair J, Cundell J, Davis J. New developments in smart bandage technologies. Adv Mater 2016.
[15] Mayet N, Choonara YE, Kumar P, Tomar LK, Tyagi C, Du Toit LC, Pillay VA. Comprehensive review of advanced biopolymeric wound healing systems. J Pharm Sci 2014;103:2211–30.
[16] Dowsett C, Blelby A, Searle R. Reconciling increasing wound care demands with available resources. J Wound Care 2014;23:552–62.
[17] Percival J. Classification of wounds and their management. Surgery 2002;20:114–7.

[18] Moore K, McCallion R, Searle RJ, Stacey MC, Harding KG. Prediction and monitoring the therapeutic response of chronic dermal wounds. Int Wound J 2006;3(2):89–96.
[19] Gurtner GC, Werner S, Barrandon Y, Longaker MT. Wound repair and regeneration. Nature 2008;453:314–21.
[20] Broderick N. Understanding chronic wound healing. Nurse Practitioner 2009;34(10):16–22.
[21] Trent JT, Kirsner RS. Wounds and malignancy. Adv Skin Wound Care 2003;16(1):31–4.
[22] Cutting KF, White RJ. Maceration of the skin and wound bed. 1: its nature and causes. J Wound Care 2002;11(7):275–8.
[23] Shahin ES, Dassen T, Halfens RJ. Pressure ulcer prevalence and incidence in intensive care patients: a literature review. Nurs Crit Care 2008;13:71–9.
[24] Posnett J, Gottrup F, Lundgren H, Saal G. The resource impact of wounds on health-care providers in Europe. J Wound Care 2009;18:154–61.
[25] Hodde J, Allam R. Submucosa wound matrix for chronic wound healing. Wounds 2007;19:157–63.
[26] Bergstrom N, Horn SD, Smout RJ, Bender SA, Ferguson ML, Taler G, Sauer AC, Sharkey SS, Voss AC. The national pressure ulcer long-term care study: outcomes of pressure ulcer treatments in long-term care. J Am Geriatr Soc 2005;53:1721–9.
[27] Voss AC, Bender SA, Ferguson ML, Sauer AC, Bennett RG, Hahn PW. Long-term care liability for pressure ulcers. J Am Geriatr Soc 2005;53:1587–92.
[28] Greenwald L. Medicare deadline spurs hospitals to prevent pressure ulcers. E-Zine. Available at: <http://ezinearticles.com/?Medicare-Deadline-Spurs-Hospitals-to-Prevent-Pressure-Ulcers&id=846302/>; 2007.
[29] Centers of Medicare and Medicaid Services. Medicare program: changes to the hospital inpatient prospective payment systems and fiscal year 2008 rates—final rule. Fed Regist 2007;72:47130–8175.
[30] Yim E, Richmond NA, Baquerizo K, et al. The effect of ankle range of motion on venous ulcer healing rates. Wound Repair Regen 2014;22:492–6.
[31] Browse NL, Burnand KG. The cause of venous ulceration. Lancet 1982;2:243–5.
[32] Falanga V, Moosa HH, Nameth AF, et al. Dermal pericapillary fibrin in venous disease and venous ulceration. Arch Dermatol 1987;123:620–3.
[33] Falanga V, Kirsner R, Katz MH, et al. Pericapillary fibrin cuffs in venous ulceration. Persistence with treatment and during ulcer healing. J Dermatol Surg Oncol 1992;18:409–14.
[34] Falanga V, Eaglstein WH. The trap hypothesis of venous ulceration. Lancet 1993;341:1006–8.
[35] Coleridge-Smith PD, Thomas P, Scurr JH, Dormandy JA. Causes of venous ulceration: a new hypothesis? Br Med J (Clin Res Ed) 1988;296:1726–7.
[36] Thomas PR, Nash GB, Dormandy JA. White cell accumulation in dependent legs of patients with venous hypertension: a possible mechanism for trophic changes in the skin. Br Med J (Clin Res Ed) 1988;296:1693–5.
[37] Abbade LP, Lastoria S. Venous ulcer: epidemiology, physiopathology, diagnosis and treatment. Int J Dermatol 2005;44:449–56.
[38] Margolis DJ, Bilker W, Santanna J, Baumgarten M. Venous leg ulcer: incidence and prevalence in the elderly. J Am Acad Dermatol 2002;46:381–6.
[39] Alavi A, Sibbald RG, Mayer D, et al. Diabetic foot ulcers: part I. Pathophysiology and prevention. J Am Acad Dermatol 2014;70(1):e1–18.
[40] Fernando DJ, Masson EA, Veves A, Boulton AJ. Relationship of limited joint mobility to abnormal foot pressures and diabetic foot ulceration. Diabetes Care 1991;14:8–11. Armstrong DG. Loss of protective sensation: a practical evidence-based definition. J Foot Ankle Surg 1999;38:79–80.
[41] Ahmed ME, Delbridge L, Le Quesne LP. The role of autonomic neuropathy in diabetic foot ulceration. J Neurol Neurosurg Psychiatry 1986;49:1002–6.
[42] Mallefet P, Dweck AC. Mechanism involved in wound healing. Biomed Sci 2008;7:609–15.
[43] Falanga V. Wound healing and its impairment in the diabetic foot. Lancet 2005;366:1736–43.
[44] Singer A, Richard AF, Clark MD. Cutaneous wound healing. New Engl J Med 1999;341:738–46.
[45] Dulmovits BM, Herman IM. Microvascular remodelling and wound healing: a role for pericytes. Int J Biochem Cell Biol 2012;44:1800–12.
[46] Stein C, Kuchler S. Targeting inflammation and wound healing by opioids. Trends Pharmacol Sci 2013;34:303–12.

[47] Clayton W, Elasy TM. A review of the pathophysiology, classification, and treatment of foot ulcers in diabetic patients. Clin Diabetes 2009;27:52–8.
[48] Karthikesalingam A, Holt PJE, Moxey P, Jones KG, Thompson MM, Hinchcliffe RJ. A systematic review of scoring systems for diabetic foot ulcers. Diabetic Med 2010;27:544–9.
[49] Meggitt B. Surgical management of the diabetic foot. Br J Hosp Med 1976;16:227–32.
[50] Oyibo SO, Jude EB, Tarawneh I, et al. A comparison of two diabetic foot ulcer classification systems. Diabetes Care 2001;24:84–8.
[51] Wagner FW. The dysvascular foot: a system of diagnosis and treatment. Foot Ankle 1981;2:64–122.
[52] Armstrong DG, Lavery LA, Harkless LB. Validation of a diabetic wound classification system. The contribution of depth, infection, and ischemia to risk of amputation. Diabetes Care 1998;21:855–9.
[53] Lavery LA, Armstrong DG, Harkless LB. Classification of diabetic foot wounds. J Foot Ankle Surg 1996;35:528–31.
[54] Dowsett C, Newton H. Wound bed preparation: TIME in practice. Wounds UK 2015;58–70.
[55] Dealey C. The care of wounds. Oxford: Blackwell Science; 2000.
[56] Dowsett C, Ayello E. TIME principles of chronic wound bed preparation and treatment. Br J Nurs 2004;13:S16–23.
[57] W Winter GD. Formation of the scab and the rate of epithelization of superficial wounds in the skin of the young domestic pig. Nature 1962;193:293–4.
[58] Moura LIF, Dias AMA, Carvalho E, de Sousa HC. Recent advances on the development of wound dressings for diabetic foot ulcer treatment—a review. Acta Biomater 2013;9:7093–114.
[59] Boateng J, Catanzano O. Advanced therapeutic dressings for effective wound healing—a review. J Pharm Sci 2015;104:3653–80.
[60] Frykberg RG, Banks J. Challenges in the treatment of chronic wounds. Adv Wound Care 2015;4: 560–82.
[61] Phillips TJ, Kehinde O, Green H, Gilchrest BA. Treatment of skin ulcers with cultured epidermal allografts. J Am Acad Dermatol 1989;21:191–9.
[62] Wainwright DJ. Use of an acellular allograft dermal matrix (AlloDerm) in the management of full-thickness burns. Burns 1995;21:243–8.
[63] Leigh IM, Purkis PE. Culture grafted leg ulcers. Clin Exp Dermatol 1986;11:650–2.
[64] Sheridan RL, Tompkins RG. Skin substitutes in burns. Burns 1999;25:97–103.
[65] Stanulis-Praeger BM, Gilchrest BA. Growth factor responsiveness declines during adulthood for human skin-derived cells. Mech Ageing Dev 1986;34:185–98.
[66] Colwell AS, Faudoa R, Krummel TM, Longaker MT, Lorenz HP. Transforming growth factor-beta, Smad, and collagen expression patterns in fetal and adult keratinocytes. Plast Reconstr Surg 2007;119:852–7.
[67] Harris PA, Leigh IM, Navsaria HA. Pre-confluent keratinocyte grafting: the future for cultured skin replacements? Burns 1998;24:591–3.
[68] O'Connor NE. Grafting of burns with cultured epithelium prepared from autologous epidermal cells. Lancet 1981;75–8.
[69] Hefton JM, Caldwell D, Biozes DG, Balin AK, Carter DM. Grafting of skin ulcers with cultured autologous epidermal cells. J Am Acad Dermatol 1986;14:399–405.
[70] Lam PK, Chan ES, To EW, Lau CH, Yen SC, King WW. Development and evaluation of a new composite Laserskin graft. J Trauma 1999;47:918–22.
[71] Green H, Kehinde O, Thomas J. Growth of cultured human epidermal cells into multiple epithelia suitable for grafting. Proc Natl Acad Sci U S A 1979;76:5665–8.
[72] Barrandon Y, Green H. Cell migration is essential for sustained growth of keratinocyte colonies: the roles of transforming growth factor-alpha and epidermal growth factor. Cell 1987;50:1131–7.
[73] Nanchahal J, Ward CM. New grafts for old? A review of alternatives to autologous skin. Br J Plast Surg 1992;45:354–63.
[74] Balasubramani M, Kumar TR, Babu M. Skin substitutes: a review. Burns 2001;27:534–44.
[75] N Hasan MY, Teo R, Nather A. Negative-pressure wound therapy for management of diabetic foot wounds: a review of the mechanism of action, clinical applications, and recent developments. Diabetic Foot Ankle 2015;6:27618.

[76] Saxena V, Hwang CW, Huang S, Eichbaum Q, Ingber D, Orgill DP. Vacuum-assisted closure: micro deformations of wounds and cell proliferation. Plast Reconstr Surg 2004;114:1086–96.
[77] Scherer SS, Pietra-maggiori G, Mathews JC, Prsa MJ, Huang S, Orgill DP. The mechanism of action of the vacuum-assisted closure device. Plast Reconstr Surg 2008;122:786–97.
[78] Isaac AL, Rose J, Armstrong DG. Mechanically powered negative pressure wound therapy as a bolster for skin grafting. Plast Reconstr Surg Glob Open 2014;2:e103.
[79] Armstrong DG, Boulton AJ, Banwell P. Negative pressure wound therapy in treatment of diabetic foot wounds: a marriage of modalities. Ostomy Wound Manage 2004;50:9–12.
[80] Banwell PE. Topical negative pressure therapy in wound care. J Wound Care 1999;8:79–84.
[81] Morykwas MJ, Simpson J, Punger K, Argenta A, Kremers L, Argenta J. Vacuum-assisted closure: state of basic research and physiologic foundation. Plast Reconstr Surg 2006;117:121S–6S.
[82] Petrie N, Potter M, Banwell P. The management of lower extremity wounds using topical negative pressure. Int J Low Extrem Wounds 2003;(2):198–206.
[83] Smith APS, Whittington K, Frykberg RG, DeLeon J. Negative pressure wound therapy. In: Krasner DL, Rodeheaver GT, Sibbald RG, Woo KY, editors. Chronic wound care 5: a clinical source book for healthcare professionals. Malvern, PA: HMP Communications; 2012. p. 271–99.
[84] Armstrong DG, Lavery LA. Negative pressure wound therapy after partial diabetic foot amputation: a multicentre, randomised controlled trial. Lancet 2005;366:1704–10.
[85] Blume PA, Walters J, Payne W, Ayala J, Lantis J. Comparison of negative pressure wound therapy using vacuum-assisted closure with advanced moist wound therapy in the treatment of diabetic foot ulcers: a multicenter randomized controlled trial. Diabetes Care 2008;31:631–6.
[86] Bollero D, Degano K, Gangemi EN, Aloj D, Malvasio V, Stella M. Long-term follow-up of negative pressure wound therapy with instillation: a limb salvage procedure? Int Wound J 2014; DOI: 10.1111/iwj.12373.
[87] Kim PJ, Attinger CE, Steinberg JS, et al. The impact of negative-pressure wound therapy with instillation compared with standard negative pressure wound therapy: a retrospective, historical, cohort, controlled study. Plast Reconstr Surg 2014;133:709–16.
[88] Saez-Martin LC, Garcia-Martinez L, Roman-Curto C, Sanchez-Hernandez MV, Suarez-Fernandez RM. Negative pressure and nanocrystalline silver dressings for nonhealing ulcer: a randomized pilot study. Wound Repair Regen 2015;23:948–52.
[89] Ellenrieder M, Redanz S, Bader R, Mittelmeier W, Podbielski A. Influence of antimicrobial coatings of vacuum-assisted closure dressings on methicillin-resistant Staphylococcus aureus growth kinetics: an in vitro study. Surg Infect 2015;16:139–45.
[90] Fong KD, Marston WA. SNaP wound care system: ultraportable mechanically powered negative pressure wound therapy. Adv Wound Care 2012;1:41–3.
[91] Bohn G. Mechanically powered ambulatory negative pressure wound therapy device for treatment of a colostomy takedown site. J Wound Ostomy Continence Nurs 2013;40:315–7.
[92] Armstrong DG, Marston WA, Reyzelman AM, Kirsner RS. Comparative effectiveness of mechanically and electrically powered negative pressure wound therapy devices: a multicentre randomized controlled trial. Wound Repair Regen 2012;20:332–41.
[93] Armstrong DG, Marston WA, Reyzelman AM, Kirsner RS. Comparison of negative pressure wound therapy with an ultraportable mechanically powered device vs. traditional electrically powered device for the treatment of chronic lower extremity ulcers: a multicenter randomized-controlled trial. Wound Repair Regen 2011;19:173–80.
[94] Brimson CH, Nigam Y. The role of oxygen-associated therapies for the healing of chronic wounds, particularly in patients with diabetes. J Eur Acad Dermatol Venereol 2013;27(4):411–8.
[95] Chambers AC, Leaper DJ. Role of oxygen in wound healing: a review of evidence. J Wound Care 2011;20:160–4.
[96] Rodriguez PG, Felix FN, Woodley DT, Shim EK. The role of oxygen in wound healing: a review of the literature. Dermatol Surg 2008;34:1159–69.
[97] Hunter S, Langemo DK, Anderson J, Hanson D, Thompson P. Hyperbaric oxygen therapy for chronic wounds. Adv Skin Wound Care 2010;23:116–9.
[98] Duzgun AP, Satir HZ, Ozozan O, Saylam B, Kulah B, Coskun F. Effect of hyperbaric oxygen therapy on healing of diabetic foot ulcers. J Foot Ankle Surg 2008;47(6):515–9.

[99] Kranke P, Bennett MH, Martyn-St James M, Schnabel A, Debus SE. Hyperbaric oxygen therapy for chronic wounds. Cochrane Database Syst Rev 2012;4. CD004123.

[100] Lairet KF, Baer D, Leas ML, Renz EM, Cancio LC. Evaluation of an oxygen-diffusion dressing for accelerated healing of donor-site wounds. J Burn Care Res 2014;35:214–8.

[101] Baker LL, Chambers R, DeMuth SK, Villar F. Effects of electrical stimulation on wound healing in patients with diabetic ulcers. Diabetes Care 1997;20:405–12.

[102] Kloth LC. Electrical stimulation for wound healing: a review of evidence from in vitro studies, animal experiments, and clinical trials. Int J Low Extrem Wounds 2005;4:23–44.

[103] McCulloch J. Electrical stimulation in wound repair. In: Yee BY, editor. The wound management manual. New York, NY: McGraw-Hill; 2005. p. 80–9.

[104] Nishimura KY, Isseroff RR, Nuccitelli R. Human keratinocytes migrate to the negative pole in direct current electric fields comparable to those measured in mammalian wounds. J Cell Sci 1996; 109:199–207.

[105] Nuccitelli R. A role for endogenous electric fields in wound healing. Curr Top Dev Biol 2003;58:1–26.

[106] Ud-Din S, Bayat A. Electrical stimulation and cutaneous wound healing: a review of clinical evidence. Healthcare 2014;2:445–67.

[107] Wendelken ME, Markowitz L, Alvarez OM. A closer look at ultrasonic debridement. Podiatry Today 2010;23:23–8.

[108] Baker KG, Robertson VJ, Duck FA. A review of therapeutic ultrasound: biophysical effects. Phys Ther 2001;81:1351–8.

[109] Young S. Ultrasound therapy. In: Kitchen S, editor. Electrotherapy: evidence-based practice. 11th ed New York: Churchill Livingstone; 2002. p. 211–30.

[110] Stanisic MM, Provo BJ, Larson DL, Kloth LC. Wound debridement with 25 kHz ultrasound. Adv Skin Wound Care 2005;18:484–90.

[111] Schoenbach SF, Song IC. Ultrasonic debridement: a new approach in the treatment of burn wounds. Plast Reconstr Surg 1980;66:34–7.

[112] Scherba G, Weigel RM, O'Brien WD Jr. Quantitative assessment of the germicidal efficacy of ultrasonic energy. Appl Environ Microbiol 1991;57:2079–84.

[113] Suchkova V, Siddiqi FN, Carstensen EL, Dalecki D, Child S, Francis CW. Enhancement of fibrinolysis with 40-kHz ultrasound. Circulation 1998;98:1030–5.

[114] Suchkova V, Carstensen EL, Francis CW. Ultrasound enhancement of fibrinolysis at frequencies of 27 to 100 kHz. Ultrasound Med Biol 2002;28:377–82.

[115] Amini S, Shojaeefard A, Annabestani Z, et al. Low-frequency ultrasound debridement in patients with diabetic foot ulcers and osteomyelitis. Wounds 2013;25:193–8.

[116] Stanisic MM, Provo BJ, Larson DL, Kloth LC. Wound debridement with 25 kHz ultrasound. Adv Skin Wound Care 2005;18:484–90.

[117] Bowler PG, Duerden BI, Armstrong DG. Wound microbiology and associated approaches to wound management. Clin Microbiol Rev 2001;14:244–69.

[118] Brook I. Aerobic and anaerobic microbiology of necrotizing fasciitis in children. Pediatr Dermatol 1996;13:281–4.

[119] White RJ, Cooper R, Kingsley A. Wound colonization and infection: the role of topical antimicrobials. Br J Nurs 2001;10:563–78.

[120] White RJ, Cutting K, Kingsley A. Topical antimicrobials in the control of wound bioburden. Ostomy Wound Manage 2006;52:26–58.

[121] Wolcott R. Economic aspects of biofilm-based wound care in diabetic foot ulcers. J Wound Care 2015;24:189–94.

[122] Hunt TK. Surgical wound infections: an overview. Am J Med 1981;70:712–8.

[123] MacMillan BG. Infections following burn injury. Surg Clin North Am 1980;60:185–96.

[124] Barillo DJ, Marx DE. Silver in medicine: a brief history BC 335 to present. Burns 2014;40:S3–8.

[125] Zhong W. Efficacy and toxicity of antibacterial agents used in wound dressings. Cutan Ocul Toxicol 2015;34:61–7.

[126] Bakker K, Apelqvist J, Schaper NC. On behalf of the International Working Group on the Diabetic Foot Editorial Board. Practical guidelines on the management and prevention of the diabetic foot 2011. Diabetes Metab Res Rev 2012;28:225–31.

[127] Diabetes UK. State of the nation 2012 – England. London: Diabetes UK, 2012. Available at: http://bit.ly/Kcg0TU.
[128] Diabetes UK. Putting feet first: national minimum skills framework. Joint initiative from the Diabetes UK, Foot in Diabetes UK, NHS Diabetes, the Association of British Clinical Diabetologists, the Primary Care Diabetes Society, the Society of Chiropodists and Podiatrists. London: Diabetes UK, 2011. Available at: http://diabetes.org.uk/putting-feetfirst.
[129] Kerr M. Foot care for people with diabetes: the economic case for change. NHS Diabetes, Newcastle-upon-Tyne, 2012. Available at: http://bit.ly/xjY7FS.
[130] Singh N, Armstrong DA, Lipsky BA. Preventing foot ulcers in patients with diabetes. JAMA 2005;293:217–28.
[131] Ramsay SD, Newton K, Blough D, et al. Incidence, outcomes, and cost of foot ulcers in patients with diabetes. Diabetes Care 1999;22:382–7.
[132] Assal JP, Mehnert H, Tritschler HS, et al. 'On your feet' workshop on the diabetic foot. J Diabet Comp 2002;16:183–94.
[133] Rathur HM, Boulton AJM. The diabetic foot. Clin Dermatol 2007;25:109–20.
[134] Margolis DJ, Bilker W, Santanna J, Baumgarten M. Venous leg ulcer: incidence and prevalence in the elderly. J Am Acad Dermatol 2002;46:381–6.
[135] Barwell JR, Davies CE, Deacon J, Harvey K, Minor J, et al. Comparison of surgery and compression with compression alone in chronic venous ulceration (ESCHAR study): randomised controlled trial. Lancet 2004;363:1854–2185.
[136] Baker SR, Stacey MC, Singh G, Hoskin SE, Thompson PJ. Aetiology of chronic leg ulcers. Eur J Vasc Surg 1992;6:245–51.
[137] Cornwall JV, Dore CJ, Lewis JD. Leg ulcers: epidemiology and aetiology. Br J Surg 1986;73:693–6.
[138] Davies CE, Hill KE, Newcombe RG, Stephens P, Wilson MJ, et al. A prospective study of the microbiology of chronic venous leg ulcers to reevaluate the clinical predictive value of tissue biopsies and swabs. Wound Repair Regen 2007;15:17–22.
[139] Trengove NJ, Bielefeldt-Ohmann H, Stacey MC. Mitogenic activity and cytokine levels in non-healing and healing chronic leg ulcers. Wound Repair Regen 2000;8:13–25.
[140] Augustin M, Brocatti LK, Rustenbach SJ, Schafer I, Herberger K. Cost-of-illness of leg ulcers in the community. Int Wound J 2014;11:283–92.
[141] Phillips T, Stanton B, Provan A, Lew R. A study of the impact of leg ulcers on quality of life: financial, social, and psychologic implications. J Am Acad Dermatol 1994;31:49–53.
[142] Lanzafame RJ. Business. Photomed Laser Surg 2007;25:371–2.
[143] Ghanassia E, Villon L, Thuan Dit Dieudonne JF, Boegner C, Avignon A, Sultan A. Long-term outcome and disability of diabetic patients hospitalized for diabetic foot ulcers: a 6.5- year follow-up study. Diabetes Care 2008;31:1288–92.
[144] O'Donnell TF Jr, Browse NL, Burnand KG, Thomas ML. The socioeconomic effects of an iliofemoral venous thrombosis. J Surg Res 1977;22:483–8.
[145] Eberhardt RT, Raffetto JD. Chronic venous insufficiency. Circulation 2005;111:2398–409.
[146] DaSilva A, Navarro MF, Batalheiro J. The importance of chronic venous insufficiency: various preliminary data on its medico-social consequences. Phlebologie 1992;45:439–43.
[147] Patel NP, Labropoulos N, Pappas PJ. Current management of venous ulceration. Plast Reconstr Surg 2006;117:254S–60S.
[148] Margolis DJ, Bilker W, Santanna J, Baumgarten M. Venous leg ulcer: incidence and prevalence in the elderly. J Am Acad Dermatol 2002;46:381–6.
[149] Phillips T, Stanton B, Provan A, Lew R. A study of the impact of leg ulcers on quality of life: financial, social, and psychologic implications. J Am Acad Dermatol 1994;31:49–53.

CHAPTER TWO

Diabetic Foot Ulcers: Assessment, Treatment, and Management

J. Cundell
School Health Sciences, Ulster University/Belfast Health and Social Care Trust, Northern Ireland, United Kingdom

2.1 INTRODUCTION

Diabetes is a chronic, debilitating, and potentially fatal illness. King et al. [1] stated that the incidence of diabetes is increasing and projected that by 2025, there would be 300 million people with diabetes worldwide. The estimated number of adults living with diabetes has since soared to 366 million, and now represents 8.3% of the global adult population. This number is projected to increase to 552 million people, or 9.9% of adults by 2030 [2]. In 2014, the United Kingdom has a diagnosed population of 3.2 million people with diabetes, an average of 6.2% of the population [3]. In Northern Ireland, in 2014, it was estimated that 81,867 adults had been diagnosed with diabetes (5.3% of the population).

In 2009, 10% of the NHS Budget (£10 billion) was spent on diabetes and its complications [4] with 87% of this expenditure being on the complications associated with foot disease—peripheral vascular disease, neuropathy, infection, and ulceration. Approximately 15% of individuals with diabetes will suffer foot problems, such as neuropathy and ulceration [5] and 1–4.1% of them will develop a foot ulcer(1) each year [6]. In the United Kingdom, 5–7% of people with diabetes currently has or has had a diabetic foot ulcer [7]. Diabetic foot ulcers are complex, chronic wounds,(2) which have a major long-term impact on patients' morbidity, mortality, and quality of life [8,9]. Such wounds can be induced by a range of aetiological factors such as trauma or pressure and are characterized by an inability to self-repair in a timely and orderly manner [10–12]. It has been suggested that the lifetime incidence of foot ulceration in those with diabetes may be as high as 25% [13,14].

Peripheral motor neuropathy leads to clawing of the toes and prominent metatarsal heads under which high foot pressures develop [15]. In the presence of sensory neuropathy with consequent insensitivity to pain, these high pressures may lead to the development of foot ulceration [16–18]. It is also believed that the claw/hammer toe deformity causes the protective submetatarsal head fat pads to displace distally due to their indirect connection

[1] An ulcer is a loss of full skin thickness with exposure of dermal, and potentially, subdermal tissue. Ulcers are associated with a loss of normal tissue viability.

[2] A wound is the disruption of the anatomic *structure* and its *function* in any body part.

to the proximal phalangeal bones that hyperextend in toe clawing [19,20]. Thus, the neuropathic foot has clawed toes, with areas for possible pressure damage and formation of callus, which can lead to ulceration, especially on the joints and tips of the toes and the metatarsal heads. The susceptibility to ulceration is further increased by the rigidity which can occur in the tissues as a result of glycation of proteins including collagen [21].

Peripheral vascular disease is very common and is probably present in all patients with long-standing diabetes [22]. The incidence of peripheral vascular disease is four times greater in patients with diabetes, and the risk of peripheral vascular disease increases with age and duration of diabetes. The resultant ischaemia not only causes ulceration, it also hinders wound healing, turning a wound into a chronic ulcer. The initial rate of tissue repair is significantly related to local cutaneous perfusion, estimated by periwound partial pressure of oxygen and carbon dioxide, and eventual ulcer reepithelialization is also related to absolute foot blood pressure [23]. Vessel wall damage and atherosclerosis cause impaired blood flow to the tissues of the extremities, primarily the foot and lower limb. This results in a reduction in the delivery of oxygen and nutrients to the cells. Disruption of the autonomic function leads to arteriovenous shunting which in turn leads to a decreased blood flow to the deep tissues and increased flow to the superficial skin [24]. This disruption of autonomic function exacerbates tissue oedema and causes relative anoxia in deep tissues.

Ulceration of the diabetic foot and consequential limb-threatening infection accounts for approximately 25% of all diabetes-related hospital admissions in the United States and the United Kingdom [13,25–29]. The development of foot ulceration precedes lower extremity amputation of between 14% and 24% of patients suffering from diabetes [30]. Such amputations become necessary when a combination of peripheral neuropathy and vascular insufficiency predisposes the diabetic foot to physical trauma and ulceration, leading to infection and gangrene [31–33]. Thus, the diabetic foot is the most common cause of nontraumatic major lower extremity amputation in the world, presenting major medical, social, and economic problems [34].

The factors which lead to amputation also inhibit healing in diabetic foot ulcers. Healing is inhibited by intrinsic factors, such as neuropathy, peripheral arterial disease, and other complicating systemic effects of diabetes, such as hyperglycaemia, and extrinsic factors, such as infection, callus formation, and the application of excessive pressure to the site. In most patients, peripheral neuropathy and/or peripheral arterial disease play a central role; hence, diabetic foot ulcers are commonly classified as neuropathic, ischaemic, or neuroischaemia(3) [35].

Impaired wound healing in diabetes is a well-established phenomenon [37–41], yet little is known of its underlying mechanism, and treatment provided for resultant diabetic

[3]Neuroischaemia is the combined effect of diabetic neuropathy and ischaemia, whereby macrovascular disease and, in some instances, microvascular dysfunction impair perfusion in a diabetic foot [36].

foot ulcers is often inadequate [42,43]. According to Lipsky et al., specific mechanisms that contribute to this chronic wound healing may include increased glycation of proteins including collagen, intracellular accumulation of sorbitol as a consequence of hyperglycaemia, abnormalities in energy metabolism, a defective inflammatory response, and an inadequate local production of polypeptide growth factors [37].

2.2 NORMAL WOUND HEALING

Wound healing can be defined as the physiology by which the body replaces and restores function to damaged tissues [44]. It is a dynamic process that involves complex mechanisms mediated by a range of growth factors [45], and entails complex interplay between connective tissue formation, cellular activity, and growth factor activation. The process of wound healing involves three activities: inflammation, proliferation, and remodeling. Although there is considerable overlap between these phases, they occur in an orderly and predictable manner during the normal wound healing process [46]. Comprehension of the effects of diabetes on wound healing, and the fact that the majority of diabetic foot wounds have impaired healing involving many complex pathophysiological mechanisms, requires an understanding of the normal wound healing processes.

2.2.1 Stage 1: The Inflammatory Phase

The inflammatory response begins immediately following injury and lasts 2–4 days. The initial injury results in bleeding and enzymatic activation of the clotting cascade, the complement cascade, and the kinin cascade; activation of plasminogen, and the aggregation and activation of platelets [47]. Within a few hours of injury, inflammatory cells invade the wound tissue. Neutrophils arrive first, followed by monocytes and lymphocytes. As described by Werner and Grose [48], they produce a wide variety of proteinases and reactive oxygen species (ROS) as a defense against contaminating microorganisms, and they are involved in the phagocytosis of cell debris [49]. Inflammatory cells are also an important source of growth factors and cytokines, which initiate the proliferative phase of wound repair. Released growth factors stimulate a further influx of white cells, fibroblasts, and cells concerned with angiogenesis (formation of new blood vessels). Lymphocyte activity follows a similar, subsequent pattern [50]. Unlike platelets, the macrophages continue to secrete growth factors to attract fibroblasts, leading to the next phase of wound healing.

Platelets are a key component of the inflammatory phase. They are anucleated blood cells, originating in the bone marrow, which present in normal circulating blood in concentrations between 1.5 and 3.0×10^{-5}/mL, where they have been principally associated with the maintenance of haemostasis [51]. Platelets consisting of α-granules contain certain growth factors. Platelet factor 4, which is a heparin-binding chemokine, contains clotting proteins, such as thrombospondin, fibronectin, and von Willebrand factor, along with dense granules which contain adenosine diphosphate (ADP), adenosine triphosphate (ATP), ionized calcium (which is necessary for several steps of the coagulation cascade), histamine, and serotonin [52].

With the formation of the clot during wound healing, platelets provide a temporary scaffold for the growth of connective tissue cells, and modulate angiogenesis through a complex and as yet undefined series of cell and growth factor mediated events [53,54]. This includes thrombin-induced changes in platelet shape, the development of pseudopodia, which promotes platelet aggregation and subsequent release of the granule content (which includes clotting factors and growth factors) [55]. In relation to wound repair, Knighton et al. demonstrated that the use of thrombin-treated platelets significantly increases the healing rate of the rabbit cornea, and that soft tissue healing directly correlated with angiogenesis [56]. Other roles of platelets include the storage of many growth factors implicated in wound healing, including platelet-derived growth factor (PDGF) and TGF-ß [57,58].

Platelets contain a range of growth factors, which participate in the inflammatory phase of wound healing by directly influencing leucocytes, for example, PDGF attracts leucocytes and fibroblasts into the wound [59]. The degranulating[(4)] platelets along with resident tissue macrophages, mast cells, and the cells damaged during wounding all lead to the release of inflammatory mediators [60]. Inflammation is the key nonspecific response to combat the establishment of infection. An individual's level of response depends on their general health, nutritional state, and the presence of any underlying disease. Down regulation of the inflammatory phase will prevent movement into the proliferative stage and, thus, is a cause of wound indolence [61].

2.2.2 Growth Factors

Growth factors are released from α-granules of platelets [62–65]. These contain storage pools of growth factors, including PDGF, transforming growth factor beta (TGF-β), epithelial growth factors (EGF), fibroblast growth factors (FGF), insulin-like growth factor I, and vascular endothelial growth factors (VEGF), as well as cytokines. Chemokines and newly synthesized active metabolites are also released [66]. According to Englert et al. the fact that platelets can secrete growth factors and active metabolites means that they can contribute to rapid healing and tissue regeneration [67,68].

Wound healing is a complex multicellular process that requires coordinated efforts by many different cell types to achieve restoration of the skin. This process is executed by a complex cellular signalling network involving numerous growth factors, cytokines, and chemokines.

[4]Cell degranulation is the process of losing cytoplasmic granules. This occurs in mast cells, basophils, neutrophils, eosinophils, and platelets when secretory products are released from the granules.

All known growth factors are pleiotropic (influencing several aspects of cell behavior) and the majority affect several target cell populations [48]. This diversity is often not reflected in their names, which are commonly derived from their first documented bioactivity or source, for example, platelets [69]. The principal growth factors believed to be involved in normal wound healing are those listed in Table 2.1 [70]. Other factors include granulocyte macrophage colony stimulating factor (GM-CSF), connective tissue growth factor, the interleukin family, tumor necrosis factor-alpha, and keratinocyte growth factor. Many of the listed growth factors have been reported to occur in abnormally low concentrations in diabetic foot wounds [71,72], making the exogenous application of additional growth factors a rationale for enhancing wound healing in this population [72,73].

The focus of this chapter is on the abnormal healing encountered in a patient with a diabetic foot ulcer, so only the following growth factors will be discussed in detail; PDGF-AB, PDGF-BB, TGFβ, and VEGF. The wider importance of growth factors and cytokines in wound healing was reviewed by Werner and Grose [48].

2.2.3 Platelet-Derived Growth Factor

PDGF was discovered in 1974, when it was found that the material released from the granules of platelets was responsible for the *in vitro* growth of cultures of many types of the serum-dependent cells [74,75].

In humans, PDGF exists principally as a heterodimer of two chains, termed A and B chains, which are of about equal size and molecular weights [74]. In humans, PDGF also exists in much lower concentrations as A–A and B–B homodimers. The physiological reasons for the maintenance of these three distinct dimeric forms remain unclear. They all express the same activities, although it has been suggested that they may bind differentially to different receptor cells, such as fibroblasts and macrophages [74]. Only PDGF-AB and PDGF-BB, however, promote contraction of collagen matrices [46] and mediate the fibroblast-dependent secretion of collagenases, noted above as important in the remodeling phase of wound healing [76].

Platelet-derived growth factor is a powerful mitogenic, chemotactic, and angiogenic factor [77–80], and according to Grageda, is the first growth factor in the wound healing cascade [81]. Its effects include: chemotactic attraction of human monocytes and T lymphocytes during the immune reaction [82]; direct induction of proliferation of microvascular endothelial cells contributing to angiogenesis; indirect proliferative effects through stimulation of smooth muscle cells and fibroblasts [83]; induction of significant angiogenic growth factors, such as beta fibroblast growth factor (b FGF) and VEGF in smooth muscle cells and fibroblasts; the significant chemo-attraction of smooth muscle cells, fibroblasts, macrophages, and leukocytes and the stimulation of collagen and matrix formation in vivo and angiogenesis [77,84].

Table 2.1 Summary of growth factors and their effects during wound healing

Growth Factor	Main stage of involvement in wound repair	Production	Known functions	Levels in acute wounds	Levels in chronic wounds	References
Platelet-derived growth factor (PDGF)	Inflammation Tissue formation Tissue remodeling	Platelets Macrophage Endothelial cells	• Attracts macrophages and fibroblasts to the zone of injury • Promotes collagen and proteoglycan synthesis • Stimulates angiogenesis • Attracts stem cells and white blood cells • Facilitates proliferation of other growth factors	Increased	Decreased	(Greenhalgh et al. [85], Ono et al. [86], Winkles [82], Heldin et al. [87])
Epidermal growth factor (EGF)	Tissue formation	Platelets macrophages	• Stimulates fibroblasts to secrete collagenase to degrade the matrix during the remodeling phase. • Stimulates keratinocyte and fibroblast proliferation. • May reduce healing time when applied topically.	Increased	Decreased	(Carpenter and Cohen [88]; Buckley et al. [89])
Trans-forming Growth Factor (TGF)	Inflammation Tissue formation Tissue remodeling	Platelets macrophages Lymphocytes hepatocytes	• TGF-a: Mitogenic and chemotactic for keratinocytes and fibroblasts TGF-β1 and TGF-β2: – Promotes angiogenesis, – Up-regulates collagen production – Inhibits degradation, – Promotes chemoattraction of inflammatorycells. – Immunosuppressant during inflammatory phase. • TGF-β3 (antagonist to TGF-β1 and β2): Has been found in high levels in foetal scar less wound healing and has promoted scar less healing in adults experimentally when TGF-β1 and TGF-β2 are suppressed. • TGF-β is chemotactic for macrophages, induces the production of procollagen type I and fibronectin, and inhibits metalloproteinases. The effect is an increased deposition of collagen.	Increased	Decreased	(Calvin [90], Yang et al. [91]; Wang et al. [92]; Barrientos et al. [72])

Vascular endothelial growth factor (VEGF)	Tissue formation	Endothelial cells	• Promotes angiogenesis during tissue hypoxia.	Increased	Decreased	(Kane et al. [93]; Kopecki et al. [94]; Papanas and Maltezos [70])
Insulin-like growth factor (IGF)	Early inflammation Cell growth	Liver	• Promotes cell growth—myoblasts and fibroblasts • Enhances collagen and matrix synthesis • MAY modulate swelling	Increased	Increased	(Clemmons [95]; Dahlgren et al. [96])
Fibroblast growth factor (FGF)	Tissue formation Tissue remodeling	Macrophages Mast cells, T-lymphocytes	• Promotes angiogenesis, granulation, and epithelialization via endothelial cell, fibroblast, and keratinocyte migration, respectively.	Increased	Decreased	(Ornitz and Itoh [97])

Source: Adapted from Papanas and Maltezos [70].

2.2.4 Epidermal Growth Factor

Epithelial cells in a wound produce EGF found in a wide variety of tissues [98,99]. Pesonen showed that EGF is released by platelets when they degranulate [100]. EGF receptors bind with the receptor cells of keratinocytes and fibroblasts, inducing a cascade of events, which result in DNA synthesis and the production of new proteins [101].

Both EGF and PDGF have been shown to act on cells in the resting state. In various models of normal repair, discussed by Arnold and West [102], the local addition of EGF, FGF, TGFβ, and PDGF has all been shown to increase the amount of granulation tissue formed early in the healing process. However, all of the above models involve experimental wounds in a variety of animals, including rats, rabbits, and pigs. Arnold and West [102] have suggested that some (or all) of the healing effects of the afore-mentioned growth factors may be due to the direct promotion of angiogenesis, but this has yet to be confirmed. Buckley et al. [89] stated that the sustained release of EGF accelerated wound repair and that EGF (and perhaps PDGF) stimulated epidermal cells to migrate and divide to cover the granulation tissue.

EGF is a potent mitogenic stimulant for epithelial cells, endothelial cells, and fibroblasts [103,104] although Falanga et al. [105] were unable to enhance healing in chronic venous stasis ulcers using EGF.

2.2.5 Transforming Growth Factor

Transforming growth factor alpha (TGF-α) is produced by epithelial cells, macrophages, platelets, and endothelial cells in the wound. This factor stimulates keratinocytes and fibroblasts in wounds [101] to form new matrix proteins and regeneration of the dermis [106].

Transforming growth factor beta (TGF-β) is a peptide growth factor found in three forms in humans—TGF-β1, TGF-β2, and TGF-β3. It is produced in the wound by epithelial cells, macrophages, platelets, and neutrophils. Depending on the wound environment, the action of this factor is either stimulatory or inhibitory [107]. In the haemostatic/inflammatory phase of tissue repair, TGF-β is released by activated platelets and acts chemotactically to attract neutrophils and macrophages to the site of injury [90]. According to Cox [101], TGF-β is also involved in the early process of the inflammatory stage of wound healing, as it stimulates macrophage action. Through its interaction with the macrophage, it also has the ability to down regulate inflammatory activity [108].

In the proliferative phase, activated macrophages produce TGF-β, which plays an integral part in angiogenesis by stimulating keratinocytes. These accelerate the rate of epithelization and produce vascular endothelial growth factor. TGF-β differs from PDGF in being able to act independently of the macrophage.

In the remodeling production of the extracellular matrix, components of fibronectin and collagen type 1 are stimulated by the actions of TGF-ß. This growth factor also controls the production of matrix metalloproteinases (MMPs) and stimulates the expression of tissue inhibitors of matrix metalloproteinase, thereby promoting collagen formation [109]. Accelerated repair in response to TGF-ß has been demonstrated in several animal studies by Bernstein et al. and Beck et al. [110–112]. TGF-ß is also involved in the organization of immature collagen as it induces wound fibroblasts to differentiate into myofibroblasts, which are essential for wound contraction. This function continues in the remodeling phase. Thus, TGF-ß has an effect on the final function, strength, and appearance of the end product of the healing process—in the production of scar tissue [113].

2.2.6 Vascular Endothelial Growth Factor

As wound healing is an angiogenic-dependent process, VEGF production is essential. White blood cells and platelets contain VEGF protein and secrete it when stimulated, indicating the role of VEGF in inflammation and coagulation [114]. The term vascular endothelial growth factor encompasses five related proteins (VEGF-A, VEGF-B, VEGF-C, VEGF-D, and VEGF-E). Of these, one form of VEGF-A (VEGF-A_{165}) is biologically active, and the most potent angiogenic protein known [115,116]. Large quantities of VEGF are produced by the basal layer of the epidermis [117], with expression of this key initiator of angiogenesis peaking 7 days after cutaneous injury [118]. VEGF triggers endothelial cell division, chemotaxis, and vascular permeability [116,119–121] and promotes the production of nitric oxide, which enhances collagen deposition.

Fibroblasts are a source of VEGF, but the release of VEGF from fibroblasts is hypoxia-dependent and is regulated by the oxygen-regulated protein ORP150 [122]. Hypoxia-induced VEGF and VEGF receptor expression promote the proliferation and migration of endothelial cells. This leads to angiogenesis and the development of collateral neovascularisation in the ischaemic tissues [123]. As well as being a potent angiogenic factor, VEGF also has a role as a vasodilator and also increases vascular permeability. VEGFs do, however, have a short period of activity [124]. Researchers have dealt with this problem by using gene therapy to extend VEGFs duration of action in treating ischaemic heart disease; a vector holds and delivers VEGF to ensure continued administration for a period of 1–2 weeks [125].

Diabetes is one of the systemic disorders reported to impair VEGF expression in the lower extremities [126]. There is ongoing research using VEGF gene therapy, also referred to as therapeutic angiogenesis, not just to treat ischaemia but also to promote wound healing in diabetic and nondiabetic subjects [127]. Brem et al. [128] conducted a study on diabetic mice, in which they found ADV/VEGF was an effective accelerator of wound closure by stimulating angiogenesis, epithelialization, and collagen deposition. They conclude by suggesting in the future, local administration and sustained, controlled release of $VEGF_{165}$ may decrease amputations in patients with diabetic foot ulcers and possibly accelerate closure of venous ulcers and pressure ulcers [128].

2.2.7 Insulin-Like Growth Factor

The insulin-like growth factors (IGFs) are polypeptide hormones secreted from many different cells which share considerable peptide homology with insulin. IGF-I and IGF-II are potent stimulators of mitogenesis and they exert their functions in an autocrine, paracrine, or endocrine manner [48].

There are two principal IGFs, referred to as IGF-I and IGF-II. Structurally, both IGFs resemble insulin in having two chains (A and B) connected by disulphide bonds. IGF-II appears to play an important role in early cell development [129], whereas IGF-I is relevant at the latter point in time maximizing growth. IGF-I is a critical growth factor required by most cells to progress through division and replication. It is primarily excreted by the liver into the blood plasma [130].

IGFs, as well as leading to increased bone formation, stimulate efficient reepithelization of wounds [131]. Several studies have revealed a beneficial effect of exogenous IGF-I on wound healing, in particular in combination with other growth factors [132]. Werner and Grose [48] discussed various studies conducted on diabetic rats and mice. They concluded that the findings from the studies are likely to be important for the pathogenesis of chronic human wounds, since IGF-I protein was absent in the basal layer of the epidermis and in fibroblasts of diabetic patients but not of healthy control subjects [48]. Blakytny et al. conducted a study measuring the levels of IGF-I in biopsied skin from subjects with diabetes, "healthy" subjects undergoing surgery deemed to have "normal skin" and from the edge of foot ulcers of diabetic patients. They found that the skin of those with diabetes and those with a diabetic foot ulcer lacked IGF-1; however, they also had an increased level of IGF-2. Blakytny et al. [133] highlighted this may be important in delayed wound healing in those with diabetes.

When considered together, these studies suggest that reduced expression of IGFs and/or their receptors leads to impaired wound healing, although this hypothesis has yet to be confirmed by clinical studies [48].

2.2.8 Fibroblast Growth Factor

The FGF are a family of heparin-binding growth factors produced by fibroblasts, endothelial cells, smooth muscle cells, chondrocytes, and mast cells [134]. Originally, acidic FGF and basic FGF were the two forms of fibroblast growth factor identified, but, more recently, the family has been expanded to include seven additional forms. These are named FGF1 to FGF9 [135].

Collagen synthesis is stimulated by bFGF (FGF2) as well as wound contraction, epithelization and fibronectin and proteoglycan synthesis [136]. Owing to its release by inflammatory cells early in wound healing, FGF2 is involved in initiating granulation tissue formation [137], but it continues to be important during subsequent tissue remodeling. Animal studies have shown that topical applications of FGF2 improve the strength of ischaemic wounds [138] and accelerate their rate of closure [139]. A recently published study by Kulwas et al. [140] has shown that in patients with type 2 diabetes and a foot ulcer there is a high concentration of VEGF-A and FGF-2. They found a positive correlation between VEGF-A and FGF-2 indicated their participation in the process of angiogenesis [140].

2.2.9 Stage 2: Proliferative Phase

The proliferative phase follows and overlaps with the inflammatory phase. It is characterized by epithelial proliferation and reepithelialization by the migration of the epithelial cells over the provisional matrix formed following wounding. In the reparative dermis, the most prominent cell types present are fibroblasts and endothelial cells. They support capillary growth, collagen formation, and the formation of granulation tissue at the site of injury [141]. The granulation tissue is composed of a dense population of macrophages and fibroblasts characterized by an extensive network of new blood vessels surrounded by loosely structured collagen, elastin, and proteoglycans [142,143]. The fibroblasts bind growth factors and secrete additional growth factors (including basic fibroblast growth factor and insulin growth factor I) and extracellular matrix (ECM) molecules. Growth factors induce both autocrine and paracrine stimulation of fibroblasts and ingrowing capillaries. Simultaneously, epithelial cells start to grow inward from the wound edges to cover the wound, strengthened by collagen. The appearance of the collagen is as strands aligned parallel to the stress lines of the wound [144] rather than like the basket weave appearance it has in an unwounded dermis. This different construction is responsible for the variance in appearance between undamaged dermis and scar tissue. The growth factors at the wound site are responsible for the regulation of the collagen synthesis by the fibroblasts and there is a fine balance between the rates of synthesis and degradation of collagen [145].

This process of reepithelialization involves a number of cytokines, which are released in large quantities at the wound edge. They include EGF, TGFα, TGFß1, nerve growth factor, and keratinocyte growth factor [146].

2.2.10 Stage 3: Remodeling Phase

The remodeling phase is also known as maturation. During remodeling, the water content of the wound reduces, and the collagen laid down during proliferation is gradually replaced by a more stable interwoven type III collagen. The amounts of connective tissue and capillaries are reduced, with wound contraction and scar formation. Remodeling is regulated by a variety of growth factors, primarily TGF- ß, PDGF, and FGF, which are stimulated during tissue injury and repair. The role of growth factors in scar formation is not fully understood, but TGF-ß is thought to be important [147,148]. This factor is known to inhibit procollagenase production and enzyme activity by increasing the synthesis of tissue inhibitors of metalloproteinase (TIMPs) leading to an increased collagen deposition [78,149].

Over a period of up to 2 years following injury, a continuing process of fibroblast-induced collagen synthesis, breakdown by collagenases, and regression of inflammatory cells occurs, gradually remodeling the wound into a mature scar [69].

2.3 THE CHRONIC WOUND

Not all wounds heal in the normal way, with many becoming "stuck" in either the inflammatory or proliferative phases, thus becoming chronic wounds.

Trengove et al. [150] defined chronic wounds as "those that have failed to proceed through an orderly and timely reparative process to produce anatomic and functional integrity of the injured site". Martinez-Zapta et al. [151] went further and defined the chronic wound as a visible break in the surface of the skin that does not heal, and/or recurs, or takes longer than 6 weeks to heal. Other definitions, such as that provided by the American Diabetes Association, suggest "failure to heal within four weeks" [152].

Unlike acute wounds, chronic wounds appear to be "stuck" in the inflammatory/proliferative process, allowing for repeated injury, infection, and inflammation, all of which impair full wound closure. A number of studies have shown that true chronic wounds are biochemically different from acute wounds, differing in their expression of growth factors, MMPs, and various proteins [152–155].

While chronic wounds may result from different underlying pathologies, they are considered biochemically similar, in that they are characterized by persistent inflammatory stimuli [156]. Persistent inflammatory stimuli can stimulate cytokine inflammatory mediators, in turn elevating protease concentrations, with increased protein degradation, resulting in the breakdown of growth factors that promote cell proliferation and granulation tissue formation. These processes lead to a shift in the wound equilibrium toward destructive processes, effectively suspending the wound in the inflammatory phase of healing [157].

2.3.1 Diabetes and Wound Chronicity

All of the processes of normal wound healing are altered in patients with diabetes and contribute to the poor healing of diabetic foot ulcers. Abnormalities in cellular function, notably the fibroblasts and neutrophils, have been reported in patients with diabetes.

Diabetic foot ulcers are always accompanied by hypoxia [158]. Prolonged hypoxia may be the result of insufficient perfusion and inadequate angiogenesis, both of which are detrimental to wound healing. Hypoxia can intensify the early inflammatory response of normal healing and, thereby, increasing the levels of oxygen radicals, which prolong tissue damage [159]. According to Vincent et al. [160], hyperglycaemia can also add to the oxidative stress when the production of ROS exceeds the antioxidant capacity. *In vitro* atypically high sugars may be toxic to fibroblasts and neutrophils; therefore, in those with diabetes it may result in a greater susceptibility to infection [161].

In addition to these factors, it has also been noted that high blood glucose concentrations impair granulocyte and neutrophil function, and chemotaxis. Resulting in an increase risk of infection [162] and impaired wound healing [163,164] due to the breakdown of the function of intrinsic healing, coupled with the disordered participation of the cellular components of healing [165]. There are changes in the cellular infiltrate and extracellular matrix, with a prolonged expression of fibronectin, fewer T cells, and more macrophages persisting beyond the initial stages of healing [166].

The role of insulin in the regulation of energy metabolism, protein synthesis, cell differentiation, and growth suggests that it may also play an essential role in regulation of wound healing [167]. There is evidence, from several decades ago, suggesting a positive effect of systemic insulin replacement on diabetic wound healing [168,169], but reports on topical insulin administration in diabetic wound healing have given conflicting results [170,171]. Topical insulin improved healing in chronic foot ulcers in both diabetic and nondiabetic mice [170], but topical insulin therapy failed to improve healing of decubitus ulcers [172]. The exact mechanism by which insulin reverses impaired wound healing is unknown [173].

Lima et al. [174] used an insulin cream in a small randomized control trial involving subjects with diabetic foot ulcers. In this study, the wound healing was so "impressive" that those treated with the placebo cream ($n = 12$) for 8 weeks were then treated with the insulin cream. Their final analysis, therefore, included all 22 subjects treated with the insulin cream. All 22 subjects had healed in 15 weeks, suggesting that topically applied insulin enhances wound healing [174].

Trengove et al. [175] demonstrated elevated levels of MMPs in the fluid from chronic wounds, which results in increased proteolytic activity and inactivation of the growth factors, essential for normal wound healing. High levels of MMPs are a feature of diabetic foot ulcers, with levels almost 60 times higher in chronic wound fluid than in acute wound fluid. This increased protease activity inhibits the normal repair process and causes tissue destruction [159,176].

The inactivation of growth factors through various cellular defects also contributes to wounds becoming chronic. Loots et al. [166] showed that some extracellular matrix proteins (fibronectin and tenascin) are deposited in diabetic foot ulcers in higher concentrations and persist for weeks or months longer than in normal (acute) wounds. Extensive debridement can remove some of this excess matrix material as well as cells that are no longer capable of appropriately responding to the signals from growth factors necessary for wound repair [177]. A number of researchers have reported that healing arrest is paralleled by reduced growth factor activity [178–180] or reduced concentrations of growth factors [181]. For example, Cooper et al. [178] demonstrated that supernatant fluid from chronic pressure ulcers showed decreased concentrations of growth factors compared to the values of acute wound supernatant. Jude et al. [182] suggested

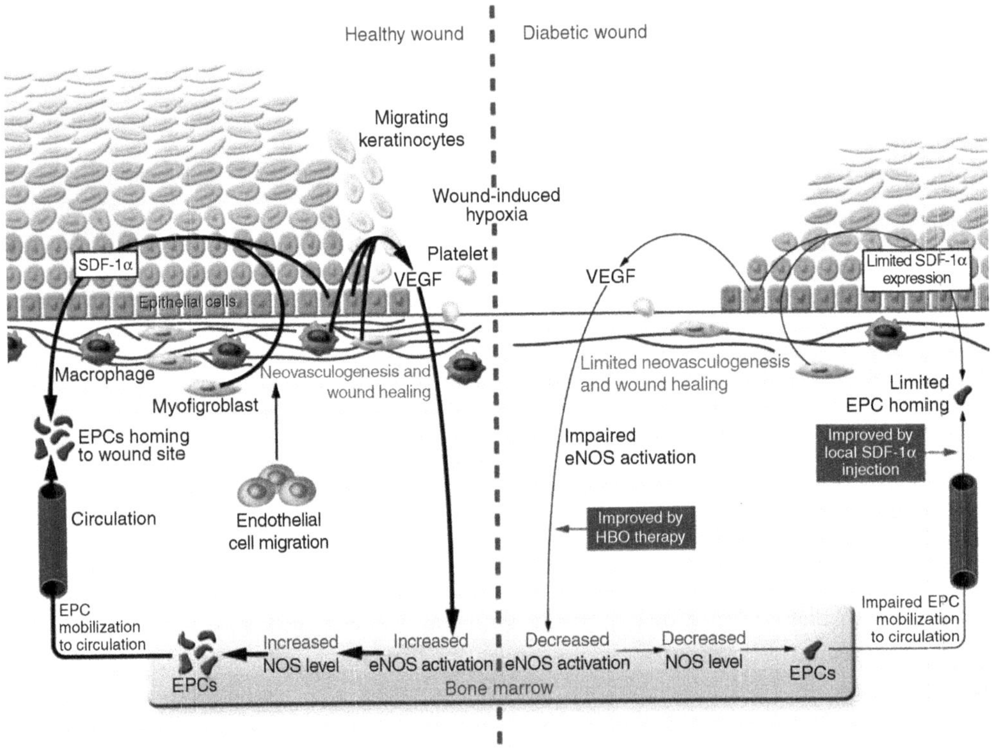

Figure 2.1 ***Mechanisms of wound healing in healthy people compared to people with diabetes [184].***

that reduced levels of TGF-ß1 and increased levels TGF-ß3 contributed to the chronic nature of venous and diabetic foot ulcers.

As already mentioned, hypoxia is a contributing factor in the impaired healing of diabetic foot ulcers. Diabetic wounds exhibit inadequate angiogenesis [183], with several studies showing the levels of VEGF are decreased [184,185].

In summary, impaired healing associated with diabetes involves hypoxia, fibroblast dysfunction, impaired angiogenesis, high levels of MMPs, reduced levels of growth factors, damage from ROS, and an immunopathy. The influence of these factors on wound healing was summarized figuratively by Brem and Tomic-Canic [184] in Fig. 2.1.

2.4 GROWTH FACTORS—A THERAPEUTIC OPTION FOR THE DIABETIC FOOT

Pierce et al. [77] observed that most of the cell types which enter a wound during healing are capable of synthesizing PDGF and are also activated by PDGF. These observations led to the hypothesis that exogenous application of PDGF could increase its proliferative effect, thus making it a potential therapeutic agent for wound healing. A series of animal studies by Pierce et al., Greenhalgh et al., and Mustoe et al. found PDGF was used as a successful treatment in animal models, in that wound healing was accelerated and the healed wound had an improved tensile strength [85,186,187]. These findings in the aforementioned studies led to clinical trials, which were performed on pressure sores, which initially indicated that PDGF had a therapeutic value in accelerating healing. However, work by Mustoe et al. [188] did not confirm these conclusions. In the last two decades, there has been considerable interest in the therapeutic potential of growth factors after two trials on diabetic foot ulcers showed some potential benefits in such therapies [189,190].

The first successful commercially available growth factor product available as a clinical means of enhancing wound healing in the chronic nonhealing diabetic neuropathic foot ulcer was Regranex. Regranex is a becaplermin gel containing 100 g of rhPDGF-BB [191]. Steed [189] investigated the efficacy and safety of recombinant human platelet-derived growth factor (rhPDGF-BB) in a double-blind, placebo-controlled, multicenter study of patients with chronic diabetic ulcers and demonstrated that 29 (48%) of 61 patients randomized to the rhPDGF-BB group achieved complete wound healing during the study, compared with only 14 (25%) of 57 patients randomized to the placebo group ($p = 0.01$). The subsequent study by Wieman et al. [190] enrolled 382 patients with chronic diabetic foot ulcers in a multicenter, double-blind, and placebo-controlled study. They demonstrated healing with becaplermin gel (rhPDGF-BB) was 43% above that of good wound care alone [190].

The efficacy of becaplermin gel treatment was evaluated in four published multicenter prospective randomized control trials, which led to its FDA approval. A total of 922 patients were treated with becaplermin gel (rhPDGF-BB) in the four published clinical trials [189,190,192,193], and the primary population was analyzed by an intention-to-treat analysis.[5] This population was defined as the group of patients, who were randomly assigned to the treatment, received at least one dose of the study drug and had postbaseline data available. In the above four trials, the gel performed better than the placebo gels. However, Embil et al. [192] reported a 21% recurrence of the ulcers at 6 months. Adverse events noted during these four published trials included infection, cellulitis, skin ulceration, and osteomyelitis, but most were attributed to diabetes rather than the use of Regranex [192]. While the results from these studies supported the efficacy of rhPDGF-BB, Jeffcoate et al. [194] stated that the results of a European study were not published, inferring the outcomes demonstrated in the study by Wieman and colleagues in 1998 could not be replicated.

[5] Intention to treat is a method of analysis for randomized trials in which all patients randomly assigned to one of the treatments are analyzed together, regardless of whether or not they completed or received that treatment.

In March 2008, the FDA issued a safety alert followed by a statement in June the same year, highlighting that there was a ×5 greater risk of death from cancer in patients who had used three or more tubes of *Regranex*.

Becaplermin gel (Regranex) was clearly not the panacea clinicians had hoped for. This, along with its prohibitive costs (£250 per tube in 1998, when the product was at the height of its use), and concerns regarding the link between becaplermin and malignancies distant from the site of application, led to its use being reevaluated, and then stopped, in Northern Ireland.

More recently, a comprehensive review of clinical trials involving the use of growth factors in the diabetic foot [195] noted a significant reduction in healing times in studies using PDGF-BB. A subsequent systematic review by Buchberger et al. [196] concluded that there are indications that using growth factors as an adjunctive therapy in the care of diabetic foot ulceration is advantageous in achieving complete wound closure.

Overall, these observations provide a significant rationale for the investigation of the use of growth factor supplementation with autologous PRP as a possible means of resolving chronic diabetic foot wounds.

2.5 INFECTION AND THE DIABETIC FOOT

The chronic diabetic foot wound is a complex wound, which fails to heal for many of the reasons discussed. However, bacterial infection is another key and common reason why these wounds fail to heal. Thus, infection forms the third corner of the triad of diabetic foot disease, that is, ischaemia, neuropathy, and infection [197].

Irrespective of the specific cause of the diabetic foot wound, there are several key principles in its management [198]. The first principle is to treat any bacterial infection. The majority of such infections occur in traumatic wounds and are associated with limb ischaemia [199,200].

2.5.1 Causative Organisms

Diabetic foot wounds are frequently described in the literature as being polymicrobial, that is, marked by the presence of several species of microorganisms [201–204]. American and European studies have found that *Staphylococcus aureus* and *Streptococcus pyogenes* (β-haemolytic streptococci) are the main causative pathogens of diabetic foot infections [205–208]. These suggestions have been confirmed by other studies, although mixed infections with aerobic gram-negative bacilli or obligate anaerobes have also been frequently suggested as causing diabetic food infections [209]. Several studies have noted that 30–50% of *S. aureus* isolated from diabetic foot ulcers are MRSA [208,210–213].

2.6 SUMMARY

Currently, in the United Kingdom, local management of infected diabetic foot wounds involves the use of topical antimicrobial dressings and the administration of systemic antibiotics. However, such an approach does not provide a comprehensive solution in the management of diabetic foot ulcers.

In the past, various recombinant forms of growth factors were used as a means of topical treatment to enhance healing of diabetic foot ulceration, but this was not the panacea early research suggested it might be. The relatively greater progress in relation to the application of PRP in oral maxillofacial surgery has shown its efficacy in enhancing wound healing, and suggests these effects relate to delivery of a range of growth factors to the wound bed. This is a rather simplistic view and the gross delivery of such growth factors may not be the most effective approach in the management of diabetic foot ulcers.

REFERENCES

[1] King H, Aubert RE, Herman WH. Global burden of diabetes, 1995-2025: prevalence, numerical estimates, and projections. Diabetes Care 1998;21(9):1414–31.
[2] International Diabetes Federation (IDF). Atlas. (5e), Available at: www.idf.org/diabetesatlas ISBN: -80-2. 2011:0-2.
[3] Diabetes prevalence. Available at: https://www.diabetes.org.uk/About_us/What-we-say/Statistics/Diabetes-prevalence-/.
[4] Kanavos P, Van Den Aardweg S, Schurer W. Diabetes expenditure, burden of disease and management in 5 EU countries. LSE Heal 2012;1–113. (January).
[5] Shenaq S, Klebuc M, Vargo D. How to help diabetic patients avoid amputation. Prevention and management of foot ulcers. Postgrad Med 1994;96:177–92.
[6] Reiber G, Bowker HP. Epidemiology of foot ulcers and amputations in the diabetic foot. The diabetic foot. St. Louis: Mosby, Inc; 2001. p. 13–32.
[7] Diabetes UK. Foot care for people with diabetes: the economic case for change. 2012. Available at: http://www.diabetes.org.uk/upload/News/Factsheet Footcare for people with diabetes.pdf.
[8] Abetz L, Sutton M, Brady L, McNulty P, Gagnon D. The Diabetic Foot Ulcer Scale (DFS): a quality of life instrument for use in clinical trials. Pract Diabetes Int 2002;19(6):167–75.
[9] Diabetes in adults | quality-statement-4-blood-glucose-control | Guidance and guidelines | NICE.
[10] Lazarus GS, Cooper DM, Knighton DR, et al. Definitions and guidelines for assessment of wounds and evaluation of healing. Wound Repair Regen 1994;2(3):165–70.
[11] Reiber GE, Boyko EJ. Diabetes research in the Department of Veterans Affairs. Diabetes Care 2004;27(suppl_2):B95–8.
[12] Reiber GE, Boyko EJ, Smith DG. Lower extremity foot ulcers and amputation in diabetes. In: Harris MI, Cowie CC, Stern MP, editors. Diabetes in America. 2nd ed. Bethesda, MD: National Institutes of Health, National Institute of Diabetes and Digestive and Kidney Diseases; 1995. p. 409–28. NIH publication 95-1468.
[13] Lavery L, Armstrong D, Wunderlich R, Tredwell J, Boulton A. Diabetic foot syndrome: evaluating the prevalence and incidence of foot pathology in Mexican Americans and non-Hispanic whites from a diabetes disease management cohort. Diabetes Care 2003;26(5):1435–8.
[14] Gregg EW, Sorlie P, Paulose-Ram R, et al. Prevalence of lower-extremity disease in the US adult population > = 40 years of age with and without diabetes: 1999-2000 national health and nutrition examination survey. Diabetes Care 2004;27(7):1591–7.

[15] Young MJ, Veves A, Boulton AJ. The diabetic foot: aetiopathogenesis and management. Diabetes Metab Rev 1993;9(2):109–27.
[16] Masson EA, Hay EM, Stockley I, Veves A, Betts RP, Boulton AJ. Abnormal foot pressures alone may not cause ulceration. Diabet Med 1989;6(5):426–8.
[17] Veves A, Murray HJ, Young MJ, Boulton AJ. The risk of foot ulceration in diabetic patients with high foot pressure: a prospective study. Diabetologia 1992;35(7):660–3.
[18] Bus SA, Maas M, Cavanagh PR, Michels RPJ, Levi M. Plantar fat-pad displacement in neuropathic diabetic patients with toe deformity: a magnetic resonance imaging study. Diabetes Care 2004;27(10):2376–81.
[19] Lippmann HI. Must loss of limb be a consequence of diabetes mellitus? Diabetes Care 1979;2(5):432–6.
[20] Bojsen-Moller F. Anatomy of the forefoot, normal and pathologic. Clin Orthop Relat Res 1979;142:10–8.
[21] Fernando D, Masson EA, Veves A, Boulton A. Relationship of limited joint mobility to abnormal foot pressures and diabetic foot ulceration. Diabetes Care 1991;14(1):8–11.
[22] Torella F, Ashleigh R, Bolia A, Nasim A. The management of tibial artery disease in diabetes. Br J Diabetes Vasc Dis 2002;2(3):162–6.
[23] Pecoraro RE, Ahroni JH, Boyko EJ, Stensel VL. Chronology and determinants of tissue repair in diabetic lower-extremity ulcers. Diabetes 1991;40(10):1305–13.
[24] Flynn MD, Edmonds ME, Tooke JE, Watkins PJ. Direct measurement of capillary blood flow in the diabetic neuropathic foot. Diabetologia 1988;31(9):652–6.
[25] Pecoraro RE, Reiber GE, Burgess EM. Pathways to diabetic limb amputation. Basis for prevention. Diabetes Care 1990;13(5):513–21.
[26] Levin M, Neal L, Bowker J. The diabetic foot. 5th ed. St. Louis: Mosby Year Book; 1993.
[27] Bouter KP, Storm AJ, de Groot RR, Uitslager R, Erkelens DW, Diepersloot RJ. The diabetic foot in Dutch hospitals: epidemiological features and clinical outcome. Eur J Med 1993;2(4):215–8.
[28] Gibbons GW, Eliopoulos GM. Infection of the diabetic foot. In: Kozak GP, Campbell DR, Frykberg RG, Habershaw GM, editors. Management of diabetic foot problems. 2nd ed. Philadelphia: WB Saunders; 1995. p. 121–9.
[29] Armstrong D, Lipsky B. Diabetic foot infections: stepwise medical and surgical management. Int Wound J 2004;1(2):123–32.
[30] Consensus development conference on diabetic foot wound care. In: Cavanagh PR, Buse JB, Frykberg RG, editors. Diabetes care. Boston, MA: American Diabetes Association; 1999.
[31] Most RS, Sinnock P. The epidemiology of lower extremity amputations in diabetic individuals. Diabetes Care 1983;6(1):87–91.
[32] Fylling CP, Knighton DR. Amputation in the diabetic population: incidence, causes, cost, treatment, and prevention. J Enterostomal Ther 1989;16(6):247–55.
[33] Larsson J, Apelqvist J. Towards less amputations in diabetic patients. Incidence, causes, cost, treatment, and prevention: a review. Acta Orthop Scand 1995;66(2):181–92.
[34] Boulton AJ, Vileikyte L. The diabetic foot: the scope of the problem. J Fam Pract 2000;49(11):3–8.
[35] Edmonds M. Infection in the neuroischemic foot. Int J Low Extrem Wounds 2005;4(3):145–53.
[36] Bakker K, Apelqvist J, Schaper NC. Practical guidelines on the management and prevention of the diabetic foot 2011. Diabetes Metab Res Rev 2012;28(Suppl 1):225–31.
[37] Lipsky B, Pecoraro R, Larson S, Hanley M, Ahroni J. Outpatient management of uncomplicated lower-extremity infections in diabetic patients. Arch Intern Med 1990;150(4):790–7.
[38] Thaller SR, Lee TJ, Armstrong M, Tesluk H, Stern JS. Effect of insulin-like growth factor type 1 on critical-size defects in diabetic rats. J Craniofac Surg 1995;6(3):218–23.
[39] Bitar M. Insulin-like growth factor-1 reverses diabetes-induced wound healing impairment in rats. Horm Metab Res 1997;28(8):383–6.
[40] Hehenberger K, Heilborn JD, Brismar K, Hansson A. Inhibited proliferation of fibroblasts derived from chronic diabetic wounds and normal dermal fibroblasts treated with high glucose is associated with increased formation of l-lactate. Wound Repair Regen 1998;6(2):135–41.
[41] Moulin V, Lawny F, Barritault D, Caruelle JP. Platelet releasate treatment improves skin healing in diabetic rats through endogenous growth factor secretion. Cell Mol Biol (Noisy-le-grand). 1998;44(6):961–71.
[42] Margolis DJ, Kantor J, Berlin JA. Healing of diabetic neuropathic foot ulcers receiving standard treatment. A meta-analysis. Diabetes Care 1999;22(5):692–5.

[43] Margolis DJ, Allen-Taylor L, Hoffstad O, Berlin JA. Healing diabetic neuropathic foot ulcers: are we getting better? Diabet Med 2005;22(2):172–6.
[44] Tortora G, Derrickson B. Principles of anatomy and physiology. 12th ed. Princeton, NJ: Wiley & Sons; 2008.
[45] Ma B, Cheng D-S, Xia Z-F, et al. Randomized, multicenter, double-blind, and placebo-controlled trial using topical recombinant human acidic fibroblast growth factor for deep partial-thickness burns and skin graft donor site. Wound Repair Regen 2007;15(6):795–9.
[46] Clark R. The molecular and cellular biology of wound repair. 2nd ed. New York: Plenum Press; 1998.
[47] Weyrich AS, Zimmerman GA. Platelets: signaling cells in the immune continuum. Trends Immunol 2004;25(9):489–95.
[48] Werner S, Grose R. Regulation of wound healing by growth factors and cytokines. Physiol Rev 2003;83(3):835–70.
[49] Dovi JV, Szpaderska AM, DiPietro LA. Neutrophil function in the healing wound: adding insult to injury? Thromb Haemost 2004;92(2):275–80.
[50] McGrath MH. Peptide growth factors and wound healing. Clin Plast Surg 1990;17(3):421–32.
[51] Folkman J, Browder T, Palmblad J. Angiogenesis research: guidelines for translation to clinical application. Thromb Haemost 2001;86(1):23–33.
[52] Singer AJ, Clark RA. Cutaneous wound healing. N Engl J Med 1999;341(10):738–46.
[53] Knighton DR, Ciresi KF, Fiegel VD, Austin LL, Butler EL. Classification and treatment of chronic nonhealing wounds. Successful treatment with autologous platelet-derived wound healing factors (PDWHF). Ann Surg 1986;204(3):322–30.
[54] Perini R, Wallace JL, Ma L. Roles of platelets and proteinase-activated receptors in gastric ulcer healing. Dig Dis Sci 2005;50(Suppl 1):S12–5.
[55] Everts P, Knape J, Weibrich G, et al. Platelet-rich plasma and platelet gel: a review. J Extracorpor Technol 2006;38(2):174–87.
[56] Knighton DR, Ciresi K, Fiegel VD, Schumerth S, Butler E, Cerra F. Stimulation of repair in chronic, nonhealing, cutaneous ulcers using platelet-derived wound healing formula. Surg Gynecol Obstet 1990;170(1):56–60.
[57] Chan RK, Liu P, Lew D-H, et al. Expired liquid preserved platelet releasates retain proliferative activity. J Surg Res 2005;126(1):55–8.
[58] Zimmermann R, Reske S, Metzler P, Schlegel A, Ringwald J, Eckstein R. Preparation of highly concentrated and white cell-poor platelet-rich plasma by plateletpheresis. Vox Sang 2008;95(1): 20–5.
[59] Deuel TF, Kawahara R, Mustoe TA, Pierce GF. Growth factors and wound healing: plateley-derived growth factor as a model cytokine. Annu Rev Med 1991;42:567–84.
[60] Ferguson MWJ, Leigh IM. Wound healing. In: Champion RH, Burton JL, Burns DA, Breathnach SM, editors. Rook/Wilkinson/Ebling, textbook of dermatology. 6th ed. Oxford: Blackwell Science; 1998. p. 337–56.
[61] Cox D. Growth factors in wound healing. J Wound Care 1993;2(6):339–42.
[62] Boehlen F, Clemetson KJ. Platelet chemokines and their receptors: what is their relevance to platelet storage and transfusion practice? Transfus Med 2001;11(6):403–17.
[63] Klinger MHF, Jelkmann W. Role of blood platelets in infection and inflammation. J Interferon Cytokine Res 2002;22(9):913–22.
[64] Anitua E, Andia I, Ardanza B, Nurden P, Nurden AT. Autologous platelets as a source of proteins for healing and tissue regeneration. Thromb Haemost 2004;91(1):4–15.
[65] Stassen JM, Arnout J, Deckmyn H. The hemostatic system. Curr Med Chem 2004;11(17):2245–60.
[66] Frechette J, Martineau I, Gagnon G. Platelet-rich plasmas: growth factor content and roles in wound healing. J Dent Res 2005;84(5):434–9.
[67] Englert S, Estep T, Ellis-Stoll C, Eppley B, Pietrzak W, Blanton M. Autologous platelet gel applications during cardiovascular surgery: effect on wound healing, Journal of Extracorporeal Technology, 37. and Platelet-Rich Plasma: of Biology and Applications in Plastic Surgery. Plast. Reconstr. Surg. 2006;118(6):148–52.
[68] Thorn JJ, Sørensen H, Weis-Fogh U, Andersen M. Autologous fibrin glue with growth factors in reconstructive maxillofacial surgery. Int J Oral Maxillofac Surg 2004;33(1):95–100.

[69] Bennett NT, Schultz GS. Growth factors and wound healing: biochemical properties of growth factors and their receptors. Am J Surg 1993;165(6):728–37.

[70] Papanas N, Maltezos E. Becaplermin gel in the treatment of diabetic neuropathic foot ulcers. Clin Interv Aging 2008;3(2):233–40.

[71] Falanga V. Wound healing and its impairment in the diabetic foot. Lancet 2005;366(9498):1736–43.

[72] Barrientos S, Stojadinovic O, Golinko MS, Brem H, Tomic-Canic M. Growth factors and cytokines in wound healing. Wound Repair Regen 2008;16(5):585–601.

[73] Robson MC. The role of growth factors in the healing of chronic wounds. Wound Repair Regen 1997;5(1):12–7.

[74] Ross R, Raines EW, Bowen-Pope DF. The biology of platelet-derived growth factor. Cell 1986;46(2):155–69.

[75] Ross R, Glomset J, Kariya B, Harker L. A platelet-dependent serum factor that stimulates the proliferation of arterial smooth muscle cells in vitro. Proc Natl Acad Sci U S A 1974;71(4):1207–10.

[76] Bauer EA, Cooper TW, Huang JS, Altman J, Deuel TF. Stimulation of in vitro human skin collagenase expression by platelet-derived growth factor. Proc Natl Acad Sci U S A 1985;82(12):4132–6.

[77] Pierce GF, Mustoe TA, Altrock BW, Deuel TF, Thomason A. Role of platelet-derived growth factor in wound healing. J Cell Biochem 1991;45(4):319–26.

[78] Kiritsy C, Lynch S. Role of growth factors in cutaneous wound healing: a review. Crit Rev Oral Biol Med 1993;4(5):913–22.

[79] Reuterdahl C, Sundberg C, Rubin K, Funa K, Gerdin B. Tissue localization of beta receptors for platelet-derived growth factor and platelet-derived growth factor B chain during wound repair in humans. J Clin Invest 1993;91(5):2065–75.

[80] Falanga V. Classifications for wound bed preparation and stimulation of chronic wounds. Wound Repair Regen 2000;8(5):347–52.

[81] Grageda E. Platelet-rich plasma and bone graft materials: a review and a standardized research protocol. Implant Dent 2004;13(4):301–9.

[82] Winkles JA. Serum- and polypeptide growth factor-inducible gene expression in mouse fibroblasts. Prog Nucleic Acid Res Mol Biol 1998;58:41–78.

[83] Nicosia RF, Villaschi S. Autoregulation of angiogenesis by cells of the vessel wall. Int Rev Cytol 1998;185:1–43.

[84] Rudkin GH, Miller TA. Growth factors in surgery. Plast Reconstr Surg 1996;97(2):469–76.

[85] Greenhalgh DG, Sprugel KH, Murray MJ, Ross R. PDGF and FGF stimulate wound healing in the genetically diabetic mouse. Am J Pathol 1990;136(6):1235–46.

[86] Ono K, Bansal R, Payne J, Rutishauser U, Miller R. Early development and dispersal of oligodendrocyte precursors in the embryonic chick spinal cord. Development 1995;121:1743–54.

[87] Heldin C-H, Eriksson U, Ostman A. New members of the platelet-derived growth factor family of mitogens. Arch Biochem Biophys 2002;398(2):284–90.

[88] Carpenter G, Cohen S. Epidermal growth factor. Annu Rev Biochem 1979;48:193–216.

[89] Buckley A, Davidson JM, Kamerath CD, Wolt TB, Woodward SC. Sustained release of epidermal growth factor accelerates wound repair. Proc Natl Acad Sci U S A 1985;82(21):7340–4.

[90] Calvin M. Cutaneous wound repair. Wounds 1998;10(1):173–8.

[91] Yang X-D, Jia X-C, Corvalan J, Wang P, Davis C, Jakobovits A. Eradication of established tumors by a fully human monoclonal antibody to the epidermal growth factor receptor without concomitant chemotherapy. Cancer Res 1999;59:1236–43.

[92] Wang D, Yu X, RA C, Brecehr P. Distinct effects if *N*-acetylcysteine and nitric oxide on angiotensin II-induced epidermal growth factor receptor ohosphorylation and intracellular Ca2+ levels. J Biol Chem 2000;275:12223–30.

[93] Kane W, McCaffrey T, Olsen K. Primary parotid maligancies. A clinical and pathologic review. Arch Otholaryngol Head Neck Surg 1991;117:307–15.

[94] Kopecki Z, Luchetti MM, Adams DH, et al. Collagen loss and impaired wound healing is associated with c-Myb deficiency. J Pathol 2007;211(3):351–61.

[95] Clemmons DR. Insulin-like growth factor binding proteins and their role in controlling IGF actions. Cytokine Growth Factor Rev 1997;8(1):45–62.

[96] Dahlgren G. Levelling up (part 2): A discussion paper on European strategies for tackling social inequities in health. Liverpool; 2006.

[97] Ornitz DM, Itoh N. Fibroblast growth factors. Genome Biol 2001;2(3). REVIEWS3005.
[98] Cohen S. Nobel lecture. Epidermal growth factor. Biosci Rep 1986;6(12):1017–28.
[99] Cohen S. Epidermal growth factor. Vitr Cell Dev Biol 1987;23:239–50.
[100] Pesonen K, Viinikka L, Myllylä G, Kiuru J, Perheentupa J. Characterization of material with epidermal growth factor immunoreactivity in human serum and platelets. J Clin Endocrinol. Metab 1989;68(2):486–91.
[101] Cox D. Growth Factors in wound healing. J Wound Care 1993;2(6):339–42.
[102] Arnold F, West DC. Angiogenesis in wound healing. Pharmacol Ther 1991;52(3):407–22.
[103] McAuslan B, Bender V, Reilly W, Moss B. New functions of epidermal growth factor: stimulation of capillary endothelial cell migration and matrix dependent proliferation. Cell 1985;8(2):175–82.
[104] Nakagawa S, Yoshida S, Hirao Y, Kasuga S, Fuwa T. Biological effects of biosynthetic human EGF on the growth of mammalian cells in vitro. Differentiation 1985;29(3):284–8.
[105] Falanga V, Eaglstein W, Bucalo B, Katz M, Harris B, Carson P. Topical use of human recombinant epidermal growth factor (h-EGF) in venous ulcers. J Dermatol Surg Oncol 1992;18:604–6.
[106] Lukas N, Strieter R, Elner V. Production of cytokines, interleukin-8 and monocyte chemo attractant protein-1. Blood 1995;86:2767–73.
[107] J S. Fibroblast growth factors: at the heart of angiogenesis. Cell Biol Int Rep 1995;19(5):431–44.
[108] Lawrence WT, Diegelmann RF. Growth factors in wound healing. Clin Dermatol 1994;12(1):157–69.
[109] Krishnamoorthy L, Morris HL, Harding KG. Specific growth factors and the healing of chronic wounds. J Wound Care 2001;10(5):173–8.
[110] Bernstein EF, Harisiadis L, Salomon G, et al. Transforming growth factor-beta improves healing of radiation-impaired wounds. J Invest Dermatol 1991;97(3):430–4.
[111] Beck LS, Deguzman L, Lee WP, Xu Y, McFatridge LA, Amento EP. TGF-beta 1 accelerates wound healing: reversal of steroid-impaired healing in rats and rabbits. Growth Factors 1991;5(4): 295–304.
[112] Beck LS, Amento EP, Xu Y, et al. TGF-beta 1 induces bone closure of skull defects: temporal dynamics of bone formation in defects exposed to rhTGF-beta 1. J Bone Miner Res 1991;8(6):753–61.
[113] Douglas HE. TGF-ß in wound healing: a review. J Wound Care 2010;19(9):403–6.
[114] Salven P, Orpana A, Joensuu H. Leukocytes and platelets of patients with cancer contain high levels of vascular endothelial growth factor. Clin Cancer Res 1999;5(3):487–91.
[115] Soker S, Gollamudi-Payne S, Fidder H, Charmahelli H, Klagsbrun M. Inhibition of vascular endothelial growth factor (VEGF)-induced endothelial cell proliferation by a peptide corresponding to the exon 7-encoded domain ofVEGF165. J Biol Chem 1997;272(50):31582–8.
[116] Ferrara N. Molecular and biological properties of vascular endothelial growth factor. J Mol Med (Berl) 1999;77(7):527–43.
[117] Brown SA, Appelt EA, Lipschitz A, Sorokin ES, Rohrich RJ. Platelet gel sealant use in rhytidectomy. Plast Reconstr Surg 1992;118(4):1019–25.
[118] Kapoor M, Howard R, Hall I, Appleton I. Effects of epicatechin gallate on wound healing and scar formation in a full thickness incisional wound healing model in rats. Am J Pathol 2004;165(1): 299–307.
[119] Yamagishi S, Yonekura H, Yamamoto Y, et al. Vascular endothelial growth factor acts as a pericyte mitogen under hypoxic conditions. Lab Invest 1999;79(4):501–9.
[120] Griffoen A, Molema G. Angiogenesis: potentials for pharmacological intervention in the treatment of cancer, cardiovascular diseases, and chronic inflammation. Pharmacol Rev 2000;52(2):237–68.
[121] Brkovic A, Sirois MG. Vascular permeability induced by VEGF family members in vivo: role of endogenous PAF and NO synthesis. J Cell Biochem 2007;100(3):727–37.
[122] Ozawa K, Kondo T, Hori O, et al. Expression of the oxygen-regulated protein ORP150 accelerates wound healing by modulating intracellular VEGF transport. J Clin Invest 2001;108(1):41–50.
[123] Shweiki D, Itin A, Soffer D, Keshet E. Vascular endothelial growth factor induced by hypoxia may mediate hypoxia-initiated angiogenesis. Nature 1992;359(6398):843–5.
[124] Hoeben A, Landuyt B, Highley M, Wildiers H, Van Oosterom A, De Bruijn E. Vascular endothelial growth factor and angiogenesis. Pharmacol Rev 2004;56(5):549–80.
[125] Rico T, Marchione R, Kirsner RS. Vascular disease in psoriasis. J Invest Dermatol 2009;129(10):2327.
[126] Veves A, King GL. Can VEGF reverse diabetic neuropathy in human subjects? J Clin Invest 2001;107(10):1215–8.

[127] Schratzberger P, Schratzberger G, Silver M, et al. Favorable effect ofVEGF gene transfer on ischemic peripheral neuropathy. Nat Med 2000;6(4):405–13.
[128] Brem H, Kodra A, Golinko MS, et al. Mechanism of sustained release of vascular endothelial growth factor in accelerating experimental diabetic healing. J Invest Dermatol 2009;129(9):2275–87.
[129] Morison IM, Becroft DM, Taniguchi T, Woods CG, Reeve AE. Somatic overgrowth associated with overexpression of insulin-like growth factor II. Nat Med 1996;2(3):311–6.
[130] Rubin R, Baserga R. Insulin-like growth factor-I receptor. Its role in cell proliferation, apoptosis, and tumorigenicity. Lab Invest 1995;73(3):311–31.
[131] G K, Lake M, Gidlund M. Insulin like growth factor - 1 and - 2 and their role in the re-epithelisation of wounds; interactions with insulin like growth factorbinding protein type 1. Scand J Plast Reconstr Hand Surg 1994;28:107–12.
[132] Lynch SE, Colvin RB, Antoniades HN. Growth factors in wound healing. Single and synergistic effects on partial thickness porcine skin wounds. J Clin Invest 1989;84(2):640–6.
[133] Blakytny R, Jude EB, Martin Gibson J, Boulton AJ, Ferguson MW. Lack of insulin-like growth factor 1 (IGF1) in the basal keratinocyte layer of diabetic skin and diabetic foot ulcers. J Pathol 2000;190(5):589–94.
[134] Reed JA, Albino AP, McNutt NS. Human cutaneous mast cells express basic fibroblast growth factor. Lab Invest 1995;72(2):215–22.
[135] Gharee-Kermani M, Pham S. Role of cytokines and cytokine therapy in wound healing and fibrotic diseases. Curr Pharm Des 2001;7(11):1083–103.
[136] Steed DL. Modifying the wound healing response with exogenous growth factors. Clin Plast Surg 1998;25(3):397–405.
[137] Gibran NS, Isik F, Heimbach D, Gordon D. Basic fibroblast growth factor in the early human burn wound. J Surg Res 1994;56:226–34.
[138] Quirinia A, Viidik A. The effect of recombinant basic fibroblast growth factor (bFGF) in fibrin adhesive vehicle on the healing of ischaemic and normal incisional skin wounds. Scand J Plast Reconstr Surg Hand Surg 1998;32(1):9–18.
[139] Uhl E, Barker JH, Bondàr I, et al. Basic fibroblast growth factor accelerates wound healing in chronically ischaemic tissue. Br J Surg 1993;80(8):977–80.
[140] Kulwas A, Drela E, Jundziłł W, Góralczyk B, Ruszkowska-Ciastek B, Rość D. Circulating endothelial progenitor cells and angiogenic factors in diabetes complicated diabetic foot and without foot complications. J Diabetes Complications 2015;29(5):686–90.
[141] Moulin V. Growth factors in skin wound healing. Eur J Cell Biol 1995;68(1):1–7.
[142] Clark R, Folkvord J, Hart C, Murray M, McPherson J. Platelet isoforms of platelet-derived growth factor stimulate fibroblasts to contract collagen matrices. J Clin Invest 1989;84:1036–40.
[143] Slavin J. The role of cytokines in wound healing. J Pathol 1999;178(1):5–10.
[144] Witte MB, Barbul A. General principles of wound healing. Surg Clin North Am 1997;77(3):509–28.
[145] Slavin J. The role of cytokines in wound healing. J Pathol 1999;178:5–10.
[146] Mehendale F, Martin P. The cellular and molecular events of wound healing. 1st ed. London: Martin Dunitz; 2001.
[147] Steenfos H. Growth factors and wound healing. J Plast Reconstr Surg Hand Surg 1994;28:95–105.
[148] Amjad S, Carachi R, Edward M. Keratinocyte regulation of TGF-BETA and connective tissue growth factor expression: a role in suppression of scar tissue formation. Wound Repair Regen 2007;15(5):748–55.
[149] Penn JW, Grobbelaar AO, Rolfe KJ. The role of the TGF-β family in wound healing, burns and scarring: a review. Int J Burns Trauma 2012;2(1):18–28.
[150] Trengove NJ, Stacey MC, MacAuley S, et al. Analysis of the acute and chronic wound environments: the role of proteases and their inhibitors. Wound Repair Regen 1999;7(6):442–52.
[151] Martinez-Zapata M, Carvajal A, Exposito J, Garcia J, Marx R. Autologous platelet rich-plasma for treating chronic wounds (Protocol). Cochrane Database of Systematic Reviews Issue 1. J Oral Maxillofac Surg 2008;59:1120.
[152] Pfeffer F, von Dobschuetz E, Riediger H, Moosmann C, Hopt UT. The non-healing wound. MMW Fortschr Med 2004;146(44):45–8.

[153] Kunimoto BT. Growth factors in wound healing: the next great innovation? *Ostomy*. Wound Manage 1999;45(8):56–64.
[154] Köveker GB. Growth factors in clinical practice. Int J Clin Pract 2000;54(9):590–3.
[155] Limova M. New therapeutic options for chronic wounds. Dermatol Clin 2002;20:357–63.
[156] Mast BA, Schultz GS. Interactions of cytokines, growth factors, and proteases in acute and chronic wounds. Wound Repair Regen 1996;4(4):411–20.
[157] Harris IR, Yee KC, Walters CE, et al. Cytokine and protease levels in healing and non-healing chronic venous leg ulcers. Exp Dermatol 1995;4(6):342–9.
[158] Tandara AA, Mustoe TA. Oxygen in wound healing—more than a nutrient. World J Surg 2004;28(3):294–300.
[159] Woo K, Ayello EA, Sibbald RG. The edge effect: current therapeutic options to advance the wound edge. Adv Skin Wound Care 2007;20(2):99–117.
[160] Vincent AM, Russell JW, Low P, Feldman EL. Oxidative stress in the pathogenesis of diabetic neuropathy. Endocr Rev 2004;25(4):612–28.
[161] American Diabetes Association (ADA). Consensus Development Conference on Diabetic Foot Wound Care. Diabetes Care 1999;22(3):1354–60.
[162] Gough A, Clapperton M, Rolando N, Foster AV, Philpott-Howard J, Edmonds ME. Randomised placebo-controlled trial of granulocyte-colony stimulating factor in diabetic foot infection. Lancet (London, England) 1997;350(9081):855–9.
[163] Papanas N, Maltezos E. Growth factors in the treatment of diabetic foot ulcers: new technologies, any promises? Int J Low Extrem Wounds 2007;6(1):37–53.
[164] Humphers JM, Shibuya N, Fluhman BL, Jupiter D. The impact of glycosylated hemoglobin and diabetes mellitus on wound-healing complications and infection after foot and ankle surgery. J Am Podiatr Med Assoc 2014;104(4):320–9.
[165] Blakytny R, Jude E. The molecular biology of chronic wounds and delayed healing in diabetes. Diabet Med 2006;23(6):594–608.
[166] Loots MA, Lamme EN, Zeegelaar J, Mekkes JR, Bos JD, Middelkoop E. Differences in cellular infiltrate and extracellular matrix of chronic diabetic and venous ulcers versus acute wounds. J Invest Dermatol 1998;111(5):850–7.
[167] Apikoglu-Rabus S, Izzettin FV, Turan P, Ercan F. Effect of topical insulin on cutaneous wound healing in rats with or without acute diabetes. Clin Exp Dermatol 2010;35(2):180–5.
[168] Goodson WH, Hung TK. Studies of wound healing in experimental diabetes mellitus. J Surg Res 1977;22(3):221–7.
[169] Andreassen TT, Oxlund H. The influence of experimental diabetes and insulin treatments on the biochemical properties of rat skin incisional wounds. Acta Chir Scand 1987;153(7–8):405–9.
[170] Hanam SR, Singleton CE, Rudek W. The effect of topical insulin on infected cutaneous ulcerations in diabetic and nondiabetic mice. J Foot Surg 1983;22(4):298–301.
[171] Hennessey PJ, Black CT, Andrassy RJ. Epidermal growth factor and insulin act synergistically during diabetic healing. Arch Surg 1990;125(7):926–9.
[172] Gerber RM, Van Ort SR. Topical application of insulin in decubitus ulcers. Nurs Res 1979; 28(1):16–9.
[173] Shearer JD, Coulter CF, Engeland WC, Roth RA, Caldwell MD. Insulin is degraded extracellularly in wounds by insulin-degrading enzyme (EC 3 4. 24. 56). Am J Physiol 1997;273(4 Pt 1): E657–64.
[174] Lima MHM, Caricilli AM, de Abreu LL, et al. Topical insulin accelerates wound healing in diabetes by enhancing the AKT and ERK pathways: a double-blind placebo-controlled clinical trial. PLoS One 2012;7(5):e36974.
[175] Trengove N, Beilefeldt-Ohmann H, Stacey M. Cytokine profile of wound fluid from nonhealing and healing chronic leg ulcers. Wound Repair Regen 1996;4(2):234–9.
[176] Sibbald G, Woo K. The biology of chronic foot ulcers in persons with diabetes. Diabetesmetabolism Res Rev 2008;24(1):25–30.
[177] Steed DL, Donohoe D, Webster MW, Lindsley L. Effect of extensive debridement and treatment on the healing of diabetic foot ulcers. Diabetic Ulcer Study Group. J Am Coll Surg 1996;183(1):61–4.

[178] Cooper D, Yu E, Hennessey P, Ko F, Robson M. Determination of endogenous cytokines in chronic wounds. Ann Surg 1994;219:688–92.
[179] Pierce GF, Tarpley JE, Allman RM, et al. Tissue repair processes in healing chronic pressure ulcers treated with recombinant platelet-derived growth factor BB. Am J Pathol 1994;145(6):1399–410.
[180] Beer HD, Longaker MT, Werner S. Reduced expression of PDGF and PDGF receptors during impaired wound healing. J Invest Dermatol 1997;109(2):132–8.
[181] Bennett NT, Schultz GS. Growth factors and wound healing: Part II. Role in normal and chronic wound healing. Am J Surg 1993;166(1):74–81.
[182] Jude E, Blakytny R, Bulmer J, Boulton A, Ferguson M. Transforming growth factor-beta2,3, and receptor type I and II in diabetic foot ulcers. Diabet Med 2002;19:440–7.
[183] Guo S, Dipietro LA. Factors affecting wound healing. J Dent Res 2010;89(3):219–29.
[184] Brem H, Tomic-Canic M. Cellular and molecular basis of wound healing in diabetes. J Clin Invest 2007;117(5):1219–22.
[185] Quattrini C, Jeziorska M, Boulton AJM, Malik RA. Reduced vascular endothelial growth factor expression and intra-epidermal nerve fiber loss in human diabetic neuropathy. Diabetes Care 2008;31(1):140–5.
[186] Pierce GF, Mustoe TA, Senior RM, et al. In vivo incisional wound healing augmented by platelet-derived growth factor and recombinant c-sis gene homodimeric proteins. J Exp Med 1988;167(3):974–87.
[187] Mustoe TA, Pierce GF, Morishima C, Deuel TF. Growth factor-induced acceleration of tissue repair through direct and inductive activities in a rabbit dermal ulcer model. J Clin Invest 1991;87(2):694–703.
[188] Mustoe TA, Cutler NR, Allman RM, et al. A phase II study to evaluate recombinant platelet-derived growth factor-BB in the treatment of stage 3 and 4 pressure ulcers. Arch Surg 1994;129(2):213–9.
[189] Steed DL. Clinical evaluation of recombinant human platelet-derived growth factor for the treatment of lower extremity diabetic ulcers. Diabetic Ulcer Study Group. J Vasc Surg 1995;21(1):71–8.
[190] Wieman TJ, Smiell JM, Su Y. Efficacy and safety of a topical gel formulation of recombinant human platelet-derived growth factor-BB (becaplermin) in patients with chronic neuropathic diabetic ulcers. A phase III randomized placebo-controlled double-blind study. Diabetes Care 1998;21(5):822–7.
[191] Steed D, Wounds B, Steenfos H. Platelet-Derived Growth Factor in the Treatment of Diabetic Foot Ulcers. J Plast Reconstr Surg Hand Surg 2000;12(6):95B–98.
[192] Embil JM, Papp K, Sibbald G, et al. Recombinant human platelet-derived growth factor-BB (becaplermin) for healing chronic lower extremity diabetic ulcers: an open-label clinical evaluation of efficacy. Wound Repair Regen 2000;8(3):162–8.
[193] Robson M, Payne W, Garner W, et al. Intergating the results of phase IV (post-marketing) clinical trial with four previous trials reinforces the position that Regranex (becaplermin) gel 0. J Appl Res 2005;5(1):35–45.
[194] Jeffcoate WJ, Lipsky BA, Berendt AR, et al. Unresolved issues in the management of ulcers of the foot in diabetes. Diabet Med 2008;25(12):1380–9.
[195] Eldor R, Raz I, Ben Yehuda A, Boulton AJM. New and experimental approaches to treatment of diabetic foot ulcers: a comprehensive review of emerging treatment strategies. Diabet Med 2004;21(11):1161–73.
[196] Buchberger B, Follmann M, Freyer D, Huppertz H, Ehm A, Wasem J. The importance of growth factors for the treatment of chronic wounds in the case of diabetic foot ulcers. Technol Assess 2010;6:0–1.
[197] McNeely MJ, Boyko EJ, Ahroni JH, et al. The independent contributions of diabetic neuropathy and vasculopathy in foot ulceration. How great are the risks? Diabetes Care 1995;18(2):216–9.
[198] Jeffcoate WJ, Harding KG. Diabetic foot ulcers. Lancet 2003;361(9368):1545–51.
[199] Lavery LA, Armstrong DG, Wunderlich RP, Mohler MJ, Wendel CS, Lipsky BA. Risk factors for foot infections in individuals with diabetes. Diabetes Care 2006;29(6):1288–93.
[200] Prompers L, Huijberts M, Apelqvist J, et al. Delivery of care to diabetic patients with foot ulcers in daily practice: results of the Eurodiale Study, a prospective cohort study. Diabet Med 2008;25:700–7.

[201] Lipsky B, Pecoraro RE, LJ W. The diabetic foot. Soft tissue and bone infection. Infect Dis Clin North Am 1990;4:409–32.
[202] Pathare NA, Bal A, Talvalkar GV, Antani DU. Diabetic foot infections: a study of microorganisms associated with the different Wagner grades. Indian J Pathol Microbiol 1998;41(4):437–41.
[203] Lipsky BA, Berendt AR. Principles and practice of antibiotic therapy of diabetic foot infections. Diabetes Metab Res Rev 2000;16:42–6.
[204] Abdulrazak A, Bitar ZI, Al-Shamali AA, Mobasher LA. Bacteriological study of diabetic foot infections. J Diabetes Complications 2005;19(3):138–41.
[205] Caputo GM, Cavanagh PR, Ulbrecht JS, Gibbons GW, Karchmer AW. Assessment and management of foot disease in patients with diabetes. N Engl J Med 1994;331(13):854–60.
[206] Goldstein EJ, Citron DM, Nesbit CA. Diabetic foot infections. Bacteriology and activity of 10 oral antimicrobial agents against bacteria isolated from consecutive cases. Diabetes Care 1996;19(6):638–41.
[207] Citron DM, Goldstein EJC, Merriam CV, Lipsky BA, Abramson MA. Bacteriology of moderate-to-severe diabetic foot infections and in vitro activity of antimicrobial agents. J Clin Microbiol 2007;45(9):2819–28.
[208] Dang X, Doble BW, Kardami E. The carboxy-tail of connexin-43 localizes to the nucleus and inhibits cell growth. Mol Cell Biochem 2003;242(1–2):35–8.
[209] Viswanathan V, Jasmine JJ, Snehalatha C, Ramachandran A. Prevalence of pathogens in diabetic foot infection in South Indian type 2 diabetic patients. J Assoc Physicians India 2002;50:1013–6.
[210] Wagner A, Reike H, Angelkort B. Highly resistant pathogens in patients with diabetic foot syndrome with special reference to methicillin-resistant Staphylococcus aureus infections. Dtsch Med Wochenschr 2001;126(48):1353–6.
[211] Tentolouris N, Petrikkos G, Vallianou N, et al. Prevalence of methicillin-resistant Staphylococcus aureus in infected and uninfected diabetic foot ulcers. Clin Microbiol Infect 2006;12(2):186–9.
[212] Esposito S, Leone S, Noviello S, et al. Foot infections in diabetes (DFIs) in the out-patient setting: an Italian multicentre observational survey. Diabet Med 2008;25(8):979–84.
[213] Mendes JJ, Marques-Costa A, Vilela C, et al. Clinical and bacteriological survey of diabetic foot infections in Lisbon. Diabetes Res Clin Pract 2012;95(1):153–61.

CHAPTER THREE

History and Evolution of Bandages, Dressings, and Plasters

J. Davis, A. McLister
School of Engineering, Ulster University, Jordanstown, Northern Ireland, United Kingdom

3.1 INTRODUCTION

There have been tremendous advances in wound care in recent years and now, should someone be unfortunate enough to be injured, there are a multitude of options available to promote speedy recovery [1–3]. A browse through any pharmacy will reveal a myriad of wound dressings, ointments, sprays, and many other wonders of modern biomedical engineering all designed to improve wound healing. You will not, however, find animal manure, dried bark, cobwebs or tree resin on the shelves, or many other unmentionables, nor will you find an attending pharmacist who will be keen to recommend such materials as a wound treatment. These ingredients, however, are very much part of the history of wound dressings from the earliest ages and have had an integral part to play in the development of the medicinal products that are used to treat the smallest cuts, grazes, and burns to those wounds that are life threatening. The aim of this chapter is to explore the pathways through which bandages and wound dressings have evolved and to highlight how seemingly bizarre approaches have inspired new molecularly designed functional materials that can direct the biological processes necessary for wound repair.

New developments in wound treatment methodologies are invariably subjected to stringent assessment procedures such that their efficacy can be validated before being applied to a patient. The fundamental research that underpins such treatments, clinical trial data, and case histories are normally subject to peer review and are published within a vast array of journals targeted at scientists, engineers, and clinicians. The wealth of information that exists at present is staggering, and it is little surprise that modern healthcare relies heavily upon the storage, transmission, and retrieval of such data. A clinician or, indeed, a patient can easily, with a few taps on a keyword, clicks of a mouse, or swipe of a finger on a smart device, find a wealth of information on a particular wound dressing or treatment. It has not always been so easy and, in many of the very early cases, the rationale for choosing one approach over another will have been determined by factors which have no scientific basis and applied with no recourse to previous medical evidence. The reliance on superstition, folklore, hearsay, and some simply ridiculous and arguably random assumptions is quite startling, and it is inevitable that many of the potions and procedures will have hastened the final departure of the patient. Some wound treatments may well have been trial and error, but others may have been inspired by keen observation. This chapter highlights both and seeks to elucidate some of the thinking that may have underpinned the adoption of particular processes and materials.

3.2 BANDAGE, DRESSING, OR PLASTER?

There can often be some confusion between use of "bandage" and "dressing," whereby the former is often used as an all-encompassing term within the public's perception and reinforced by the marketing employed in many consumer products. An example is highlighted by the term "plaster," where its use as a colloquial term in the United Kingdom implies a small adhesive bandage complete with dressing. Although these terms may be used interchangeably by some, they nevertheless elude to materials that have distinct functions. A bandage is typically a material that is used to support a dressing, splint, or other medical devices, or it can be used on its own to provide mechanical support to a part of the body. The dressing is the component which is applied directly to the wound and is responsible for promoting wound healing. Depending on the composition, the dressing can function in a multitude of ways, and while traditionally they would have been used to stem bleeds, absorb exudate, and minimize contamination, they can comprise of an intricate composite with constituents designed to ease pain, combat infection, and actively promote healing through directly influencing the wound dynamics. Plasters may have a role similar to that of a wound dressing in that, historically, they would have been a paste typically spread on a support (bandage) and applied to the wound. More recently, the term plaster, when applied in a medicinal context, has become synonymous with fracture repair where the paste/bandage composite is used as a rigid cast to provide mechanical support.

3.2.1 Flax and Linen

It is impossible to pin point the first use of a bandage, but given the discovery of dyed flax fibers and textiles akin to linen that date back some 36,000 years [4], it is likely that even the very earliest of societies had the capability to manufacture and employ some form of bandage. The first indication of bandages being deployed comes from the excavation of ancient burial sites where an examination of Neolithic skeletal remains possessing arm or leg fractures was found to display evidence of advanced healing consistent with the use of splints [5–7]. It is possible to infer that these would have required a bandage binding of some form to ensure the immobility of the frame and a secure set. Excavation of later Egyptian burial sites afforded more direct physical evidence where, in one example, an adolescent with a fractured femur had been splinted with four boards still held together with linen strappings [8].

The importance of the flax plant (*Linum usitatissimum* L) in early linen textiles cannot be underestimated and its cultivation had, and continues to have, a global spread [9]. The earliest reports point toward the first domesticated use of Flax in Mesopotamia (c.5,000–4,000 BC) and it was subsequently adopted by neighboring cultures for production into linen. It has had a pivotal role in the development of bandages and its early use is arguably enshrined in the consciousness of most people through countless movies and documentaries about Egyptian mummies. Rather than being the embalmers choice for postmortem preservation, the application of linen was commonplace within medical practice. The Edwin Smith Papyrus (c.1,500–1,600 BC), one of the earliest known surgical texts, and although incomplete, describes a range of conditions for which linen bandages are prescribed for the setting of fractures through to wound management. In relation to the earlier discussion of terminology, it is worthwhile pointing out that in the burial site excavations, the linen bandages not only held the splints in place but also a dressing containing traces of blood—albeit in a rather severe state of decomposition [8].

Flax is considered to be one of the strongest of the natural fibers and possesses a complex composite structure. The bast (outer) fiber bundles are isolated from the stem by mechanical means (breaking, scutching, and hackling), resulting in bundles of fiber of around 1 m in length. Each bundle typically consists of around 10–40 elementary fibers [10,11] which have lengths of between 2 and 5 cm with diameters in the range of 5–35 μm. A schematic of the fiber structure is indicated in Fig. 3.1. The elementary fibers

H.L. Bos et al. / Composites: Part A 37 (2006) 1591–1604

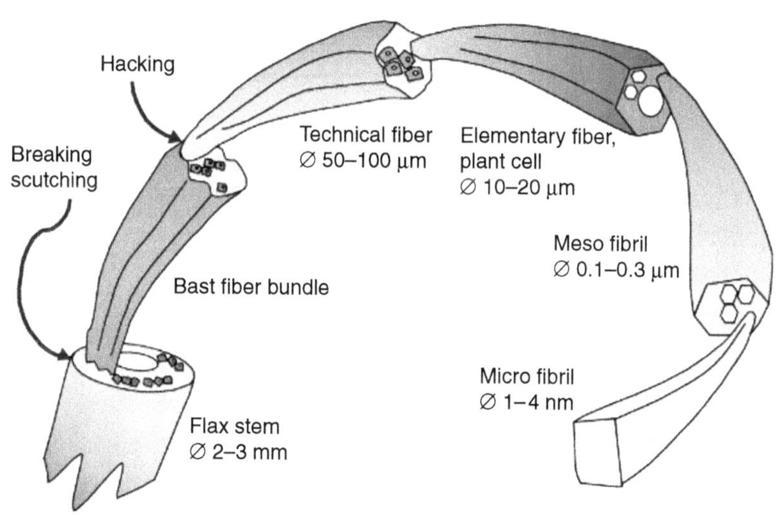

Figure 3.1 ***Schematic representation of the main components of flax.***

overlap over along the length of the primary bast bundle and are glued together by an interphase consisting of pectins and hemicelluloses. The fibers have a distinct polyhedral shape—presumably to increase the packing density with the parent bast fiber [10–13]. Although the smaller, elementary fibers are strong (c.1,500 MPa), they are generally soft and have the general appearance of bundles of blonde hair [14].

3.2.2 Lint and Charpie

The modern-day usage of the term lint tends to relate to the small accumulations of fibers originating from clothing—typically as a result of washing and drying. Historically, lint was a prepared form of flax fiber bandages in which the linen cloth was repeatedly scraped (Fig. 3.2) to provide a soft, delicate mass. The term "Charpie" originates from the French "charpir" which means "to pluck." The resulting lint can have an appearance similar in nature to that of cotton wool (and hence the association with modern-day usage) and would have typically been folded and pressed into the wound and secured by the unscraped linen cloth acting as the bandage. The production of lint could be achieved in an *ad hoc* manner and, given the ancient history of flax, probably has similarly old roots in wound healing [8].

3.2.3 New Directions for Flax Linen

The use of linen as a bandage material was slowly replaced by the introduction of cotton, which being less expensive and more elastic, proved to be more commercially attractive and clinically applicable. Nevertheless, there has been a resurgence of interest in the use of flax fibers as a consequence of genetic engineering with new improved processing qualities and the introduction of new functional properties [16–19]. Interest in the latter

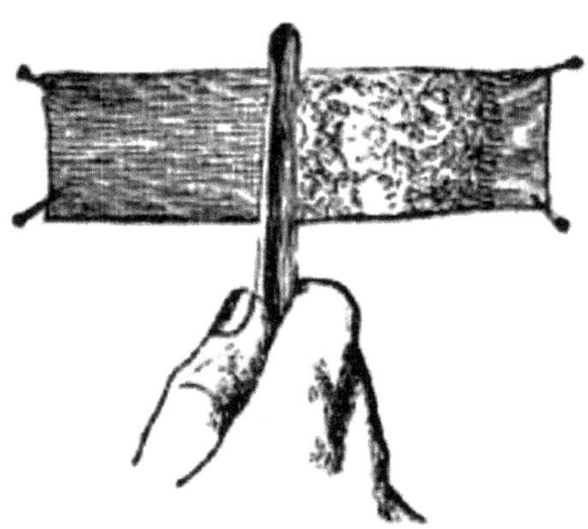

Figure 3.2 ***Historical example of lint scraping for wound dressings [15].***

is predominantly driven by the need for improved engineered structures but, it could be anticipated that the translation to biomedical contexts will inevitably follow. The incorporation of antioxidant and antimicrobial structures is of direct significance for wound healing and could mark the transformation of the linen from a simple mechanical support structure to a more active dressing [16–19]. It has also been noted that the fibers themselves can possess cannabinoid-like groups that, although such use is highly speculative, could be useful as a pain-relieving dressing [19].

3.2.4 Cotton Bandages

Cotton (*Gossypium Hirsutum)* began to replace linen in the 1800s, being less expensive to produce and easier to process than flax fibers. It is presently the most used natural fiber in the world and certainly the predominate material within simple bandage and dressing designs. The earliest evidence of cotton being used in textile manufacture relates to around 3,000 BC in India with textile artifacts of similar age being found in archaeological sites in Southern America. Cotton cultivation first spread from India to Egypt, China, and the South Pacific. Large-scale cotton cultivation in Northern America began in the 16th century [20]; however, it was not until the late 18th century that the production could be mechanized which revolutionized the spinning and weaving industry and precipitated the decline in linen as a bandage material [21].

Each cotton fiber is composed of concentric layers as indicated in Fig. 3.3. The cuticle layer on the fiber consists predominantly of wax and pectin materials [22]. The primary wall, the most peripheral layer of the fiber, is composed of cellulosic crystalline fibrils [23]. The secondary wall of the fiber consists of three distinct layers. All three layers of the secondary wall include closely packed parallel fibrils with spiral winding of 25–35 degrees and represent the majority of cellulose within the fiber. The innermost part of cotton fiber, the lumen, is composed of the remains of the cell contents. Before boll opening, the lumen is filled with liquid containing the cell nucleus and protoplasm. The twists and convolutions of the dried fiber are due to the removal of this liquid. The cross section of the fiber is bean shaped, swelling almost round when moisture absorption takes place [24]. The cotton fiber is a sequential aggregate of macrofibril, microfibril, and elementary fibrils. Elementary cotton fibrils are typically composed of 30–36 cellulose chains and regarded as the basic crystalline unit of cotton cellulose [25] and are 3–10 nm in width [26]. When aggregated into a microfibril and macrofibril, the diameters increase to 10–40 and 60–300 nm, respectively [26].

The fiber length-to-breadth ratio can range from 6,000:1 for the longest and best types, to about 350:1 for the shortest and coarsest cotton. The greater the ratio, the more readily the cotton fibers can be spun into yarn. The cotton polymer is a linear, cellulose polymer. The repeating unit in the cotton polymer is cellobiose which consists of two glucose units. The cotton polymer system consists of about 5,000 cellobiose

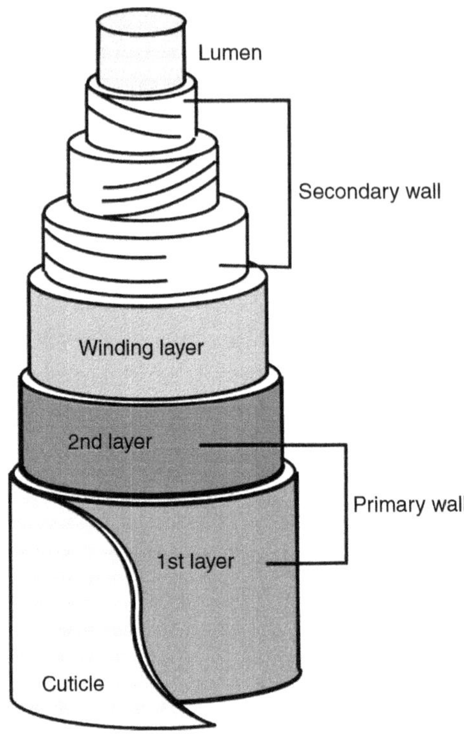

Figure 3.3 ***Structure of a cotton fiber.***

units [27,28]. Cotton is a crystalline fiber. Its polymer system is about 65–70% crystalline and, correspondingly, about 35–30% amorphous. Therefore, the cotton polymers are, in the main, well oriented and probably no further apart than 0.5 nm, in the crystalline regions.

During the late 19th century, bandages were often made and rolled by hand into a firm and compact mass. For general purposes, common calico or unbleached cotton was used due to economic viability and strength. By the end of the 18th century, it was widely accepted that bandaging was indeed a skill [29], and over the subsequent years there were many descriptions of how to actually apply the different bandages. William Northcote [30] described four different ways in which you could apply a simple bandage, as well as many different bandages designed for particular injuries or treatment purposes. The art of bandaging, however, is truly enshrined in the triangular bandage designed by Friedrich von Esmarch (1823–1908) [31]. Esmarch's contribution to surgical procedures is immense and was borne out of experience on the battlefield. He was recognized as a leading authority on hospital management and military surgery and, despite developing many techniques to aid recovery, will be best remembered for his book: "The Surgeon's Handbook on the Treatment of Wounded in War: A Prize Essay" and, of course, for the

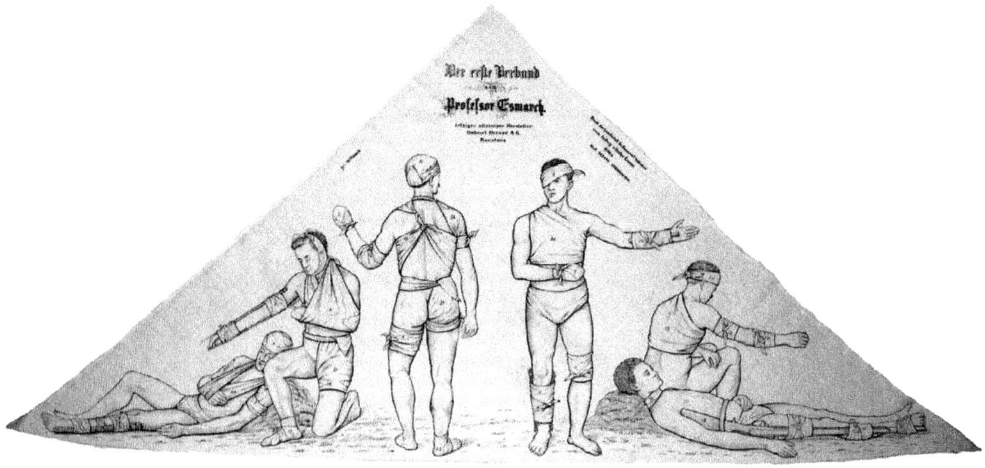

Figure 3.4 ***Esmarch's triangular bandage [32].***

development of the triangular bandage [32]. The bandage itself is a three-sided piece of linen or cotton (4 feet at the base) and, through the medical equivalent of origami, can be used folded and applied in 32 different ways. The triangular bandage (highlighted in Fig. 3.4) begun life as a key component in the German Army's first aid [33].

Cotton still remains as the principal bandage material with cotton gauze being the most common and readily found within any pharmacy as indicated in Fig. 3.5. The gauze bandage is a simple woven strip of material which has been steadily refined over the years and, in its present-day incarnation, more often than not, comes modified with an absorbant coating that minimizes the risk of the gauze itself adhering to the wound and causing further damage upon its removal.

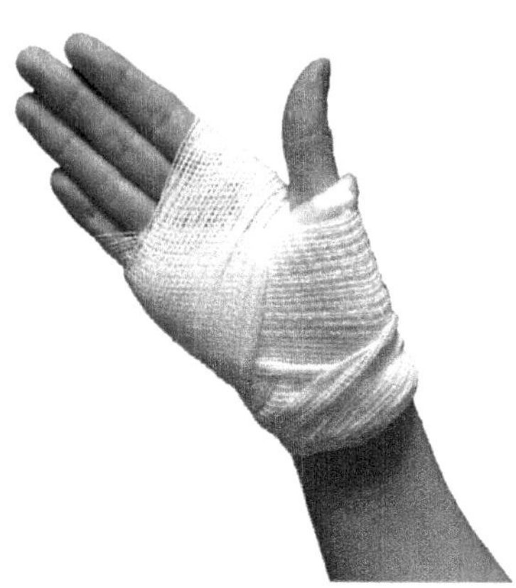

Figure 3.5 ***Cotton gauze bandage.***

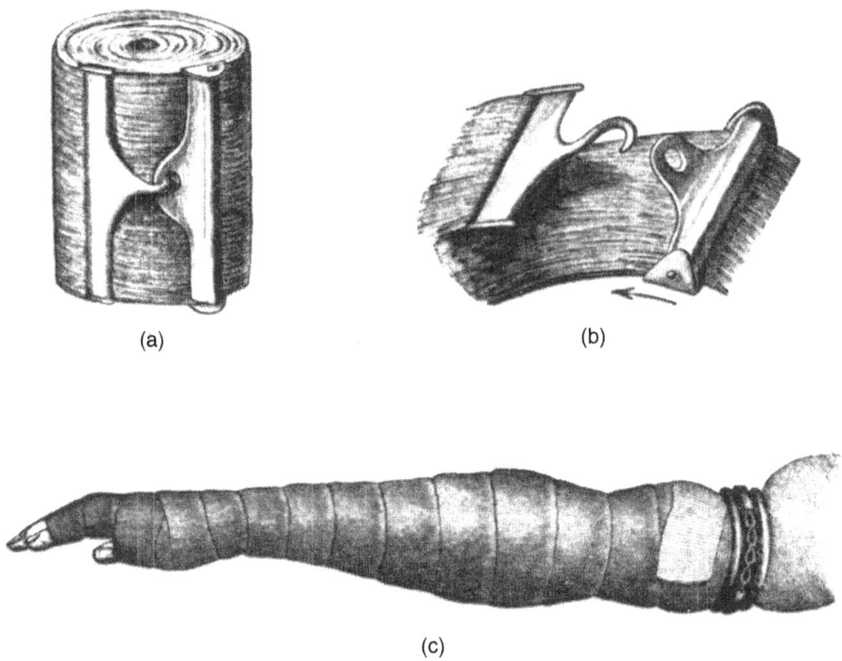

Figure 3.6 ***Esmarch elastic bandage.*** (a) Elastic constrictor; (b) clamp buckle; and (c) elastic bandage and constrictor [34].

3.2.5 Elastic Bandages

Esmarch inventions did not stop at the triangular bandage and he was one of the first people to recommend the use of elastic bandage during operations to prevent haemorrhaging. In 1874, Esmarch described his method in which to compress the limb (Fig. 3.6) before amputation surgery, which meant that it transferred all the blood back into the body and therefore minimize the amount of blood lost during surgery [31,32]. It was Robert Liston who employed the use of elastic bandages to give support in for sprains. To do so, he applied the elastic bandage over a thin stocking [33]. By the late 19th century, the use of fine pliable rubber bandages for varicose veins became a general practice toward the end of the 19th century.

In 1922, the first official specification for dressings was issued in the second supplement to the British Pharmaceutical Codex (B.P.C.), 1911, which included a number of bandages, all of which are still in use. Examples of the bandages included in the supplement are listed in Table 3.1, including the additional 1952 supplement to the B.P.C, 1949.

3.3 DRESSINGS

It is generally acknowledged that our ancestors will have had a variety of plants and materials at their disposal and, it is likely that acute observation and an inevitable trial-and-error approach is liable to have furthered the knowledge of wound treatment.

Table 3.1 List of bandage material outlined in the British Pharmaceutical Codex [35]

Listed in 1922	**Addition in 1952**
Calico	Cotton crepe elastic adhesive
Crepe	Diachylon elastic adhesive
Domette	Cotton and rubber elastic
Flannel	Zinc paste and ichtammol
Muslin	Rayon and rubber elastic
Open wove	Cotton and elastic net bandage
Plaster of Paris	

It is important to remember that human societies have had many thousands of years to observe the effects and therein select which substances and techniques possess properties conducive to wound healing. Due to the abundant nature of plants, their use within wound healing is thought to have occurred from the very earliest of times. There is an old adage that "what does not kill you makes you stronger" and this is particularly pertinent to early wound treatments. Some of the more bizarre ingredients that have found their way into wound dressings are highlighted in Table 3.2, but the list is far from comprehensive and it is impossible to imagine the full range of materials that may have been investigated.

There can be little doubt that magic and superstition were prevalent in early medical practices, and it is likely that, while there may have been advances in treatment through observation and experimentation, the lack of communication and dissemination would have been a major impediment. Much would have been done through the word of mouth and even then, it would have been passed through specific individuals such as shaman. The first documented medical manual detailing information on wound

Table 3.2 Topical wound treatments from ancient or primitive societies

Bile	Bark	Alum
Blood	Dyes	Antimony
Butter	Fruit	Arsenic
Cobweb	Herbs	Clay
Cochineal	Honey	Copper salts
Egg-white	Leaves	Lead salts
Faeces	Oils	Mercury salts
	Moss	
Lard or grease	Resins	Potassium salts
Meat	Sap	Tar or pitch
Milk	Sugar	Zinc salts
	Turpentine	
	Wine or vinegar	

Source: Adapted from Forest [36].

treatment has been attributed to clay tablets found in Mesopotamia, around 2,500 BC, which are a far cry from the wireless tablet systems employed in modern clinical settings. These tablets bring a new perspective to the notion of a "hard copy" but they nevertheless represented a vital step forward in documenting approaches to healthcare. It was postulated by Majno [37] that wounds were washed with water or milk and were dressed with honey or resin, probably conifer [38]. In the Mesopotamian culture, a traditional approach to wound healing was to:

> *"Pound together fur-turpentine, pine turpentine, tamarisk, daisy, flour of inninnu strain; mix in milk and beer in a small copper pan; spread on skin; bind on him and he shall recover" [39].*

These raw ingredients are far from random and it is possible to gleam some rationale behind their use. The use of acids, alcohol, honey, and resin would certainly have served as potent antimicrobials which would undoubtedly have improved the chance of recovery.

3.3.1 Egyptian Wound Management

The Ebers Papyrus (1,500–1,600 BC) is widely accepted as the oldest complete Egyptian medical treatise and contains a multitude of references to the treatment of wounds—often in considerable detail. This marks a significant step forward from cave paintings and clay tablets to a format where the information could be readily copied and disseminated, the Ebers Papyrus is itself alleged to be but a copy of an older manuscript. In terms of clinical development, it would appear that the Egyptians essentially built on the knowledge of the Mesopotamians. They appeared to have learned that a closed wound heals faster than an open wound and, in doing so, they were arguably the first to invent an adhesive bandage by applying gum or heated resin to fine linen strips and using these to draw wounds together [36]. Their experience in the intricate embalming process of bodies and the fabrication and application of bandages no doubt influenced the methods used for wound management and, in doing so, minimised the propensity for wound infection [38–40].

The Edwin Smith Papyrus (1,500–1,600 BC) mentioned the use of splints for fractures and recorded that wounds were being treated with fresh flesh (debridement of wounds), which were kept in place for the first day by bandages, after which dressings of fat and honey were applied. The agents used in Egypt at the time would have been ones that were readily available, such as combinations of honey, lard or resin, and lint. Lint, made from flax fiber, probably aided in the drainage of the wound, while grease made from animal fat acted as a barrier to bacteria. The grease would also have helped to prevent the bandage from sticking minimizing the possibility of reopening a wound upon redressing [38]. These elements have much in common with present-day "advanced" dressings where absorption of exudate, low adherence, and an occlusive antibacterial layer are key factors in their design (Fig. 4.1).

The triple antibiotic paste is not dissimilar to the ointments that can be found in pharmacies today and used to treat minor cuts, scrapes, or burns. It is clear from the papyri that the effectiveness of honey was well recognized and is the predominant ingredient in Egyptian medicine of the period. Although unbeknown to the ancient doctor, the aseptic, antiseptic, and antibiotic properties of honey are ideal for wound treatment and it is little surprise to find commercial dressings still employing the same ingredients [38,39,41,42].

The scarcity of trees in Egypt would have made resin difficult to obtain, resulting in myrrh being imported in large quantities. The exact reason as to why resins were used in the development of dressings is still unclear. It has been postulated that it may have been down to superstition, whereby there is the belief that resin does not decay and therefore the same logic could be applied in this situation and prevent further corruption of the wound. It is also possible that the fact that resins are produced when a tree is injured and ooze from the opening to fill and seal it as they congeal may have been used as inferential evidence. Nevertheless, the fragrance of resin, in particular frankincense and myrrh, is likely to have been of considerable benefit to patient and practitioner when dealing with particularly foul, malodorous sores [36].

It is noteworthy to highlight the degree to which superstition impacted on the practice, with the use of castor oil advocated for external application to septic wounds and burns and the use of hartshorn "to drive out painful swellings" or as fumigation "to expel demons" [35]. Another pertinent example of superstitious serendipity in the discovery of those agents liable to promote healing is typified by the use of green copper pigments (malachite and chrysocolla)—a color assumed to represent life—and which was applied to wounds much like a paint. Fortuitously, the copper complex provides a powerful antiseptic and astringent action which reduces the propensity toward infection. It is worthwhile noting that such pigments are, in many respects, the ancient fore runners of the present-day interest in copper complexes as antimicrobial additives within new dressing designs [43–45].

3.3.2 Asian Influences

Indian and Chinese medicines have similarly ancient beginnings as those of Egypt, and would appear to have developed independently and, in both cases, there are extensive written records of herbal folklore. Chinese medicine is thought to extend far back in time, with the legendary emperors, Yu Hsiung who compiled the Nei Ching and Shen Nung, who concocted the first herbal, the Pen-tsao, around the time of 2,800 and 2,600 BC [36]. The Indian Vedas, epic poems documenting Indian society around 1,500 BC, have been found to be rich in detail regarding herbal medicines. The Sushruta Samhita and the Charaka Samhita, however, were two collections that documented Hindu medicine in detail, though there is considerable debate as to their date. One particular advance in wound treatment and described by Sushruta did not however originate from

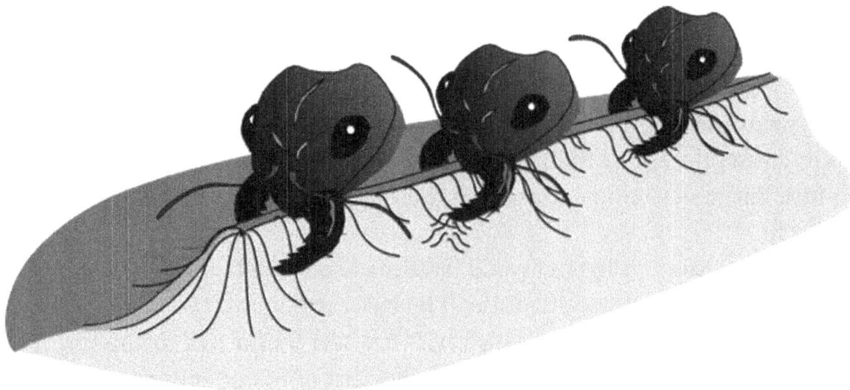

Figure 3.7 ***Ant sutures.***

plants. Surgical stitching was notoriously problematic and, particularly dangerous in the case of intestinal surgery. The suture thread acted much like a wick—drawing fecal matter through the wall of the newly sown bowel resulting in infection and death. A wholly innovative solution was developed and served as the forerunner of modern stapling. Rather than the clips being of an inanimate material, the Indian surgeons used live ants. The mandibles of latter are known to have a vice-like grip on most objects they come into contact with and hence were employed to grasp and close the cut edges of the patient's intestine. The ants, when placed in series around an incision or join, were found to seal the wound much more effectively than conventional thread. Decapitation of the ants left the head still gripping the tissue with the irreversible nature of the clasp action allowing the surgeon to close the abdominal wound as described by Sushruta (Fig. 3.7):

> *"Large black ants should be applied to the margins of the wound and their bodies then severed from their heads, after these have firmly bitten the part with their jaws. [46]"*

It can be assumed by the time the patient's immune system had attacked and processed the ant heads, the intestinal wounds would have healed—a very ancient form of biodegradable staple. The ant mandible approach to wound closure was applied through numerous periods and geographical regions and was used up until the 1900s.

3.3.3 Hippocrates and Greek Medicine

The earliest Greek medical references are found in Homer's Iliad from around 800 BC, and it appears that the Greek army had their own surgeons during the time of the Trojan War. However, at this stage they had still not managed to master the skill of cautery or ligatures to prevent bleeding, they instead referred to casting incantations after washing and dressing wounds. The Greeks recognized the importance of cleanliness, by recommending washing the wound with clean water, vinegar, and wine. As well as this they also differentiated between acute and chronic wounds.

Hippocrates (460–377 BC) enabled the advancement in medicine by describing disease and their natural history. He suggested that contused wounds should be treated with salves to promote suppuration, remove necrotic material, and reduce inflammation. He did not, however, postulate that pus was necessary, as would be suggested later. His preference was to leave wounds dry. This runs counter to the moist wound approach used today but it must also be noted that the dry wound theory persisted well into the 1900s. Once the wound had dried, Hippocrates recommended the use of wine or vinegar for washing. He also stipulated that Mother Nature's own remedies such as honey and oil, as well as wine, would be the best at healing wounds. Again, the acidity of the treatments would have had some benefit in terms of reducing bacterial growth but it is inevitable that the patient would have found the process far from painless.

Although Hippocrates advocated that the majority of wounds should be kept dry, this did not prevent wounds being covered with fat and oil-based ointments after being washed in wine or vinegar. In these respects, the treatment was not far removed from the strategies employed by Egyptian clinicians before him. The use of verdigris (a green pigment derived from the action of acetic acid on copper) also has echoes of Egyptian practice, but it has been postulated that these were stronger than either malachite or chrysicikka.

By the 5th century, bandaging had become an art form, and surgeons began to recognize that bandaging too tightly could cause gangrene. Hippocratic teaching foreboded against the over indulgent use of bandages, which further engrained the humoral theory of disease in the minds of physicians as was all philosophers. The imbalance of the body's humors (ie, blood, phlegm, yellow, or black bile) was considered to cause disease and the bad humor should be relieved if the illness was to be cured. Hippocratic teaching considered that wounds in themselves were diseases, and therefore, by analogy, humoral imbalance prevented healing. Venesection was a common practice in the ancient world and was also advocated in the treatment of wounds—including fresh wounds to remove the stagnated blood that was thought to pool round the wound. Thus, a vessel near the wound would be exposed to allow the corrupt blood out. The remainder of the bad humors could be removed by purging, and the implementation of a strict diet would prevent the production of more bad humor. Even the strongest patient would have been severely drained by this treatment, and one who had lost any quantity of blood must have been at severe risk of death. There is little doubt that Hippocrates was ahead of his time he predicted methods of antiseptic by using tar for dressing wounds as well as advising surgeons to keep their nails short and their hands clean during operations [35].

3.4 PLASTERS

Modern-day usage of the word plaster brings an image of a solid, inflexible material which, even when considered in a medical context, suggests a cast for broken bones. Historically, usage of the term plaster was much more "flexible" and while they could be of a solid nature, they were also regularly applied as pastes, ointments, or poultices—all of which served as a dressing:

> *"A plaster is said (to be made) when many different things [such] as powder, gums and fats, tallow and oil are melted together until they become hard and are made into gobetis [gobbets] and kept; and then made abroad [spread] upon leather, and laid on the place ... as diachylon [a lead plaster], apostolicon [an ointment containing 12 ingredients, hence called the 'Apostles'], oxycroceum [a plaster compounded of olive oil and crocus], etc" [47]*

In order to stiffen the plaster, many different agents were used. One of the earliest mentions is by the Persian pharmacist, Abu Mansur Muwaffaq, who in "Pharmacological Principles" in 975 described the use of plasters for bone fractures [47]. Lister recommended the use of bandages steeped in waterglass (a mixture of silicates of soda and potash) "*wound round the limb as it lies in the splint (Gooch'd) so as to ensure absolute immobility*." However, Lister highlighted that the use of waterglass, glue, gummed, and other fixed bandages took longer to dry, harden, and stiffen than plaster of Paris, and less durable, especially if the plaster of Paris was coated in a "gummed bandages."

Plasters were formulated for not just open wounds, but for a number of ailments. The concoction that plasters consisted of centuries ago would be unheard of today. For example, one recipe calls for a plaster constructed from pitch, honey, and bean flour; another for a plaster derived of dried goat's dung moistened with strong vinegar for the treatment of sciatica [47]. Equally unpleasant is the recommendation of one raw egg and bole, spread upon linen cloth and bound over the eye for cataracts. These clearly deviate from a modern-day expectation of a plaster.

Plasters were generally a combination of a variety of ingredients, with the resultant mixture being spread either directly onto the affected area of skin or applied to the wound after being distributed on an intermediate piece of material (bandage). Lanfrank's "entreet" is of particular interest as it was created by melting white rosin and wax together with a strong vinegar and straining through a cloth in cold water. The mixture was then kneaded in a quite ceremonious manner, by the physicians whose hands were anointed with oil of roses. Once the necessary kneading was carried out, the mixture was spread onto cloth and laid directly upon the wound until the formation of new connective tissue, resulting in a scar. Interestingly, there are two formulas provided for this mixture, which appear to be season dependent. For summer, equal parts of rosin and wax were combined, while in winter the ratio shifted to four parts rosin to five parts wax, which was said to produce a mixture that is more manageable in the colder temperatures [47].

Diachylon plaster was said to be first used by the physician to the Roman Emperor Tiberius. He described plaster as a glutinous mass made chiefly from mucilaginoud seeds or roots such as linseed and marshmallow [47]. The name "diachylon" was then applied the mucilaginous plaster and continued to be used for several centuries afterward. A critical point to note is the term "Diachylon" which is retained for some dressings today but, which will not have the "red lead oxide" present. The use of lead (PbO) compounds in dressings has a long historical legacy and it is surprising to note that the use of lead continued well into the 1900s where there are references to the "spirit of lead" being applied to cuts and grazes. Obviously, given the toxic nature of the material such ingredients are no longer present. There have been several scholars who have posited that the fall of the Roman empire may have been due to the presence of lead in the wine that was produced at the time which would have had considerable impact on normal behavior. It could be added that the addition of lead compounds to wounds, an aggressive biological matrix, could have been equally effective as a long-term poison. There have been chemical analyses of body remains (typically bone and hair) to determine heavy metal concentration and the assumption is water poisoning or murder but could it have been more to do with medical malpractice?

The significance of using plasters for treatment during the 16th century is highlighted in the entry recorded at the St Bartholomew's Hospital, London, during August 1555;

> *"This day yt ys orderyd that Garlop the surgyn shall have the chamber that ys empty in the dorter to dryie and make his plasterys" [47]*

Christopher Wirtzung (1598) noted the kind of medicaments used for the preparation of the three most common plasters highlighted in Table 3.3.

The use of plasters was widespread and, in the 17th century, John Woodall specified that within a surgeon's chest the means to prepare plasters should be included. This typically involved a small board and paper or leather skins upon which the plasters should be spread. In regards to the plaster box, it should be equipped with at least a spatula to spread the unguents on lint and the surgeon's needles. Of course, these were not the only

Table 3.3 Examples of types of plasters including their application [47]

Type		**Ingredients**	**Application**
Plaster	Burns Scalds	Oil Wax Litharge Nightshade	As an ointment for new burns Spread upon linen and used as a plaster if the burn was 2 or 3-day old
Soft plaster	Staunch blood	Egg white Bole Dragon's blood Bloodstone Frankincense	Spread upon town before being applied onto the wound. An unusual material to spread a plaster mass
Corn plaster	Shoemaker wax	"Diachilon Magnum" Pitch	Spread upon cloth and applied

materials suggested by Woodall; in addition to the plasters and their accompaniments, other materials were suggested which, in turn, could have been used as plasters such as gum elemi, galbanum, common pitch, and burgundy pitch. These were reportedly useful for causing an abscess to ripen and "commence to suppurate" [47].

3.4.1 Adhesive (Sticking Plasters)

The origins of the "sticking" plaster are hard to pinpoint with any certainty though, one of the first documented applications can be attributed to William Northcote who, in 1770, commented upon the different types of sutures, describing a "dry suture" as one made of diachylon or diapalma plaster mixed with turpentine and spread upon leather. This was then cut into strips and placed at a small distance from each other and was found to adhere to the skin [47]. In Gray's "Supplement to the Pharmacopia," the plaster is described as a solid tenacious compound which is usually adhesive at the heat of human body [48] and documents an extensive list of preparations some of which are highlighted in Table 3.4. The presence of the high wax content presumably aids in the adhesion. The plasters were applied in strips about ¼ inches apart, keeping the wound edges closed but leaving sufficient space to allow blood to drain away and thereby promoting straightforward healing [35]. John Hunter also promoted the use of sticking plaster as a dry suture, saying that it was more general in its application and for many

Table 3.4 Plaster recipes

Ammoniacum	Mercury
Ammoniacum with mercury	Minimum
Aromatic	Mucilage
Assa foetida	Opium
Belladona	Oxycroccum
Cantharides	Palm
Court	Paracelsus'
Cumin	Pitch
Delacroix's agglutinative	Poor Man's
Frankincense	Prestat's Adhesive
Galbanum	Red Lead
GUm	Resin
Iron	Soap
Isinglass	Soap Cerate
Liston's Isinglass	Strengthening
Kirland's volatile	Verdigris
Ladanum	Warming
Lead	Wax
Meliot	

purposes preferable to a uniting bandage [47]. Adhesive plasters have an advantage over stitches, in bringing a larger surface of the wound together and did not inflame the parts to which they were applied or, as stitches did, produce suppuration or ulceration. Notes by William Buchan provide more information on the formulation of plasters where a "common wax plaster" used over deeper wounds consisted of yellow wax, white resin, and mutton suet [47]. The latter was widely used as a cerate, an unctuous solid preparation, harder than an ointment, containing sufficient wax to prevent it from melting when applied to the skin.

3.4.2 Baynton Plaster

Toward the end of the 18th century, Thomas Baynton, an army surgeon, noted that leg ulcers were a great cause of invalidism in the army. In an attempt to minimize this, he strapped an adhesive plaster over a patient's leg ulcer, he melted the common plaster (diachylon) with yellow resin in an iron ladle over a slow fire, stirring it until it began to cool, whereupon it was spread thinly upon strips of smooth porous calico. The plaster was then cut into pieces of 2–3 inches wide and of sufficient length to be wrapped around the limb, allowing for a 4-inch spare end. Baynton preferred the use of calico to linen for his plasters as he considered the former more porous and elastic, as noted previously, giving support without undue stricture. For the covering bandage he used calico rather than linen or flannel; calico was softer and therefore more accommodating than linen, cooler, less cumbersome, and cleaner than flannel [35]. The plaster was reputedly a great success and a significant step forward in the treatment of venous leg ulcers [47].

3.4.3 Belladona Plaster

Edward Garnett Taylor is the inspiring inventor of the Belladonna plaster which was targeted as a wound aid for the poor. The basis of the plaster revolved around mixtures of oil, fat, and litharge (lead oxide) to which he would then add the extract of belladonna. The final mixture was then spread upon sheets of paper. His wife would then distribute these plasters free of charge to those in need. Over time, the demand for these plasters grew so strong that the Edward Taylor Limited company arose to enable the manufacture of the plaster in bulk [35].

The recipe on which Taylor based his mixture was thought to originate from the Pharmacopia in usum Noscomii Mancuniensis. Interestingly, although the pharmacopeia contained a number of plasters, not one contained belladonna. In Taylor's own copy of the work, there appears to be a note in pencil, which mentions the use of the belladonna [47]. Belladonna has a long history in herbal medicine and is noted for it use as a pain reliever, muscle relaxer, and anti-inflammatory—all of which would have been pertinent to the wound dressing.

3.4.4 Isinglass/Ladies Sticking Plaster

Isinglass plaster was historically produced from "Turlington's balsam" or "balsamum traumaticum" and water [47]. Isinglass is a substance traditionally obtained from the dried swim bladders of fish and is a form of collagen used in various food and drink industries but can be processed into a paste for gluing purposes. The balsams were so-called "patent medicines" and, as such, little is known of their exact composition. Nevertheless, the three components were melted together and spread "while yet fluid with the heat" onto silk by means of a brush. The isinglass plaster was held in high regard by Robert Liston, as it did not irritate the wound and recommended its use in place of the common adhesive plaster. One failing of the latter was that its adhesiveness could be gradually lost through permeation of the wound exudate. It was also typical for the adhesive plaster to heat the wound causing erythema. Liston's recipe consisted of a solution of isinglass in spirit, which was then spread upon slips of ribbon, linen, or oiled silk, glazed on the reverse side [47]. The system was readily adopted and, on occasion, applied to a membrane so thin that they were almost transparent and could almost be considered as the forerunner of the transparent films that are in use today. The plaster itself could be cut to fit and was adhered to the body by being moistened beforehand using a hot sponge. In this way, the adhesive matter was dissolved before immediate application which resulted in a sufficient hold of the bandage that was reported to the last duration of the cure. Moreover, due to the transparent nature of the bandage, any fluid collecting beneath the plaster could be clearly seen and, if needs be, a hole could be cut out to drain away the excess fluid.

In 1880, a new application for the isinglass plaster was reported by Fairlie Clarke. The proposed use was for after skin graft surgery by the method devised by Jacques Louis Reverdin (1842–1929). In his process, a minute piece of skin is raised with forceps, cut off with scissors, placed upon the granulating surface, and secured into position by a pad of dry lint and a strip of the plaster [47]. Transparent isinglass plaster was recommended as particularly apt alternative.

3.4.5 Rubber Adhesive Plaster

In the early 19th century one of the earliest antiseptic plasters was the "lac plaster," which was made from phenol and shellac (a resin secreted by the female lac bug and hence the name granted to the plaster) which was spread onto calico and painted with a solution of gutta percha in benzene. Gutta percha was obtained from a variety of guttiferous trees throughout the Pacific Rim and the material is probably the whole residue from the latex, dried after collection from whichever tree was its source. Unfortunately, the plaster itself did not adhere effectively enough to the skin so as to prevent drainage and was quickly abandoned. The product was arguably ahead of its time and certainly one of the forerunners of the adhesive plasters (band-aids) that adorn the shelves of pharmacies worldwide [47].

One of the first companies to start a more systematic investigation into the use of rubber in adhesive plasters was probably the manufacturer, Mitchells. This new type of plaster quickly took off and it was not long until the Manchester-based Edward Taylor began to make rubber-based plaster on tin spools, under the name of "Savars" for the Liverpool-based Evans, Son, Lescher & Webber. One of the main advantages of using rubber adhesive plasters is that they will adhere to the skin freely, without the need to precondition it by either warming or moistening [47]. Today, most adhesive plasters are made of cohesive modifiers, tackifiers, plasticizers, and fillers. The cohesive materials are normally water-white crepe rubber, Brazilian para rubber, high-quality smoked sheet rubber, or a synthetic rubber; a typical tackifier is colophony resin. The mass is manufactured by breaking down the rubber using mechanical knives, and then milled, along with other ingredients under carefully controlled conditions. Any vulcanising materials, such as moisture or sulfur, must be avoided along with any heat—otherwise the properties of the material will be compromised. Today, self-adhesive plasters come in a wide range of selections from spread on elastic or nonelastic cotton or rayon cloth, linen, plastic film, or on wool felt [35] (Fig. 3.8).

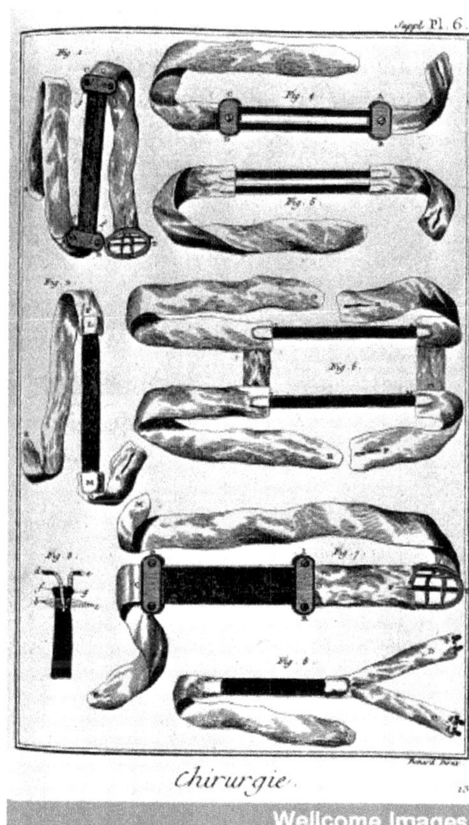

Figure 3.8 ***First use of rubber in bandages (Wellcome Library, London) [49].***

3.5 BAND-AID DISCOVERY AND COMMERCIALIZATION

The invention of the Band-Aid began with a presentation by Dr Joseph Lister, a renowned surgeon, to a medical congress based in Philadelphia in 1876. His address focused on the necessity of implementing more sanitary procedures in the operating theater. Lister's theory that serious infections found in postoperative patients, which were often fatal, were a result of the presence of invisible airborne germs. This theory was received with a great deal of scepticism from a majority of surgeons present and, it must be noted that Pasteur's seminal work on the germ theory of disease would still have been relatively new and controversial at that period. Due to the lack of knowledge and understanding of the science of bacteriology of the time, it is perhaps understandable as to why Dr Lister's theory garnered this kind of response. It should also be noted that sweepings from the mill floor were regularly procured for use in surgical dressing with little thought as to the possibilities of contamination.

Robert Johnson, coowner of the Brooklyn pharmaceutical firm Seabury & Johnson, did not share the opinion of the conference and was among the first to appreciate the significance and consequences of Lister's theory of "invisible assassins" proliferating within the unsanitary conditions found within the surgical environment. Johnson became a firm advocate of the "Listerian way" and initiated the development of a Lister-inspired antiseptic surgical dressing. Designed around a cotton gauze, the dressings were individually sealed in a germ-resistant package that could be shipped to the most remote areas of America and became one of the first products produced by Johnson & Johnson. This was followed by breakthroughs in sterilization techniques and new, zinc oxide, adhesive tape. The commercial success that followed the initial release of the self-adhesive bandage, led to the company developing a diverse range of products. The original BAND-AID was a revolutionary product, the brainchild of Earle Dickson, a cotton buyer from the company's purchasing department. Dickson's inspiration is often accredited to his accident-prone wife, Josephine. Dickson's desire was to create a convenient, at-home, dressing for minor cuts. In doing so, his proposition to the company was a version of a bandage using a strip of adhesive surgical tape and placing a gauze pad in the middle of the thin strip [50].

3.6 WOUND PACKING

Not all wounds, especially the ones created in the midst of war or by gunshots, are simple small and cleanly cut. On many occasions, due to a number of reasons, tissue lost leaves behind a vast area of dead space. To minimize the disruption to the healing process of the wound, this dead space may be packed, typically with gauze. It is important to loosely fill dead space within the wound to facilitate the removal of exudate and debris but, just as importantly, to encourage the growth and granulation of tissue from the base of the wound which may otherwise undergo premature closure resulting in abscess formation [51].

James Gamgee was the first to use the gauze as a covering for cotton wool to make pads for wound dressings. In collaboration with Robinson and Son of Chesterfield, Gamgee carried out experiments involving bleaching the gauze, which resulted in it becoming more absorbent. This rapidly led to the production of absorbent pads, leading to rolls of cotton wool-covered gauze, and subsequently to the production of the well-known Gamgee tissue which is still used today [52].

One of the main suppliers manufacturing absorbent cotton gauze was Johnson and Johnson, who were so inspired by its qualities that they wrote:

> *"Owing to the peculiar adaptability of cotton gauze cloth for wound dressing, it has come into general use during the present of era of surgery... A good quality of gauze cloth has numerous and obvious advantages over any other material used for this purpose. It is highly absorbent, pliable, with an open texture that is firm and strong. It is entirely free from the loose fibres irritating particles found in unspun cotton; it is cool and light and readily shaped into the required forms" [53]*

In terms of manufacturing the gauze, it is not to say that it did not experience any difficulty. In 1898, Mr Charles Stonham suggested that the use of a ribbon gauze, with a uniform 2' width and an edge which cannot fray and was supplied by the Galen Manufacturing Co. However, it was not until 1923 that the first official description of this type of dressing appeared in the B.P.C. monograph. In this edition, this absorbent ribbon gauze was it could be "used for packing cavities as its edges do not fray."

In terms of medicated gauzes, the first carbolized gauzes were used by Lister in 1871. He experimented with the absorbent antiseptic dressing by using a cheap muslin gauze and saturated it in carbolic resin, which he reported to be an "elegant and convenient form of oakum" [52]. Aside from carbolic gauze, at the time iodoform (CHI_3) gauzes appeared to be the most popular dressing by the end of the 19th century. Although, in 1900, Herbert Spencer published a paper discussing his support for the use of iodoform gauze as a uterine packing, exception was taken on grounds of potential poisoning by the iodoform and carbolise, salalembroth, and cyanide gauzes were used instead as alternatives [52]. Another variation of historical gauze use was in a constant antiseptic vapor dressing, which in 1885 J.C. Voigt described as

> *"A dressing which throws a constant antiseptic steam into the wound can be prepared. Plain ordinary gauze, unimpregnated with any other antiseptic material can be kept soaking in pure eucalyptus oil. Before being put on the wound, which is to be, dressed, strips of this eucalyptus gauze are squeezed as dry as possible and then steeped in eucalyptus and olive oil. Thus prepared the strips of gauze are put on the wound, and immediately over the are applied some folds of ordinary absorbent cotton wool, which have been freshly wrung out of the pure eucalyptus oil... [54]."*

Again, the 1923 B.P.C monograph listed a total of 11 different types of medicated gauzes. However, by 1959 only the double cyanide of mercury gauze stood the test of time, and of the unmedicated type, only absorbent and ribbon gauze remained [52].

3.7 FIELD DRESSING—NECESSITY AND INVENTION

It has often been postulated that if it were not for the experience gained and the observations made on the battlefield, the advancement of wound treatment would not have been as prolific. A perennial problem often faced on the battlefield is the prompt, if not urgent, and efficient application of wound dressings to stabilize the patient and aid their subsequent recovery. Historically, wounds would have been treated some time after the event and the injured party would have been left until it was safe to remove them from the field of action. The introduction of the first field dressing is reported to have been devised by the German military surgeon, Friedrich von Esmarch (Section 3.1), during the Franco–Prussian War. Esmarch's triangular bandage has been previously described in Section 3.2.4 and was incorporated as an integral component of the Germany army first aid pack, alongside two compresses of sublimate gauze, and an antiseptic bandage—all of which were all wrapped in a rubber cloth, with a grand total weight of 100 g. A comparison of the first aid kits deployed in a military capacity is given in Table 3.5.

The first aid kit adopted by the British Army in 1891 consisted of an outer gray linen cover, with a thin waterproof layer inside that being rendered airtight by cementing the edges together. Although these first aid kits were a step in the right direction, it soon became apparent that an ideal first aid kit for the field must be:

1. Simple in its construction, to be applied efficiently by unskilled hands, and with the least possible delay.

Table 3.5 Comparison of military first aid kits [35]

Year	Nationality	Contents of first aid kit
1880s	French	• One impermeable fabric • One small cushion of sublimated jute • A sublimate gauze compress and bandage • Two safety pins • Iodoform used for both as gauze and as powder to dust over wound
1891	British	• Two safety pins • A 12″ × 6″ piece of waterproof cambric • ½ yards long gauze bandage • 17″ × 13″ piece of gauze • A 160 grains weight of compressed flax charpie between two layers of gauze
1893	German	• Sublimate gauze bandage 5 m in length • Two compresses of the same material • A safety pin that was wrapped in a waterproof linen cloth and sewn inside the tunic of the uniform of the officers

2. The dressing material employed must not interfere with the free evaporation of the wound secretion.
3. The dressing material must be hygroscopic, and not only aseptic but also antiseptic.
4. The antiseptic must not be nonvolatile and resistant to chemical changes for a long time.
5. It must contain a fixative material to prevent displacement of the dressing after it had been applied.
6. All dressing materials must be kept ready for use in a waterproof cover [55].

Most of these features were common in a first field dressing, details of which were published in the *Training Manual of the British Red Cross (*1911), and which was repeated up to August 1915 [56]. In July 1928, the International Commission in Geneva was held to discuss the steps needed to initiate the standardization of medical materials. Colonel Thomann, the chief pharmacist to the Swiss Army, proposed an alternative to the use of Iodoform, which was currently being used in the Swiss army as the principal antiseptic. The issues surrounding the use of this antiseptic were its lack of stability and odor. Therefore, in the search for a better alternative, the Swiss medical service carried out a number of trials on a number of antiseptics and concluded with the recommendation of the "Vioform," which in the presence of a secreting wound will slowly release iodine. In addition to Thomann's proposed recommendation, Dr Chausse and Professor Demolis reported that war wounds were often prone to infection; therefore, it was a necessity that a dressing must not only be an antiseptic but also be sterilized [57].

It must be noted that, when in a moment of crisis, it is not always possible to obtain the most appropriate dressing material and a degree of ingenuity can be required. This is especially true during conflicts where supplies of particular raw materials may become scarce and there is a need to improvise. The casualty rates during the First and Second World Wars are apt examples where demand can significantly outstrip supply—at which point textiles of wide description and composition were suddenly being recycled to aid the war effort. Arguably, the most ingenious approach to finding an alternative to conventional linen or cotton dressing was adopted by the Japanese during the Russo–Japanese War (1904–1905) where sphagnum moss was used as a dressing. Contrary to first impressions, it is, in principle, an ideal material as it has an excellent absorption capacity and, rather than causing infection, possesses antiseptic properties which prevented the onset of gangrene [35].

3.8 WINTER'S REVOLUTION IN WOUND MANAGEMENT

Traditional dressings such as gauzes, which are nonocclusive, had a tendency to dry out and when that occurred they would adhere to the wound bed. Even if they did not dry out, there was a possibility that granulating tissue would grow into the dressing structure [58], which would inevitably result in the adherence of the dressing to the fresh tissue. This would cause additional trauma to the wound, effectively setting the healing back and would inevitably cause pain to the patient [59].

It was not until 1962 that the medical community began to reappraise and question the supposed merits of dry wound management. Dr George Winter published his landmark *Nature* paper "Formation of the scab and the rate of epithelisation of superficial wounds in the skin of the young domestic pig" in *Nature* in 1962 and, in doing so, effectively set in motion the quest for interactive dressings that rely on a moist wound environment [60]. It can be argued that such dressings had been discovered and implemented from ancient times and, as noted in the preceding sections of this chapter, that is certainly the case, albeit in a sporadic manner. What is significant with Winter's paper, however, is that he effectively brought the argument for actively maintaining a wet wound to the fore and clearly demonstrated that under such conditions wounds healed faster. Winter formed multiple partial thickness wounds on the backs of pigs, half left open to the air and half covered with a polymer film to keep them hydrated. The latter wounds healed faster, as measured by the migration of new epithelium on the wound bed. This work began the evolution of modern wound dressings that promote moist wound healing [61–65].

The initial interactive dressings based on Winter's findings were constructed from polyurethane which simply adhered to the surrounding skin and maintained moisture within the wound environment. The principal effect was to prevent dehydration of the wound through forming an occlusive covering. An important side benefit was that it reduced pain by bathing the exposed nerve endings in physiological wound secretions. However, it was found that the adhesive used to adhere the dressing to the wound area could cause trauma upon removal [66]. Due to the strong adhesive bonds of the dressings, this can result in tears on skin, unless the adhesive bond is compromised by stretching the dressing laterally and parallel to the wound surface before trying to remove the dressing at a 90 degree angle above the wound area. Although these precautions may minimize the incident of skin tears, another problem is still at hand, nonabsorbency. When the fluid accumulates at the surface of the wound it often resulted in a break in the dressing seal and exposed the wound to the external environment which facilitates bacterial proliferation [59]. This is still very much an issue today and has given rise to silicone contact layers which are much more friendly to the periwound skin [67].

3.9 THE IDEAL DRESSING

It is clear from the discussion that dressings must perform a variety of roles and, over the years, many suggestions for what would constitute the "Ideal Dressing" have been proposed. Scales et al. [68] were among the first to put forward the key characteristics that should be present and also described some of the tests that could be used to gauge the appropriateness of possible contenders to the title of Ideal dressing. These are listed in Table 3.6 and reflect their understanding of wound healing and the materials available at the time. In addition to composing these ideal properties, they also understood the necessity that not one dressing alone would be suitable for every wound, accepting that;

> *"The properties which the dressing should possess depend upon the extent of the loss of the epidermal cell layer and of any damage to the dermis, and the events that occur following injury and during healing of the wound [68]."*

Indeed, they were also aware of the current limitations in terms of available materials, stating that;

> *"With present materials it is impossible to produce the ideal dressing and it seems likely that future dressings will be a compromise… Plastic film dressings have a certain advantages over traditional fabric dressings but they also possess certain undesirable features – for example, the occlusive waterproof dressing causes maceration of the skin surrounding the wound and an increase in bacterial flora of normal skin. Both nylon and cellophane are insufficiently permeable and flexible [68]."*

The remainder of the publication was focused on the description of a first aid dressing that consisted of new microporous plasticized polyvinylchloride film backing layer, bearing an absorbent pad located centrally in the middle of the dressing. This was subsequently commercialized by Smith and Nephew and was swiftly rebranded to the now familiar Elastoplast Airstrip [68].

Among the acknowledgments in Scales' publication, is a reference to the "invaluable technical help of Mr G.D. Winter" who was based within the same department. Therefore, it is not a surprise that in a later publication (19 years later), Winter revisited Scales' 10 point "ideal" dressing requirements, and modified and enhanced them to create his own 18 requirements for wound dressings. These are compared alongside Scales' original recommendations in Table 3.6. At the time of Scales' publication, the majority of dressings and gauze that were in common use met roughly 10 of Winter's 18 requirements. Since the original publication there has been a steadfast pursuit toward the production of dressings that meet most of the requirements. This drive, together with a greater understanding of wound dynamics, has led to the evolution of the definition of the ideal dressing or dressing system, and now reflects the need for a combination of different components required to produce the optimum healing environment for any given wound. In addition, it also factors in the progression of wounds and the need for the optimal conditions to adapt with the changing wound environment. Thomas has proposed a modified definition of wound healing as follows:

> *"The ideal dressing or dressing system provides an environment within the wound in which the objectives of the current phase of treatment may be achieved in a timely and cost effective manner without compromising either the patient's safety or quality of life, or adversely affecting the integrity of the periwound skin or the final cosmetic appearance of the healed wound where this is relevant [70]."*

Table 3.6 Comparison between the "ideal" properties postulated by Scales [68] and Winter [69]

Comparison of the "ideal" properties of a dressing

Scales [68]	Winter [69]
1. It should have a high porosity to water vapor, preferably at least 1,400 g, per square meter per 24 h, measured at 37°C with a relative humidity of 75% (P.A.T.R.A. (1948) tentative standard method) 2. It should not adhere either to blood clot or to granulating surfaces, nor should it allow the penetration of capillary loops. It must however, absorb free blood or exudate and give "protection" to the wound 3. It should be a barrier to the passage of microorganisms 4. It should be capable of following the contours around a joint during movement—for example flexing of a finger 5. It should be unaffected by domestic or industrial fluids—for example, detergent and oils 6. It should not produce a tissue reaction when applied to normal skin or granulating surface, nor a state of allergy or hypersensitivity[a] 7. It should be noninflammable 8. It should be capable of being sealed to the skin 9. It should be capable of being sterilized 10. It should be available at a low cost	• Constant in performance over a range of temperatures and humidities • Able to create ideal microclimate for most rapid and effective healing (prevents dehydration and is permeable to oxygen)[a] • Nonadherent[a] • Capable of providing good absorption of blood and exudate • Capable of providing mechanical protection to wound[a] • Capable of protecting against secondary infection[a] • Tear resistant • Conformable to anatomical contours • Soil resistant[a] • Nonallergenic • Nontoxic • Nonflammable • Fiber-fast (does not shed loose material into wound)[a] • Sterilizable • Cost effective[a] • Of small bulk (hospital storage problem) • Stable with a long shelf life • Able to accept and release medicaments[a]

Note: Those highlighted with an "a" were requirements generally not met by the bandages at the time of Winter's publication.
Source: Adapted from Thomas [70].

This definition applied not only to the dressing itself but also to the products designed to achieve debridement, combat odor, or infection, or promote granulation, or epithelialization. In addition, it also follows that for some wounds, optimal management may involve the sequential application of a number of different "ideal" dressings, which are selected according to the condition at which they present on the day of application.

A revision of the list of requirements for dressings used in modern-day healthcare is highlighted in Table 3.7 and is split into primary and secondary categories. Primary requirements are those that are common to most wound management materials, whereas secondary requirements relate to the specific types of wounds or wounds that are in a particular stage of healing or condition. In addition, the performance of these categories

Table 3.7 Performance requirements of the "ideal dressing"

Primary requirements	**Design feature/ wound related**
Maintains the wound and the surrounding skin in an optimum state of hydration (this implies the ability to absorb exudate effectively under compression)	DF + WR
Provides protection to the periwound skin from potentially irritant wound exudate and excess moisture	DF + WR
If self-adhesive, forms an effective water resistant seal to the periwound skin, but is easily removable without causing trauma or skin stripping	DF
Forms an effective bacterial barrier (effectively contain exudate or cellular debris to prevent the transmission of microorganisms into or out of the wound)	DF
Conforms well to wound and limb	DF
Produces minimal pain during application or removal as result of adherence to the wound surface	DF + WR
Free of toxic or irritant extractables	DF
Does not release particles or nonbiodegradable fibers into the wound	DF
Requires minimal disturbance or replacement	DF + WR
Maintains the wound at optimum temperature and pH	DF + WR
Secondary requirements	
Possesses antimicrobial activity—capable of combating localized infection	DF
Has odor-absorbing/combating properties	DF
Has ability to remove or inactivate proteolytic enzymes in chronic wound fluid	DF
Possesses haemostatic activity	DF
Exhibits effective wound-cleansing (debriding) activity	DF + WR

Source: Adapted from Thomas [70].

has been subdivided into those that are determined principally by the design and construction of the dressing, over which the clinician has little or no control, and those in which the ability of the product to perform in a particular fashion is significantly influenced by the nature and condition of the wound.

Even from a quick glance at this review table, it is clear that it is unlikely for one dressing, or dressing system to be capable of possessing all the required properties for every type of wound, a view which still rings true a half century later following the work of Scales.

3.10 SUMMARY

The first attempts at wound treatment and management may not have appeared too convincing from the patient's perspective, given the seemingly random assortment of materials and approaches that will have been used. Despite such beginnings, knowledge of the wound dynamics and the interaction of materials (good and bad) have clearly informed more modern approaches. There has been a gradual recognition of the importance of wound dressing and the functions that they need to perform to aid in the healing process. The concept of an "ideal dressing" now directs much of the research into new materials and their applications, and it is clear that present and future generations will benefit from the hard-won experiences of previous approaches to wound management.

REFERENCES

[1] Frykberg RG, Banks J. Challenges in the treatment of chronic wounds. Adv Wound Care 2015; 4(9):560–82.
[2] Boateng J, Catanzano O. Advanced therapeutic dressings for effective wound healing—a review. J Pharm Sci 2015;104(11):3653–80.
[3] Mayet N, Choonara YE, Kumar P, et al. A comprehensive review of advanced biopolymeric wound healing systems. J Pharm Sci 2014;103(8):2211–30.
[4] Kvavadze E, Bar-Yosef O, Belfer-Cohen A, et al. 30,000-year-old wild flax fibers. Science 2009;325(5946):1359.
[5] Macknin JB. The history of orthopedics. In: Mazloom S, Parvizi J, editors. Orthopedic residency guide. New Delhi: Jaypee Brothers Medical Publishers; 2014.
[6] Woods M, Woods MB. Ancient medicine: from sorcery to surgery. Minneapolis, MN: Runestone Press; 2000.
[7] Prioreschi P. A history of medicine: primitive and ancient medicine. Horatius Press; 1996.
[8] Smith H. Minor surgery: or hints on the every-day duties of the surgeon. Philadelphia, PA: E. Barrington & G. D. Haswell; 1850.
[9] FU Y. Genetic evidence for early flax domestication with capsular dehiscence—Agriculture and Agri-Food Canada (AAFC). Genet Resour Crop Evol 2011;58(8):1119–28.
[10] Mussig J, Martens R. Quality aspects in hemp fibre production—influence of cultivation, harvesting and retting. Ind Hemp 2003;8(1):11–32.
[11] Schnegelsberg G. Handbuch Der Faser – Theorie Und Systematik Der Faser. Frankfurt: Deutscher Fachverlag; 1999.
[12] Bos H, van den Oever M, Peters O. Tensile and compressive properties of flax fibres for natural fibre reinforced composites. Mater Sci 2002;37:1683–92.
[13] Bos H, Donald A. In situ ESEM study of the deformation of elementary flax fibres. Mater Sci 1999;34:3029–34.
[14] Sfiligoj Smole M, Hribernik S, Kleinschek KS, Kreže T. Plant fibres for textile and technical applications. Adv Agrophys Res 2013;369–98.
[15] Smith, H.H. Minor surgery; or, hints on the every-day duties of the surgeon. Philadelphia: Ed. Barrington & Geo. D. Haswell; 1843.
[16] Skorkowska-Telichowska K, Zuk M, Kulma A, Bugajska-Prusak A, Ratajczak K, Gasiorowski K, Kostyn K, Szopa J. New dressing materials derived from transgenic flax products to treat long-standing venous ulcers—a pilot study. Wound Rep Regen 2010;18:168–79.
[17] Silva C, Matamá T, Kim S, et al. Antimicrobial and antioxidant linen via laccase-assisted grafting. React Funct Polym 2011;71:713–20.
[18] Kulmaa A, Skórkowska-Telichowskad K, Kostyna K, et al. New flax producing bioplastic fibers for medical purposes. Ind Crops Prod 2015;68:80–9.
[19] Styrczewska M, Kulma A, Ratajczak K, Amarowicz R, Szopa J. Cannabinoid-like anti-inflammatory compounds from flax fiber. Cell Mol Biol Lett 2012;17:479–99.
[20] Tortora P, Collier B. Understanding textiles. 5th ed. Prentice-Hall; 1997.
[21] Kadolph S, Langford A. Textiles. 8th ed. Prentice-Hall; 1998.
[22] Polyutov AA, Gal'braikh LS, Byvshev AV, Pen RZ, Kleiner YY, Irklei VM. Cotton cellulose: ecological and resource-saving raw material for production of viscose fibres. A review. Fibre Chem 2000;32(1):6–11.

[23] Duckett K. Surface properties of cotton fibers. In: Schick M, editor. Surface characteristics of fibers and textiles. Marcek Dekker; 1975. p. 67.
[24] Kassenbeck P. Structure of cotton fibers as revealed by enzymatic degradation. Text Res J 1970;40: 330–4.
[25] Peterlin A, Ingham P. Morphology of secondary wall firbils in cotton. Text Res JV 40 1970;345–54.
[26] Ulman's. Encyclopaedia of industrial chemistry. 5th ed. New York:VCH Publishers; 1986.
[27] Sekhri S. Textbook of fabric science: fundamentals to finishing. New Delhi: PHI Learning Privates Limited; 2011.
[28] Timár-Balázsy Á, Eastop D. Chemical principles of textile conservation. Butterworth-Heinemann; 1998.
[29] Gooch B. . Surgery 1972;I:144.
[30] Northcote WN. Mar Pract Physic Surg 1770;1:264.
[31] Herzenberg JE. Johann Friedrich August Von Esmarch: his life and contributions to orthopaedic surgery. Iowa Orthop J 1988;8:85.
[32] von Esmarch F. The surgeon's handbook on the treatment of wounded in war: a prize essay. Marston, Searle & Rivington; 1878.
[33] Elliott IM, Elliott JR. Bandages. A short history of surgical dressings. London: Pharmaceutical Press; 1964. p. 28–34.
[34] Esmarch F, Kowalzig E. Surgical technic: a textbook on operative surgery [Grau LH, Sullivan WN, Trans.]. New York: Macmillan Co.; 1901.
[35] Elliott IMZ, Elliott JR. A short history of surgical dressings. London: Pharmaceutical Press; 1964.
[36] Forrest RD. Early history of wound treatment. J R Soc Med 1982;75(3):198–205.
[37] Majno G. The healing hand: man and wound in the ancient world. Cambridge, MA: Harvard University Press; 1975.
[38] Shah JB. The history of wound care. J Am Col Certif Wound Spec 2011;3(3):65–6.
[39] Yardley P, editor. A brief history of wound healing. Oxford: OrthoMcNeil Pharmaceutivals and Janssens-Cilog; 1998.
[40] Ackerknecht E. A short history of medicine. Baltimore, MD: John Hopkins University Press; 1982.
[41] Farrar G, Krosnick A. Wound healing. Clin Ther 1991;13:430–4.
[42] Brown H. Wound healing research through the age. Wound healing biological and clinical aspects. Philadelphia, PA: W.B. Saunders; 1992.
[43] Zhao S, Li L, Wang H, et al. Wound dressings composed of copper-doped borate bioactive glass microfibers stimulate angiogenesis and heal full-thickness skin defects in a rodent model. Biomaterials 2015;53:379–91.
[44] Borkow G, Okon-Levy N, Gabbay J. Copper oxide impregnated wound dressing: biocidal and safety studies. Wounds Compend Clin Res Pract 2010;22(12):301–10.
[45] Klinkajon W, Supaphol P. Novel copper (II) alginate hydrogels and their potential for use as antibacterial wound dressings. Biomed Mater 2014;9(4):045008.
[46] Muffly TM, Tizzano AP, Walters MD. The history and evolution of sutures in pelvic surgery. J R Soc Med 2011;104(3):107–12.
[47] Elliott IMZ, Elliott JR. Plasters and protectives. A short history of surgical dressings. London: Pharmaceutical Press; 1964. p. 63–73.
[48] Gray SF. Gray's supplement to the pharmacopoeia: being a concise but comprehensive dispensatory and manual of facts and formulae, for the chemist and druggist and medical practitioner. Longman and Company; & Highley, Simpkin and Company; John Churchill; Henry Bohn; and Henry Renshaw; 1848.
[49] Diderot D, D'Alembert J. First use of rubber in bandages. Encycl. ou Dict. Raison. des Sci. des arts, métiers. Wellcome library, London; 1777:133.
[50] Fucini J, Fucini S. Johnson & Johnson health care products. Entrepeurs the men and women behind famous brand names and how they made it. Boston: G.K. Hall & Co; 1985. p. 34–6.
[51] Columbia B, Nursing P, Committee W, Technique A, Procedure:. Wound packing. Columbia Br Nursing Prov Committee Wound Tech Aseptic 2015;(June):1–5.
[52] Elliott IMZ, Elliott JR. Muslin, gauze and sponges. A short history of surgical dressings. London: Pharmaceutical Press; 1964. p. 80–9.
[53] Johnson & Johnson. Gauze dressings in surgery. New Brunswick, NJ: Johnson & Johnson; 1895.

[54] Voigt JA. Constant antiseptic vapour dressing. Lancet 1885;I:793.
[55] Senn N. J Assoc Military Surg. 1903:331–47.
[56] First Field Dressings. 1911:155.
[57] Report of the third session of the International Commission on the Standardisation of Medical Materials. Genva; 1928.
[58] Rogers AA, Walmsley RS, Rippon MG, Bowler PG. Adsorption of serum-derived proteins by primary dressings: implications for dressing adhesion to wounds. J Wound Care 1999;8(8):403–6.
[59] Queen D, Orsted H, Sanada H, Sussman G. A dressing history. Int Wound J 2004;1(1):59–77.
[60] Winter GD. . In: Harkiss K, editor. Healing of skin wounds and the inflenece of dressings on the repair process. Bradford: Bradford University Press; 1971.
[61] Nemeth A, Eaglstein W, Taylor JLJP, Falanga V. Faster healing and less pain in skin biopsy sites treated with an occlusive dressing. Arch Dermatol 1991;127(11):1679–83.
[62] Foertsch C, O'Hara M, Stoddard F, Kealy G. Treatment-resistant pain and distress during pediatric burn-dressing changes. J Burn Care Rehabil 1998;19(3):219–24.
[63] Gates J, Holloway G. A comaprison of wound environments. Ostomy Wound Manage 1992; 38(8):35–7.
[64] Junker JPE, Kamel RA, Caterson EJ, Eriksson E. Clinical impact upon wound healing and inflammation in moist, wet, and dry environments. Adv Wound Care 2013;2(7):348–56.
[65] Wodash AJ. Wet-to-dry dressings do not provide moist wound healing. J Am Coll Clin Wound Spec 2012;4(3):63–6.
[66] Campbel K, Woodbury M, Whittle H, Labate T, Hoskin A. A clinical evalutaion of 3M no sting barrier film. Ostomy Wound Manage 2000;46(1):24–30.
[67] Burge T. Removing adhesive retention dressings. Br J Plast Surg 2004;57(1):93.
[68] Scales J, Towers A, Goodman N. Development and evalutaion of a porous surgical dressing. Br Med J 1956;2(4999):962–8.
[69] Winter GD. . In: Turner TKRB, editor. Methods for the biological evaluation of dressings. Cardiff: Surgical Dressing Research Unit; 1975.
[70] Thomas S. Surgical dressings and wound management. Cardiff, South Wales: Medetec Publication; 2010.

CHAPTER FOUR

Passive and Interactive Dressing Materials

J. Davis, A. McLister
School of Engineering, Ulster University, Jordanstown, Northern Ireland, United Kingdom

4.1 INTRODUCTION

The application of a dressing is a common and critical aid to wound management. There is a myriad of commercial dressings available to the healthcare practitioner and they come in a wide variety of forms and compositions. The more common include hydrocolloids, hydrogels, xerogels, foams, films, and, in more recent times, tissue-engineered grafts [1,2]. The traditional forms of lint and gauze still have a role within modern-day wound management, but they have become secondary to the advanced dressing materials that are designed to be interactive and stimulate wound healing. The great diversity of wound dressings that are presently available reflects, in large part, the huge variability of wounds where differences in type, shape, position, stage of healing, composition, and underlying condition will require different approaches to be taken to promote healing. As a consequence, there is a requirement for the dressing to possess tailored physicochemical properties that can perform specific roles. The various functions that wound dressings need to provide are summarized in Fig. 4.1 and reflect the ideal dressing characteristics originally proposed by Winter [3].

Debridement of the wound area, as noted in the previous chapters, is a vital function that removes necrotic tissue and bacterial biofilms resulting in a clean surface that is, in principle, primed to commence healing [1]. The removal of the dead and decaying tissue is critical as it would otherwise significantly impede the healing process through aiding the proliferation of bacteria, prolonging inflammation, and preventing reepithelization. The physical presence of necrotic tissue alone is a significant barrier to wound closure and, in some instances, healing can be reinitiated once such material has been removed [4]. Many of the dressings discussed here can facilitate autolytic debridement, whereby the retention of moisture at the wound bed can help soften and liquefy the accumulations of dead cells and fibrinous deposits. These can be characterized as slough (white/yellow) or necrotic (black) and their removal is a necessary step toward healing. Debridement can be achieved using a variety of methods, but the use of an occlusive or semiocclusive dressing can be a relatively painless approach which only removes dead tissue.

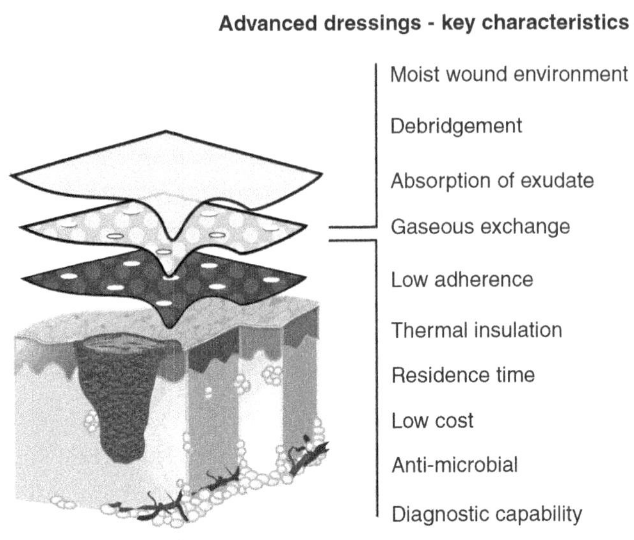

Figure 4.1 ***Characteristics of the ideal dressing.***

The relevance of providing a moist wound environment as a means through which to enhance and accelerate the healing process was noted by Winter [3], but it is only in recent times that it has been adopted as a standard requirement [1,5]. It has been recognized that a sufficiently moist wound can provide a suitable matrix for the transport of growth factors across the wound bed that encourages increased fibronolysis, accelerated angiogenesis, and the synthesis of connective tissue [6,7]. Dressings that promote a moist environment will clearly aid the rehydration of the tissue and, as a consequence, the increased fluidity can significantly help to reduce the pain associated with movement and dressing changes [8].

The production of exudate is the wound's natural approach to maintaining a moist environment and this will occur to varying degrees throughout the various healing stages [9]. Exudate is, however, responsible for much more than simply preventing the wound microenvironment from dehydrating and, as part of the normal inflammatory response, it facilitates the diffusion of immune and growth factors, assists autolysis, and functions as a transport medium for essential nutrients in cell metabolism [9]. Damaged cells release a variety of cytokines and histamine that induce vasodilation and increased capillary permeability. As a consequence, the passage of large moieties such as phagocytic white blood cells is possible which, along with proteolytic enzymes, serve to remove pathogens and the remnants of devitalized tissue. The origins of exudate can be inferred from the Latin, "exsudare," which means to "ooze out like sweat" [10]. It is no surprise to find that the exudate is a complex medium rich in both biochemical and cellular components, and although its production is a normal response to support wound healing, it can become problematic when its production becomes excessive. There is a "Goldilocks" issue with wound hydration in that too little, and too much are both nonideal situations. Maintaining the correct balance, and one which is therapeutically advantageous, is a considerable challenge and there is no algebraic formula or algorithm which allows the healthcare professional to gauge the optimum level of exudate. An excessively moist wound can all too easily impede wound healing and induce maceration of the surrounding tissue [11]. The application of a dressing that can absorb excess exudate will therefore have a key role in wound management and the capacity of the various materials to achieve such is dependent on both chemical composition and the format in which they are presented to the wound.

The ability of the dressing to absorb exudate does not however simply relate to the removal of moisture, but also the components held within it. It must be remembered that exudates contain a large variety of bioactive species that, while having an initial function in wound regeneration, can outstay their welcome and impede the progression toward closure. Excessive concentrations of tissue degrading enzymes such as metalloproteases that block tissue proliferation and break down extracellular scaffolding will clearly be deleterious within a wound trying to build new structures and, therefore, their removal by a suitable dressing can certainly improve the opportunities for healing.

The longer the wound remains unhealed, the greater the propensity for infection and, if not identified and treated sufficiently early, the possibility of limb or life-threatening events is markedly increased. In one study surveying the outcomes for patients suffering from a diabetic foot ulcer (DFU), it was found that some 56–58% of outpatients presenting with a new ulcer were infected [12,13]. More worryingly, the risk of hospitalization and lower extremity amputation is some 56–155 times greater for those diabetics with an infected wound than those without [13]. The moist and chemically rich environment provided by wound fluid is almost ideal for bacteria [14–16]. In the past, the prime function of the dressing was to physically protect the wound from contamination and infection. More modern approaches to the design and implementation of dressings center on another critical balancing act, where the intention is to create and maintain an environment that is conducive to the host's repair mechanism while being hostile (or at least unfavorable) to the growth of microorganisms [17]. There is an ever-increasing interest in developing materials that can fulfil these requirements and an overview of some of these approaches is detailed in the subsequent sections of this chapter. A far more detailed inspection of the role of dressings in combatting microbial colonization and infection is however reserved for discussion in Chapter 6.

The provision of oxygen to the tissue is another key factor that must be considered in the design of dressings, particularly as it is an essential feedstock for cell metabolism. There are a host of cellular processes (ie, epithelization and fibroblast formation) that are dependent on its availability and hence the dressing must be capable of gaseous exchange [18]. The physical form of the dressing can impart a raft of properties, but it is also

Table 4.1 Adhesion categories of common dressings

Class	Examples
Adherent	Cotton gauze
Low adherent	Polyurethane Foam
Non adherent	Hydrogels, Hydrocolloids
Atraumatic	Silicone dressings

important that the system can be removed without disrupting the healing processes that have been initiated as a consequence of its original placement (Table 4.1). The dressing must afford low adherence to the tissue to prevent pain and further injury. The hydrogel systems, in particular, have been recognized for their ability to morph to the contours of the wound site and can easily be removed but, they are seldom placed on the wound by themselves. There will be a bandage or film of some form to secure the dressing, and it is important to remember that even here, there needs to be caution where the removal of the supporting material does not affect the neighboring wound tissue.

4.2 DRESSING DESIGN

While gauze dressings and cotton wool have traditionally offered wounds a degree of protection from contamination and were adept at absorbing exudate, they offered no active route through which to promote healing. Modern wound dressings are increasingly being designed as platforms through which to provide structures amendable to tissue reconstruction and which can deliver bioactive molecules to the wound in a controlled manner. There is an abundance of topical medicants that can be applied to the wound—whether in the form of solutions, sprays, creams, or ointments, but their effectiveness can often be questioned [19]. They absorb fluid from the wound bed and thereby lose their rheological properties which in highly draining wounds lead to their removal [19]. The use of dressings and macromolecular frameworks (hydrocolloids, hydrogels, foams, and films) can offer greater control over the release of the therapeutic agents and can promote prolonged residence time within the wound [19–22]. These agents (growth factors or antimicrobials) can play an active role in the various stages of healing combatting infection, cleansing the wound, or stimulating fibroblast activity to aid tissue remodeling. This is particularly significant in the management of chronic wounds where they typically persist for many months [23,24], and the ability to achieve sustained concentrations of a bioactive agent is important. It is also important to note that during the lengthy healing process, the wound will remain susceptible to infection, and, therefore, dressings loaded with antibiotics will enable wound site dosages that are higher than those achievable (or recommended) through systemic circulation. These have a range of merits and also some considerable limitations and it must be appreciated that their effective deployment is reliant on the expertise of the healthcare professional.

Table 4.2 Dressing Classifications

Type	Role	Polymer
Natural	Structural	Cellulose derivatives
		Chitin
		Silk fibroin
	Bioactive	Chitosan
		Hyaluronic acid
		Alginate
		Dextran
		Fibrin
		Elastin
		Collagen
		Gelatin
		Honey
Synthetic	Structural	Poly(vinyl alcohol)
		Poly(ethylene oxide)
		Poly(ethylene glycol)
		Poly(vinyl pyrrolidine)
		Polyurethane
		Poly(hydroxyethylmethacrylate)
		Poly-L-lactic acid
		Silicone

There are a large number of papers which have reviewed the present state of the art in terms of dressing design [19–22,25]. The aim of this chapter is to provide a synthesis of the core approaches and to highlight the structural elements and their impact on the various processes associated with wound healing. Moura et al. [25] have previously provided an excellent survey of modern approaches to wound healing and this chapter builds on their foundation and seeks to update and extend its remit. The following discussion breaks the dressing types down into their base components (as indicated in Table 4.2), and again many of these are used in mixed formulations to exploit and combine individual properties into a more effective clinical aid.

There are four broad classes within which dressings tend to be placed, but it must be acknowledged that they are seldom used in isolation and composite assemblies tend to predominate. These are discussed in turn and followed by the polymers that are blended in these structural categories.

4.2.1 Hydrocolloids

Hydrocolloid is a broad term given to a class of dressings that are, in essence, intricate polymer composites and are among the most widely used dressings in clinical practice. The more common ingredients found in dressings are sodium carboxymethylcellulose, gelatin, pectin, collagen along with various elastomers and adhesives [26–28]. As the

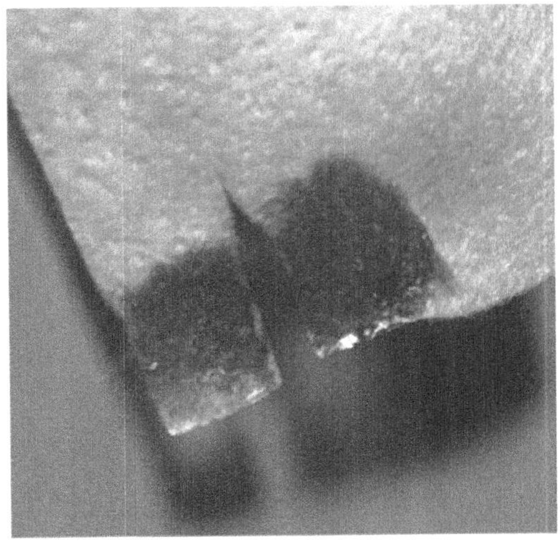

Figure 4.2 ***Aquacel hydrofiber sheet during exposure to water.***

"hydro" component of the name implies, the underpinning rationale is to create and maintain a moist wound environment. The principal components are typically colloidal particles that, upon contact with wound exudate, form a gel which retains the moisture. The components are mixed and formulated into thin films, mesh, or foams. An interesting property of many hydrocolloids is that they adhere to both moist and dry sites [1]. In many cases, the chemical functionality of the polymers contained within the formulation can be manipulated such that chemical cross links are introduced. Such modifications will obviously affect the physical properties of the material in terms of processing, but it will also have an impact on the resulting gel formed from absorbing wound exudate [28,29]. The hydrocolloids can also be produced as a nonwoven fiber mat (Hydrofibre©, Convatec) which can be applied as a flat sheet that conforms to the wound morphology. The latter is particularly hydrophilic and will form a thin soft gel (Fig. 4.2) on exposure to wound fluid and can be useful for absorbing excessive exudate [28,29]. They are usually deployed as part of a larger assembly—through incorporation within a polyester mesh or as part of a film or foam dressing, and known to induce autolytic debridement which, as noted previously, efficiently aids the elimination of dead tissue [28,29].

4.2.2 Hydrogels

Research publications focusing on hydrogels abound within the literature as they have found particular use within drug delivery technologies [20–22]. In general, they represent a broad class of polymer which form a gel-like network whose structural properties can be manipulated through ionic and covalent cross linking [6,30,31]. The structures can be subdivided into two groups: physical and chemical gels. Physical gels, often referred to as reversible, typically rely on the spaghetti-like disordered tangle of the polymer chains with secondary, intra and inter, chain bonding involving ionic, hydrogen or hydrophobic interactions lending additional structural support. The reversible nature of the gels is attributed to the fact that it is often possible to "detangle" the structure through changing the environmental conditions in which the gel was formed [20–22]. Thus, manipulating pH or temperature can often affect their dissolution and hence their attractiveness as a drug delivery system. In contrast, chemical gels are considered to be "permanent" as the chains are held together through covalent bonds between the chains. These cross links are normally introduced during the processing of the gel rather than in situ [32]. Irrespective of whether they are reversible or not, they can be noncharged or charged depending on the functional groups that are present within the polymer backbone. The latter tend to exhibit a degree of swelling in response to pH or in response to an applied electrical field and it is the subsequent structural changes that enable the release of drugs [33].

It has been suggested that the hydrogels closely resemble natural living tissue as a consequence of their high water content, porosity, and relatively soft nature. One particular advantage of their application in wound healing relates to the fact that they are inherently flexible (Fig. 4.3) and can be removed with relative ease without causing undue damage to the underlying wound bed [26,34]. As mentioned, a common feature is the high water content which can be ideal in terms of a wound application where it is necessary to maintain a moist environment [34,35]. There is, of course, a delicate balance between therapeutically moist and excessive moisture where the latter can cause maceration of the wound which can further impede the healing processes [36]. The hygroscopic nature of the base materials can be exploited as a means of actually removing excess moisture [35].

The loose structural framework inherent to most hydrogels, when coupled with the ability to incorporate a huge array of therapeutic agents within the network, can significantly enhance their influence on the healing processes. This creates a degree of interactivity when compared with the more passive dressings in that the gel structures can, to some degree, respond to stimuli such as pH or temperature which cause the

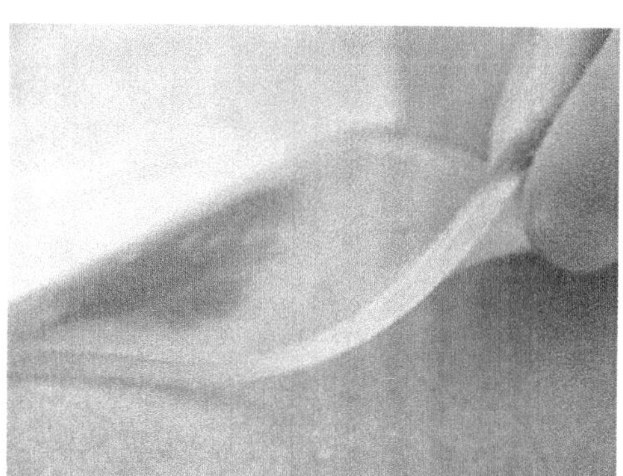

Figure 4.3 ***Hydrogel dressing.***

structures to swell or shrink. The latter are key features of a controlled release system and this characteristic has been widely exploited for the delivery of entrapped agents [30,31].

In contrast to the hydrocolloid dressing, hydrogels do not need the addition of wound fluid to create the gel and, as such, are suitable for dry wounds [37]. The latter is often described as a "moisture donor effect" and can aid autolytic debridement and, in turn, facilitate collagen production [38]. Despite being "pregelled," they can still absorb and retain exudate within the inner gel framework through expansion of the cross-linked chains. This can facilitate the isolation of contaminants (bacteria, proteases) and thereby aid the restimulation of the healing processes.

4.2.3 Foams

Foam dressings can be used as a complementary layer or as a direct alternative to the hydrocolloids and are regularly applied to high draining wounds [39]. This category contains a diverse range of polymers with an equally varied range of structural forms [34]. As the name suggests, they can readily adhere to the contours of the wound site and can provide a cushioning/protective effect which goes beyond the simple ability to absorb exudate [34,40]. As the thickness can be manipulated, large capacity dressings can be left on the wound for longer durations minimizing disruption to the wound and this is a particular characteristic that has proven attractive in the treatment of chronic ulcers [39–41]. It is common for the foams to be used in combination with a thin porous contact layer (typically silicone), as indicated in Fig. 4.4. The contact layer serves as the main interface between the wound and the absorbent foam and is engineered in such a way

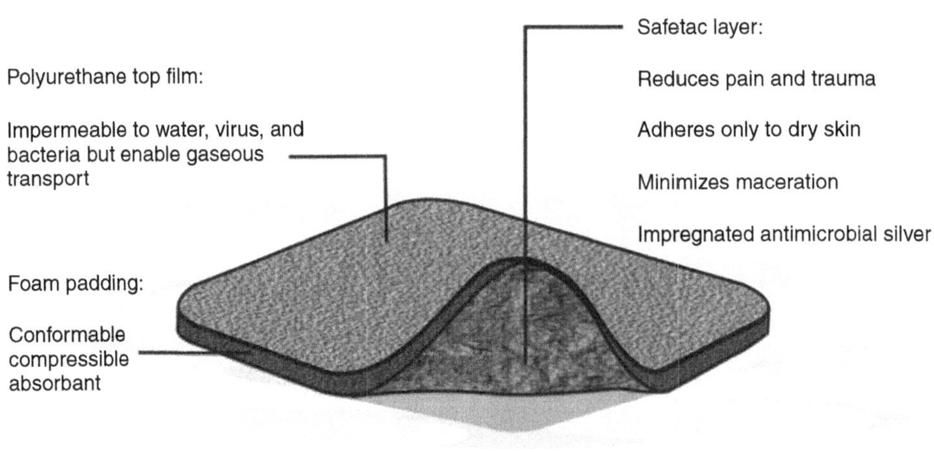

Figure 4.4 ***Multilayer foam dressing.***

so as to direct the exudate vertically—toward the foam-preventing lateral flow toward the undamaged skin [42,43].

4.2.4 Films

These are typically thin layers which are applied to wounds with low exudate and are generally used as a primary or secondary dressing and as complementary layer within the other systems mentioned previously [44]. The original form of the dressings was based on polyethylene and had little permeability of gases or moisture and was essentially occlusive [45]. The films themselves possess no capacity for the absorption of exudate and could, if left unchecked, serve to increase the possibility of bacterial growth and infection [45,46]. Semipermeable films, in contrast, provide a much more favorable environment for healing through allowing gaseous exchange while retaining moisture within the wound bed. These films are typically prepared as an interpenetrating network (IPN) in which two or more polymeric networks are mixed in a way that they cannot be separated once formed. The crucial aspect of this process is that two component chains are distinct and not chemically bonded to one another—merely entangled within each other. Varying the nature of the polymers through introducing crosslinks or different functional blocks can alter the properties of the resulting film and therein the permeability toward gases/moisture etc. The resulting films are combined with an adhesive layer and applied as a sheet across the wound site [47] and are typically used for superficial wounds or as a protective layer for other dressings [34,40,48]. They are used in some aspects of chronic wound management where they can protect the wound bed with the transparency of the film enabling visual inspection [49–51].

4.2.5 Dressing Selection—Practical Application

There are a great many commercial dressing available to the clinical staff and most will come with a variety of marketing claims, but it can be difficult to interpret whether the claims made on a particular trial for one particular type of wound are liable to be applicable to the wound presented by the patient at the time of consultation. The physical form of the dressing may have a generic shape which may not always be appropriate, and it is possible to induce more damage through the deployment of an ill-fitting system. In most cases, the selection of the dressing will come down to the expertise of the practitioner who can take into account the needs of the wound and of the patient. The selection process will always commence with a visual inspection of the wound and patient assessment but the main factors to consider are:

- Wound location
- Size/depth
- Exudate—amount and nature
- Wound bed tissue

Table 4.3 Summary of dressing applications

Type	Characteristics	Wound application
Hydrocolloid	AE, AD	Moderate exudate
Hydrogel	RW, MC, AB, CT, LA	Dry/low exudate
Foam	AE, MC, CWB, LA	Moderate/high exudate, cavity filling, fragile Skin
Film	MC, TL, PL	Primary dressing: low exudate. Secondary dressing: hydrogels/foam

AD, autolytic debridement; AE, absorbs exudate; CT, cooling; CWB, conforms to wound bed; LA, low adhesion; MC, moisture control; PL, permeability; RW, rehydrating; TL, transparency.
Source: Adapted from [22].

- Periwound skin condition
- Compatibility
- Risk of infection
- Pain and trauma due to dressing changes
- Patient life style/well-being

The capabilities of the different dressings are considered in Table 4.3 and the selection process for different wound states is summarized in Table 4.4.

It is important to consider the physico-chemical properties of the dressings and what they are designed to achieve. Among the main queries are: duration of placement, stability, potential for leakage, possibility of odor, sensitivity, comfort. It must also be noted that, in each of the categories within Table 4.1, there will be an antimicrobial variant employing some form of antimicrobial (silver, iodine, etc). As always, it will be necessary to consider the cost effectiveness of employing a particular dressing. This may be a concern where a silver-impregnated dressing is used, yet there is no sign of infection and hence a simpler system may be more appropriate.

Table 4.4 Selection of dressing type depending on wound condition

Tissue type	Exudate	Role of dressing	Primary dressing	Secondary dressing
Necrotic	Dry	RH, AD	Hydrogel	Film
Slough	Dry/low	RH, MC, AD	Hydrogel	Film
Slough	Moderate/high	AB, MC, AD	Hydrocolloid/Foam	Bandage or film
Granulating	Dry/low	MC, PT	Hydrogel/Film	
Granulating	Moderate/high	MC, PT	Hydrocolloid/Foam	
Epithelializing	Low	PT	Hydrocolloid/Film	
Infected	Low/High	MC, OC, AM	Antimicrobial Dressing	

AD, autolytic debridement; AE, absorbs exudate; AM, antimicrobial; MC, moisture control; OC, odor control; PT, protect new tissue; RW, rehydrating.
Source: Adapted from [22].

4.3 POLYMERIC WOUND DRESSINGS OVERVIEW

It is clear from the previous discussions that the effectiveness of the wound treatment depends on a large number of factors such as the wound type, stage, the extent and nature of injury, the morphology of the wound, and the tissues involved as well as a myriad of possible therapeutic agents—either employed topically to the wound or systemically. Selection of the dressing is therefore only one factor, but it is nevertheless a critical protagonist as it can directly influence the cellular dynamics at play. The wound can be treated using passive or, what has become loosely termed, interactive dressings [52]. The former are usually employed for acute wounds where there is only a need to protect the wound from the external environment and absorb exudate. The underlying wound and the natural biochemical processes can be effectively left to themselves to bring about healing and wound closure. The interactive dressings are usually applied to slow-healing wounds where there is often a need to perform some form of intervention to stimulate the healing processes. This can be to simply maintain a moist environment or the dressing can impart some form of treatment to enhance/accelerate the healing. The latter can be achieved through the incorporation of therapeutic agents or antimicrobials within the materials [20–22]. Alternatively, it could be to exploit the inherent chemical properties such as to regulate the pH of the environment to facilitate particular enzymatic and cellular processes conducive to healing [40]. There has been considerable activity related to the modification of existing polymers and the design of new systems and composite assemblies and a bewildering array of chemical structures and functionalities have arisen in recent years—each variant professing to offer new advantages in wound treatment [53,54]. The polymers employed in the design of new dressing materials can be divided into two categories: natural and synthetic. There are of course a multitude of systems that bridge the two and composite formulations exploiting the properties of two or more different polymers are increasingly common. An examination of the core structures can however offer some insights into dressing design and application.

4.4 DFU DRESSINGS BASED ON NATURAL POLYMERS

Polymers that can be considered natural can arise from a multitude of sources but tend to either possess a protein or polysaccharide backbone [55]. The core advantages of these systems relate to the similarity of the components to, and potential compatibility with, the wound environment and the extracellular matrix (ECM) in which they will be in contact when in the form of a dressing. One of the critical issues with their adoption however is the variation in their composition as a consequence of their origin. Natural materials tend to exhibit much larger heterogeneity and batch variation when compared to purely synthetic alternatives [56,57]. There has been a considerable increase in the patient's desire for all things natural but, within the medical sphere, acquiescing to such requests can be significantly tempered by the associated risk of infectious agents being transmitted or the presence of immunogenic motifs as a consequence of the origins of the materials—particularly in the case where the material has arisen from animal sources [56].

Stability and variable mechanical properties are also potential limitations [58] though it must be appreciated that the imposition of manufacturing processes and rigorous quality control can go some way to counter the issues—albeit at additional economic cost [59]. In some instances, it is more favorable to consider the possibility of composite manufacture where the natural components are incorporated within a synthetic blend. This is a compromise which enables a greater degree of production conformity while retaining the inherent functionality of the natural material that would otherwise be difficult to mimic synthetically [60]. The natural polymers that are presently employed within wound dressings are discussed in turn in the following sections, and, in each case, critical overviews of the structure-function relationships and the potential clinical merits are presented.

4.4.1 Chitin and Chitosan

Chitin is derived from the exoskeleton of arthropods, crustaceans, and molluscs and is essentially a large chain polysaccharide [61]. It can be extracted from the shells of common shrimps and crabs and its ready accessibility has rendered it commercially attractive for use in a host of biomedical applications [62,63]. Chitin is a linear polysaccharide of N-acetyl-D-glucosamine (2-acetylamino-2-deoxy-D-glucose) units linked by β-(1-4) glycosidic bonds [64–66] and the basic structure is detailed in Fig. 4.5.

Chitin is not soluble in aqueous solutions, hence its use as an exoskeleton, and therefore it is usually processed through deacetylation into chitosan as indicated in Fig. 4.5 [67,68]. The resulting chitosan is still a linear copolymer of D-glucosamine and of N-acetyl-D-glucosamine but a key factor in the versatility of the chitosan, in comparison to its parent, is the availability of the primary amino group through which the base polymer can be extensively manipulated.

The term chitosan is a relatively broad classification and is typically used to describe a series of chitin derivatives having different degrees of deacetylation which are defined in terms of the proportion of primary amino groups in the polymer backbone and of their average molecular weights [68]. Both aspects are significant as the functional properties of the polymer have been shown to be directly dependent on the extent to which the acetate groups have been removed [58]. The key advantages of the system, in relation to its use as a wound dressing, lie in the fact that it is a natural product, is biodegradable, nonantigenic, and nontoxic. More recently, it has been shown to demonstrate considerable antimicrobial properties which is a significant factor when

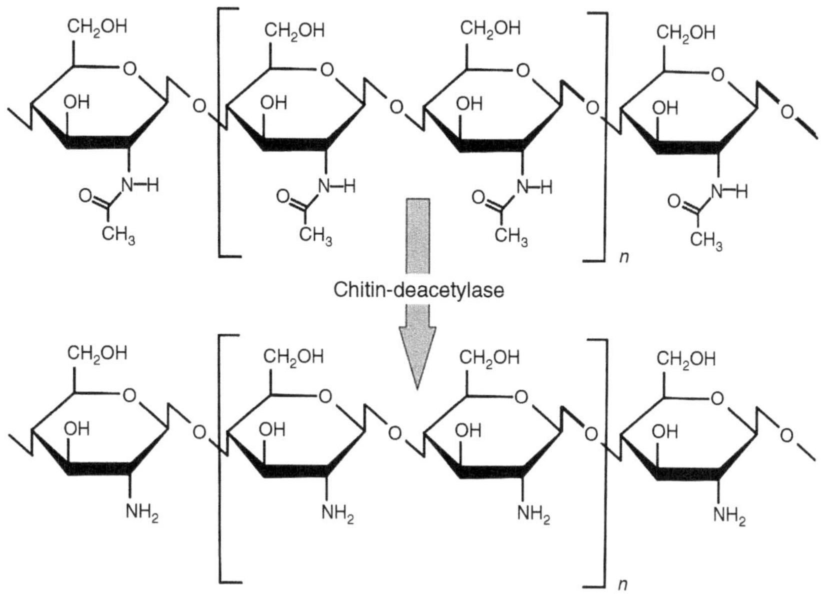

Figure 4.5 ***Conversion of chitin to chitosan.***

considering the duration over which a chronic wound can exist and the propensity for infection [58,60,61].

The polymer can be readily modified through a variety of routes such as chemical hydrolysis or enzymatic processing [65,66]. Moreover, both the amino and the hydroxyl groups on the chitosan chain can be functionalized with a myriad of chemical substituents, and this partly explains the large number of derivatives which abound within the research literature. Chitosan itself is cationic by virtue of the deacetylation process yielding primary amino groups (Fig. 4.5), and while such groups are ideal for chemical modification, the subsequent amide formation can reduce the overall cationic activity. Chitosan in its native form is therefore a weak poly-base and, as such, it exhibits some interesting pH-sensitive properties—it dissolves at relatively acidic pH while being insoluble under neutral and alkaline conditions and therefore possesses the ability to swell when protonated [61,69]. The latter has stimulated considerable interest in its ability to control the delivery of pharmaceuticals, and it is easy to comprehend how such a property can be particularly apt for use in dressings [61,70–72]. In terms of materials processing, its solubility in organic acids can allow the production of particles, membranes, fibers, and sponges [63,73]. The cationic nature of the polymer backbone at normal physiological pH enables electrostatic interaction with a range of anionic species within the wound fluid and tissue [6,74].

Chitosan and its various derivatives have been shown to present a wide variety of properties that have been found to be particularly advantageous when considering their application in wound dressings: cationic at typical wound pH values, film-forming, exhibits mild gelation and has strong wound tissue adhesive properties. They have also been shown to demonstrate an ability to enhance coagulation and thereby aid healing [59,65,67]. They have been reported to enhance the inflammatory response of polymorphonuclear leukocytes, macrophages, and neutrophils to an appropriate trigger [75].

Chitosan has also been used as copolymer in a number of hydrogel systems—particularly those based on alginate where it functions as a cross linker to improve the structural integrity of the macromolecular network. It has been frequently postulated that through the hybrid approach, it should be possible to tailor the designs to enhance healing performance. This could involve improving exudate absorption capacity, exploiting the antibacterial function, or stimulating angiogenesis and the reepithelization of the skin tissue [59,65].

4.4.2 Hyaluronic Acid and Other Glycosaminoglycans

Hyaluronic acid (HA) is found in the connective tissues such as cartilage, eye vitreous humor, umbilical cord, and synovial fluid [6,56]. However, it is also produced on a large scale through microbial fermentation which offers greater quality control and can avoid the issues associated with its extraction from animal sources [76,77]. It is a linear polysaccharide of alternating disaccharide units of α-1,4-D-glucuronic acid and β-1,3-N-acetyl-D-glucosamine linked by β(1-3) glycosidic bonds [69], as shown in Fig. 4.6. A key factor in its use within wound dressings relates to the fact that it is nonallergenic and biocompatible. It is often referred to simply as hyaluronan due to the fact that in vivo it exists as a polyanion [76]. It is relatively water soluble and possesses unique viscoelastic properties, whereby it can form three-dimensional structures through hydrogen bonding [76].

Hyaluronic acid has been utilized in a large number of wound dressings—typically in the form of foams or gels. The exact role of the biomaterial is very varied and can perform a number of important physiological functions ranging from structural

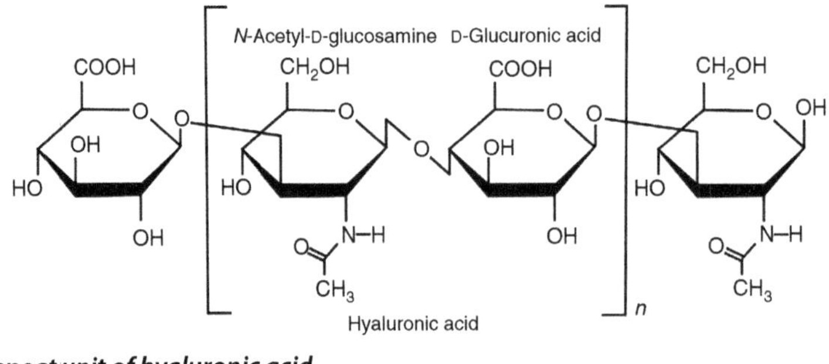

Figure 4.6 ***Repeat unit of hyaluronic acid.***

support through to lubrication and ECM water sorption/retention [78,79]. In particular, dressings composed of the material have been shown to encourage mesenchymal and epithelial cell migration and differentiation which, in turn, enhance collagen deposition and angiogenesis [76,80]. The ability of the polymer to aid wound healing has been attributed, at least in part, to its degradation profiles where its action can be strongly dependent upon its molecular weight. It has been suggested that the high molecular weight polymer variants have a structural role while the lower weight degradation products are the key factors that stimulate the wound-healing processes noted previously [79–82].

4.4.3 Cellulose and Its Derivatives

Cellulose, as many will recall from their secondary education studies, is the principal component of plant cell walls and that it is by far the most abundant organic polymer on Earth. In the pursuit of green and sustainable technologies, it is a renewable biomaterial, easily acquired and at low cost [56]. Moreover, it is an excellent feedstock for conversion into a range of derivatives that have found extensive use within a range of commercial applications across the biomedical sector. It is regularly modified and there is a rich literature base on the characterization and application of its derivatives for wound dressings. Cellulose-based material are widespread across the biomedical sector and their prevalence can be attributed, at least in part, to their inherent biocompatibility (especially when combined with other natural polymers such as collagen) as they have shown reduced inflammatory responses [83,84]. In addition, the resorption of cellulose within the tissues does not occur since cells are not able to synthesize cellulases necessary for its hydrolysis [84]. The core polymer itself is a linear chain consisting of β-1,4 linked D-glucose subunits which are joined to form cellobiose repeating units as indicated in Fig. 4.7 [85].

Cellulose glucan chains are arranged in a parallel formation—packed side-by-side. These form an array of microfibrils that, while stabilizing the structure, minimize its flexibility. There is extensive hydrogen bonding within the composite structure which confers the high degree of stability and rigidity (as evidenced by its use in nature) but, ironically, makes them water insoluble despite the apparent hydrophilicity of the component groups. Cellulose derived from microbial sources has been found to be significantly different from that arising principally from plant origin. Although crystalline, it has been shown to possess a unique nano fibrillar structure that has a high capacity for water retention [49,83], and hence, in terms of moisture control alone, it has been shown to have considerable potential for wound healing [49,50].

The chemical and physical characteristics of particular cellulose systems are dependent on the degree of polymerization and the internal structure and interaction of the constituent chains. These will thereby influence the processing of the base material and

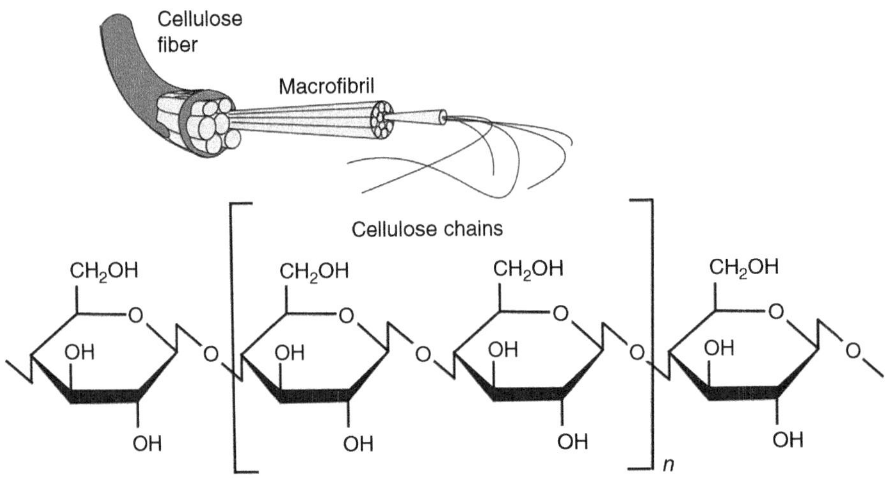

Figure 4.7 ***Cellulose microstructure.***

its suitability for particular applications [51]. Cellulose can be relatively resistant to most chemicals but is slowly degraded by microbial action (as evidenced by fungal rotting processes) which can markedly improve its water solubility [83,85]. It must be noted, however, that some cellulose derivatives (predominantly ether systems) such as methyl cellulose, hydroxypropyl cellulose, hydroxyethyl cellulose, hydroxyethyl methyl cellulose, hydroxypropyl methyl cellulose, and carboxymethyl cellulose are partially soluble. Carboxymethylcellulose, in particular, has become one of the most common components of hydrocolloid dressings. These systems are also notable in that they offer a number of advantages in terms of processing/manufacture such as solubility in nonaqueous solvents. They have also been shown to possess thermoplastic characteristics and, from a wound dressing perspective biosurface activity.

Cellulose ester derivatives (acetate and sulphates) can be formed as fiber or film-like materials and, through controlling their molecular weights, their aqueous viscosities and gelation characteristics have been finely tuned and exploited across a range of different biomedical or pharmaceutical applications [50,82]. It has been shown that cellulose can stimulate the wound-healing processes through the release of therapeutic levels of a number of growth factors (ie, PDGF, epidermal growth factor (EGF), and FGF) directly at the wound site. Moreover, it has been found that dermal fibroblast migration and proliferation are similarly promoted [51,86,87]. There have been numerous studies that indicate considerable ability for inhibiting bacterial growth which, given the duration of chronic wounds, is a particularly significant characteristic. A typical example of a commercial cellulose-based dressing is Aquacel Hydrofiber Wound Dressing (ConvaTec, USA). This is a carboxymethyl derivative of cellulose (hydrocolloid) which absorbs wound fluid to generate a local gel that maintains a

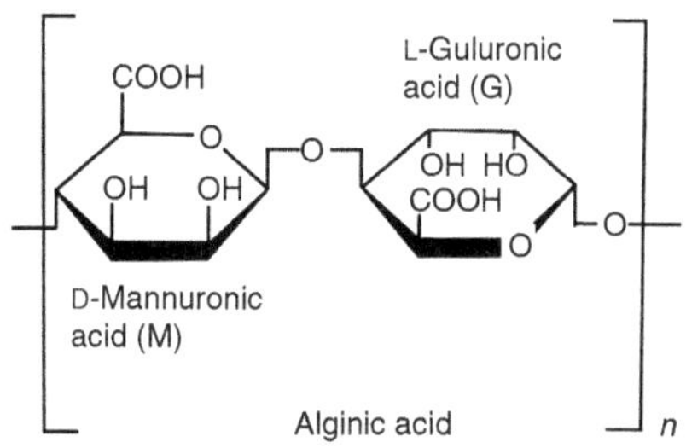

Figure 4.8 ***Repeat units of alginate highlighting the G and M residues.***

moist environment that, as with Winter's recommendations, should help promote wound healing.

4.4.4 Alginates

Alginate (or alginic acid) is derived from the marine algae (Laminaria hyperborean, Ascophyllum nodosum, and Macrocystis pyrifera) and, to a lesser extent, from some soil bacteria. There is an extensive industrial base devoted to its processing for use in tissue engineering and a raft of drug delivery applications have emerged in recent years [56]. It is a polysaccharide composed of β-D-mannuronate (M-residues) and α-L-guluronate (G-residues) as indicated in Fig. 4.8 and these are covalently linked in different alternating or random sequences [56,85,88].

A key property of the alginate polymer is the ability to form reversible hydrogels through the interaction of the carboxylic acid functional groups with metal cations. The latter are typically divalent species (Ca^{2+}, Mg^{2+}, Ba^{2+}, etc.) which can serve to cross-link the G residues in adjacent chains, as indicated in Fig. 4.9 [88].

A more recent approach to controlled crosslinking has been to exploit the differing affinities of the G residues for ferric/ferrous cations [89,90]. The ferric (Fe^{3+}) state is traditionally regarded as a "hard" cation which will preferentially bind to the carboxyl groups within the alginate and thus effectively holds the structure together. In contrast,

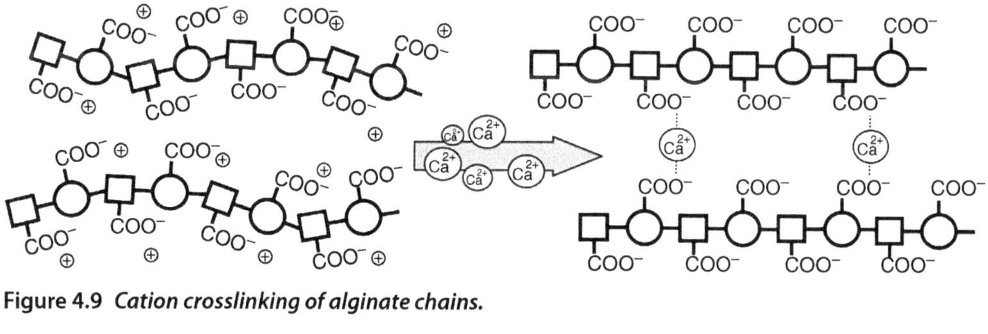

Figure 4.9 ***Cation crosslinking of alginate chains.***

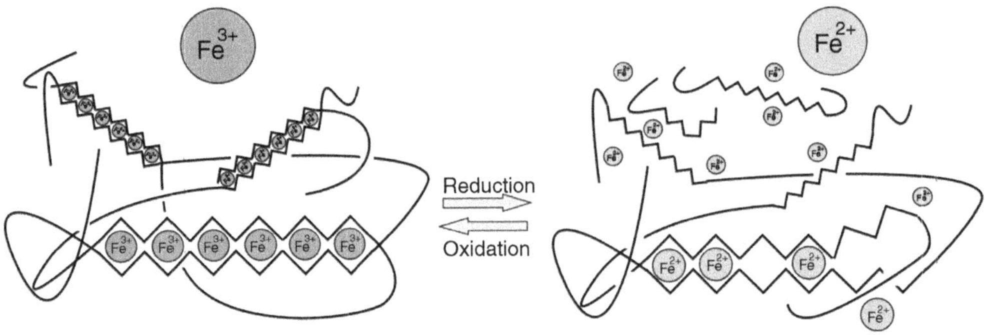

Figure 4.10 ***Influence of iron redox state on the integrity of an alginate hydrogel.***

the ferrous (Fe^{2+}) state is a "soft" cation that tends to bind neutral ligands (typically nitrogen and sulphur moieties) and thus redox cycling between the two forms can lead to the formation/dissolution of the cross links and hence the dissolution of the large three-dimensional hydrogel network as indicated in Fig. 4.10. This approach has considerable applications for drug release systems [89,90], but it could be envisaged that it could find its way into smart dressing applications (Chapter 5).

There are several key advantages to the use of alginate in wound dressings: high biocompatibility, low toxicity, and good muco-adhesive properties [56,85,91]. The hydrogels are pH sensitive and this is a feature that has been proposed as a route through which bioactive substances could be released in a controlled (stimuli responsive mode) from a wound-based hydrogel [88]. It must be noted that there can be issues of reproducibility in their operation, especially when considering the high degree of compositional variability that can be encountered within a wound environment. The main issue relates to degradation of the network through either enzyme hydrolysis of the loss of the cross linker [91]. One approach to countering this weakness has been to replace the metal counter ion cross-linker with copolymers possessing the ionic functionalities that can interact directly with those on the alginate. A diverse range of systems have been investigated and include: gelatin [92], heparin [93], polyvinyl alcohol [94], and chitosan [95].

Calcium alginate based dressings are now commonplace, particularly in the treatment of diabetic foot ulcers where their hygroscopic nature can efficiently absorb wound exudate while facilitating debridement. There have been numerous studies where their application has been shown to accelerate wound healing [39,96,97].

4.4.5 Collagen

Collagen represents 25% of the total protein body content and can be found in skin, bone, cartilage, tendon, and ligaments [30,31,57,98,99]. Its primary function is to

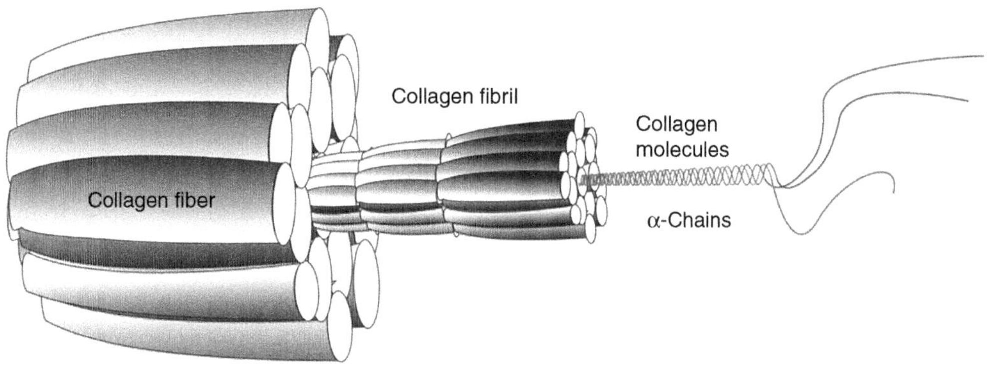

Figure 4.11 ***Structural assembly of collagen fibers.***

provide strength to the tissue matrices [100], but it is far being a passive structural support and can interact with cells and aid essential cell signalling associated with a host of functions. These can include cell anchorage, migration, proliferation, differentiation, and survival [56,100]. It provokes little in the way of inflammatory and cytotoxic responses and hence its attractiveness toward wound applications [57]. Collagens are typically rod-type proteins with typical molecular weights in the region of 300,000 g/mol [56,101], and there are some 27 types of collagen with Type 1 being the most abundant protein present in mammals and, as a consequence, the most commonly investigated for biomedical purposes [56,85]. The basic structure of collagen is shown in Fig. 4.11.

As it is protein, it degrades enzymatically within the body through the action of various proteinases [102]. Although fibers are relatively stable, their mechanical, degradation, and water absorption properties can be significantly improved through chemical manipulation—typically involving cross-linking through the use of glutaraldehyde (targeting amino groups) [103] or carboiimide (targeting carboxyl moieties) [104]. Alternative approaches to enhancing the fiber stability can be achieved through the use of physical methods (freeze drying) [105] or through the incorporation of the material as a copolymer is a composite network (ie, hydrogels) such that the additional components shield the peptide from enzyme hydrolysis [106,107].

Given the fact that collagen is a major constituent of human ECM, it is widely regarded as a core substrate for tissue engineering and wound dressing. Historically, there have been concerns over the extraction of collagen from animal sources from moral and ethical viewpoints but also from the scientific perspective of initiating foreign body responses [101,102]. The latter can be addressed through the introduction of enzyme purification techniques to remove the immunogenic sequences [108], but this clearly adds another complex step to the overall processing overhead. This is not an inconsiderable issue as collagen can be difficult to process to the grade required for biomedical consistency and applicability. There is also the issue of sterilization where many of the methods that are presently employed inadvertently result in further chemical and physical modifications of the collagen substructure [102]. Nevertheless, collagen is frequently used as a component in wound dressing materials and has been successfully employed in a diverse range of forms that include gels, pads, particles, pastes, powders, sheets, or solutions.

4.4.6 Gelatin

Gelatin is obtained through the irreversible hydrolysis of collagen but, in contrast to its parent, offers more processing avenues and this is reflected in its use in a diverse range of pharmaceutical and biomedical applications. Gelatin is obtained through the processing of collagen as indicated in Fig. 4.12, which, depending on whether acid or alkaline approaches are taken, will give two different types of end product [109]. The different pH

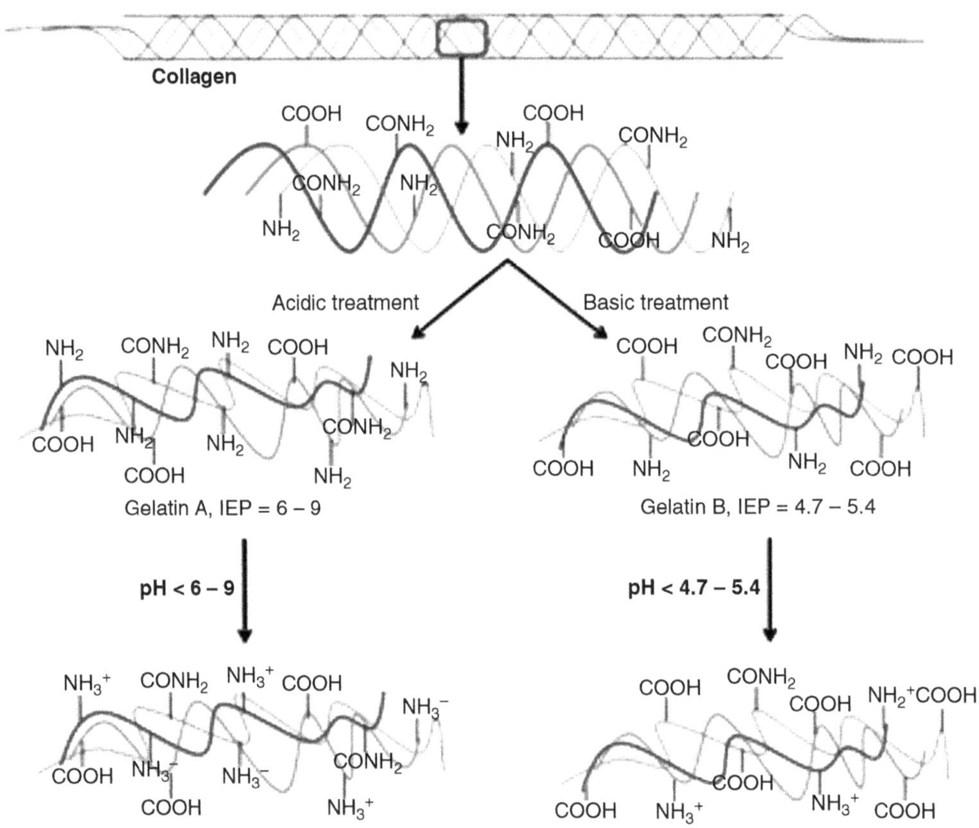

Figure 4.12 ***Processing of collagen to yield acidic or basic gelatin*** *[109].*

regimes affect the isoelectric point [56] which has the advantage of enabling the gelatin to be tailored to different applications enabling its complexation with either positive or negatively charged biomolecules [110].

In contrast to the collagen from which it is derived, gelatin has been shown to elicit a very low level of antigenicity due to the fact that the protein has been effectively denatured during the processing stages [57]. The protein is commonly used as a component in hydrogels and particularly in those biomedical applications where there is a need for a controlled or sustained release of a therapeutic agent [56,111]. The release profile of a compound contained with a gelatin matrix is generally determined by the enzymatic degradation of the polymer network and, in a similar approach to that used in collagen, the rate of release can be finely tuned through controlling the degree of cross linking between the polymer chains [112]. The cross links can be inserted through similar chemistries to those employed in the manipulation of collagen with carbodiimides [113], glutaraldehyde [114]. Physical crosslinking as a consequence of polyion interactions or through combination with other gelating polymers is also possible [92,115].

A number of studies have demonstrated the ability of collagen and gelatine-based dressing to significantly affect the healing dynamics of the wound through reducing infection and by promoting the formation of granular tissue that can encourage improve healing rates [116–118]. The polymolecular framework created by the gels also enables other species to be encapsulated which can confer additional functionality toward the healing processes. Examples include glucose oxidase whose reaction with endogenous glucose can provide a sustained release of reactive oxygen species (peroxide) as well as natural compounds (such as polyphenols, growth factors), antibiotics (such as doxycycline and levofloxacin), and ionic silver as an antimicrobial agent [117,119,120].

4.4.7 Fibrin

Fibrin is a key factor in the clotting of blood and therefore interest in its use in wound-healing application probably comes as little surprise. Fibrin is a fibrous, non-globular protein which arises through the action thrombin (a protease) on fibrinogen upon activation of a wound event. The basic scheme is highlighted in Fig. 4.13. The soluble fibrinogen is converted into fibrin at the wound site, whereupon it polymerizes forming long strands of tough insoluble protein that, through crosslinking, incorporates platelets into a mesh and eventually forms a plug that completes the clotting process [57,121]. It has been found that the fibrin molecules contain specific domains that may be useful in improving cell binding and thus, there have been extensive studies of fibrin as a biomaterial for improving cell adhesion, spreading, migration, proliferation, and tubule formation [56,121,122]. These characteristics are ideal for tissue engineering

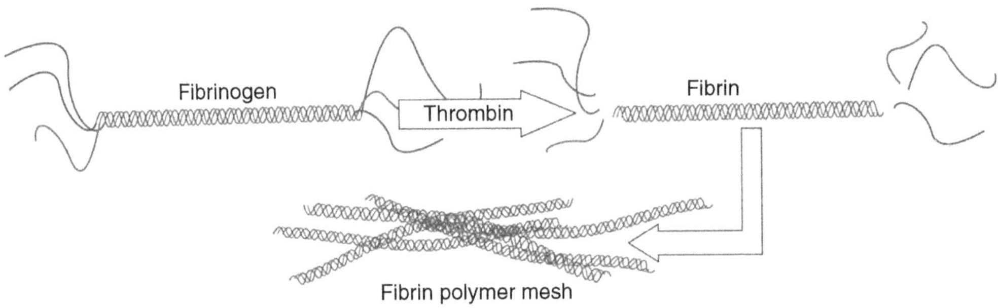

Figure 4.13 ***Production of fibrin.***

applications, whereby the incorporation of the fibrin within a hydrogel can serve as a tissue scaffold. One issue however is that the structural integrity of the hydrogels is relatively poor—suffering from low mechanical rigidity and it is possible that degradation can occur before the acquisition of any substantial engineered tissue [121]. The use of fibrin as an adhesive has found considerable practical application—especially in surgical procedures (possessing hemostatic, chemotactic, and mitogenic properties) [56] and has been shown to aid the fixation of skin grafts as well as limiting the risk of infection in chronic wounds [123].

Fibrin gels are generally obtained by the enzymatic cross-linking of fibrinogen with thrombin as would be the case in its natural application. The structure of the resulting gel is dependent on a host of factors and can be manipulated through varying the concentrations of fibrinogen and thrombin, the local pH, ionic strength, and the calcium ion concentration [124]. As with gelatin, gels formed from fibrin are capable of holding a range of other components which can impart varying functionality to the wound dressing and serve to improve wound healing. In a similar approach to that mentioned previously, the incorporation of inhibitors (for COX-2, iNOS) suppresses nitric oxide produced such that the inflammatory response could be reduced and the wound healing accelerated [125].

4.4.8 Silk Fibroin

Fibroin protein isolated from the silkworm (Bombyx mori or Antheraea mylitta) has gathered some considerable interest from the biomedical research communities as a consequence of the material's properties: biocompatibility, hemocompatibility, slow degradability, water vapor, and gas permeability [126,127]. Silk fibers are a core shell structure which is composite polymer composed of a fibrous protein (fibroin) core encapsulated by a glue-like protein (sericin) as indicated in Fig. 4.14. In the case of *B. mori*, there are two core brins of fibroin which, when coated with sericin, yields fibers with diameters in the range of 20 μm. Electron microscopy of the silk microstructure has

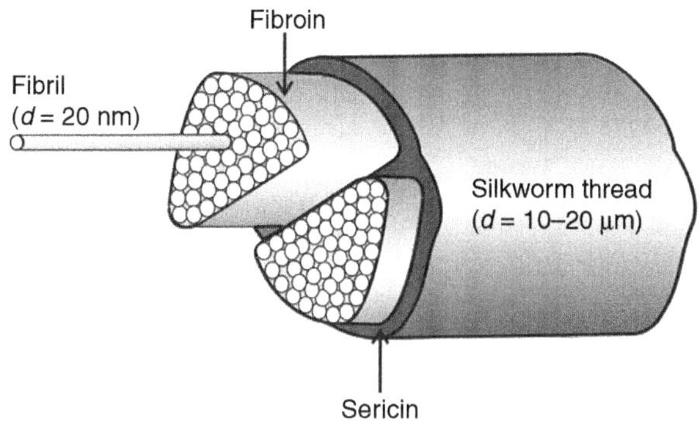

Figure 4.14 ***Structural components of silk fibroin from B. mori.***

indicated that the silk fiber is composed of bundles of oriented nanofibrils [128–133]. Initial studies have suggested that the sericin acts as an encapsulant, but more recent investigations have indicated that the coating may also have fungicidal or bactericidal activity [134].

The structure of the fibroin fibers extracted from *B. mori* is reported to be composed of a highly repetitive $(Gly\text{-}Ala)_n$ sequence adopting antiparallel β-sheet conformation. The β-sheet crystallite is the molecular network constructed by crosslinking-sheet conformation of the molecular structures within several neighboring silk protein molecules [135]. It has been shown that the silk fiber is composed of almost a 50:50 ratio of amorphous to crystalline regions [136]. Silk fibroin has been shown to support epidermal cells and promote fibroblast attachment and proliferation which can aid wound healing [56].

4.4.9 Dextran

Dextran is a hydrophilic, highly soluble polysaccharide polymer which is inert in biological systems and, as with other polysaccharide chains, is readily functionalized through its reactive hydroxyl groups [137,138]. Each chain is composed of α(1,6)-linked D-glucose residues with a degree of branching via α(1,3) linkages, as indicated in Fig. 4.15. The material is obtained from various bacterial strains via the action of dextransucrase [56,85].

Dextran is biodegradable, biocompatible, resists protein adsorption and does not affect cell viability and, as such, has found numerous healing applications within bone, dermal, and subcutaneous healing [56,138]. It has been found to facilitate inflammatory cell infiltration and promotes angiogenic cell migration into the wounds to promote healing [139]. Dextranomer, a dextran polymer, has been assessed in diabetic patients presenting with an ulcer or an infected wound, whereby the polymer was applied directly to the wound and covered with gauze or a non occlusive bandage. The study involved 15 patients presenting with wounds and, of those, 12 were found to have healed

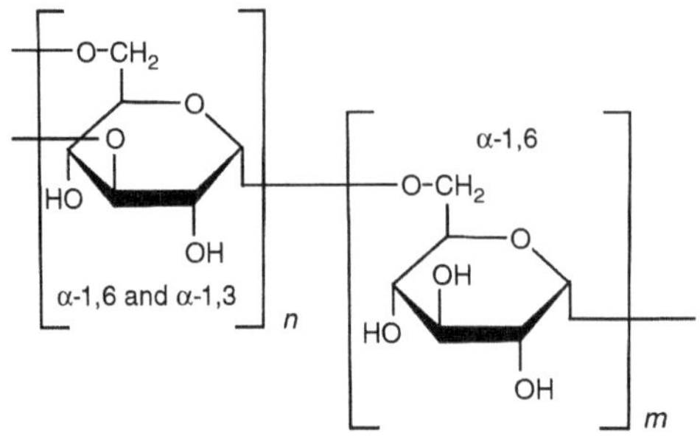

Figure 4.15 ***Repeat units of dextran.***

completely [140]. The effect of the wound preparation on infected wounds was found to be dramatic and, it has been reported, there was a clear and indeed remarkable decrease in the inflammatory response from the outset with the formation of granulation tissue within a few days. One explanation that has been postulated relates to the capacity of the dextranomer to cleanse the wound by absorbing the exudate, protein degradation products, prostaglandins, bacteria, and other contaminants. This would have the net effect of reducing inflammation and improving healing [140].

4.4.10 Elastin

Native Elastin is a major constituent of skin but is characterized as being highly insoluble and consequently very difficult to process from a manufacturing perspective [141,142]. Precursor forms and derivatives such as tropoelastin (Fig. 4.16), α-elastin (an oxalic acid derivative of elastin), and elastin-like polypeptides are more soluble and amenable to manipulation and, as such, have found much broader applications as elastin-based biomaterials [142,143]. These have found to elicit favorable cellular interactions and enhanced

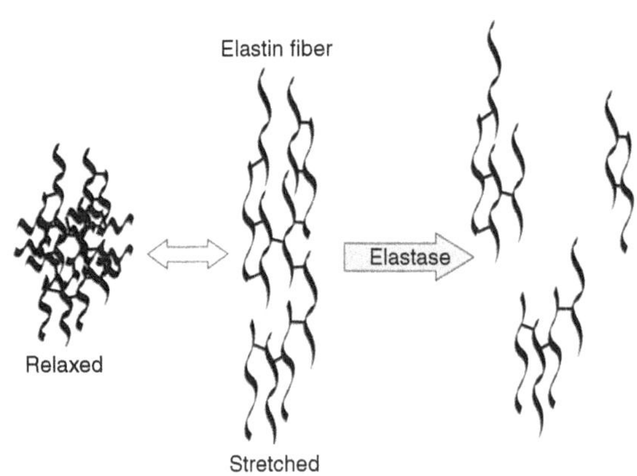

Figure 4.16 ***Formation of elastin fibers.***

tissue regeneration through increased chemotactic activity, fibroblast proliferation, and collagenase synthesis [144].

The difficulties associated with the extraction and subsequent processing of soluble elastins have meant that there is a relatively small literature base through which to compare the effectiveness of their use in wound dressings. Nevertheless, it has been demonstrated that a gel consisting of elastin-like peptides loaded with keratinocyte growth factor (KGF) enhanced the reepithelialization and granulation of wounds in diabetic mice [142]. It should be noted that in common with the other protein-based biomaterials—the wealth of functionality associated with the substituent groups on the peptide chain can enable modification through chemical [145,146], enzymatic [146], and physical processes [147]. This could enable further modification but, at present, the use of elastins within the design of dressings remains at the curiosity stage.

4.5 DFU DRESSINGS BASED ON SYNTHETIC POLYMERS

The chemical modification of natural polymers is an obvious approach to create new functionalities and capabilities and allow new interactive dressings tailored to particular applications. However, there are practical limitations to what can be achieved given that the base polymer is preformed and its manipulation will be subsequently be hindered by processing issues. Designing a polymer from the bottom up, however, can overcome many of these issues and there is a vast range of monomers through which to consider new designs. While once it may have been thought that synthetic polymers would be inferior to the biocompatible/bioactive properties of natural systems, advances in polymer synthesis have enabled the production of polymers with biocompatible and biodegradable functionality that compete and outperform many of the natural analogues [137]. Improvements in manufacturing and processing enable a high degree of control over the composition and properties which are in stark contrast to the concerns that plague natural products [111]. Moreover, the possibility of biological contamination is minimized though there are obvious issues over the possible toxicology of degradation products or processing additives. The following sections consider the main classes of synthetic polymers which are prevalent within wound-healing applications, but, as mentioned previously, very often dressings arise out of complicated arrangements of more than one material and there are often composites composed of multiple synthetic and synthetic-natural hybrids.

4.5.1 Poly(Vinyl Alcohol)

Poly(vinyl alcohol) (PVA) is a hydrophilic, nontoxic, noncarcinogenic, and relatively biocompatible polymer obtained from the polymerization of vinyl acetate (Fig. 4.17) by means of alcoholysis, hydrolysis, or aminolysis [30,31,122,148]. PVA is a robust and easily processed polymer which is found in a vast array of applications but which has niche

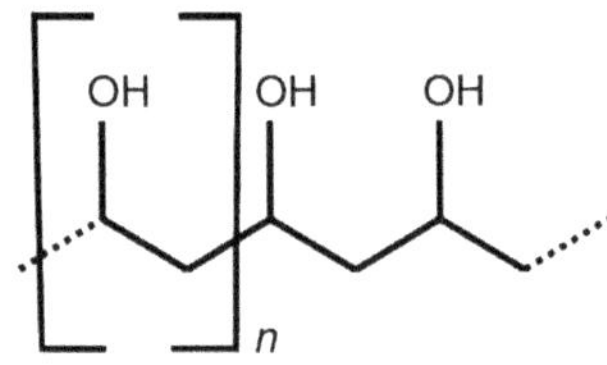

Figure 4.17 ***Repeat units of PVA.***

applications in tissue engineering and drug delivery technologies. The key properties are its hydrophilicity and water absorption capabilities and are processed into particles, fibers, textiles, sponges, and films. Its synthetic nature engenders good resistance to enzyme degradation and it has reasonable chemical stability, though it has been noted to exhibit poor thermal stability. Although there are also limitations in terms of its mechanical properties (strength and flexibility) [149–152], it must be noted that it is seldom used on its own and these limitations can be successfully mitigated through its incorporation as a copolymer (typically with chitosan, gelatin, dextran, and hyaluronic acid) in a hydrogel [153,154]. While PVA is susceptible to chemical or enzymatic degradation in vivo, structures based solely on it may erode through gradual dissolution and thus its applicability as a long-term dressing is questionable [122]. The PVA polymer stability can also be enhanced through chemical or physical crosslinking of the hydroxyl groups [148,150]. Chemical cross-linking can be achieved through employing succinyl chloride [148], adipoyl chloride [152], and sebacoyl chlorides [155].

There are many instances in which PVA and its derivatives have been used in wound healing—within dressing for acute and chronic wounds [156]. There are several notable applications whereby the PVA has been used as a matrix (or carrier) for exogenous agents that can stimulate the healing processes and protect against complications (particularly infection) in chronic wounds [156,157]. The polymer has also been incorporated with dextran to aid swelling capacity on contact with wound exudate.

Hydrogels based on PVA can be stabilized through chemical crosslinking but it is more common for them to rely on hydrogen bonding. This is a weaker interaction involving the creation of crystalline junction points that can still confer a significant degree of structural integrity, as indicated in Fig. 4.18. Repeated freeze–thaw cycles increase the hydrogen bond interactions between chains, increase the junction points, and produce a more robust gel.

4.5.2 Poly(Ethylene Glycol)/Poly(Ethylene Oxide)

Poly(ethylene glycol) (PEG) is a polyether which is also, confusingly for some, interchangeably used with the terms poly(ethylene oxide) (PEO) and poly(oxyethylene) (POE) and are produced through the polymerization of ethylene oxide [122,158]. As a constituent for use in wound dressings, this class of materials has a number of core advantages: they

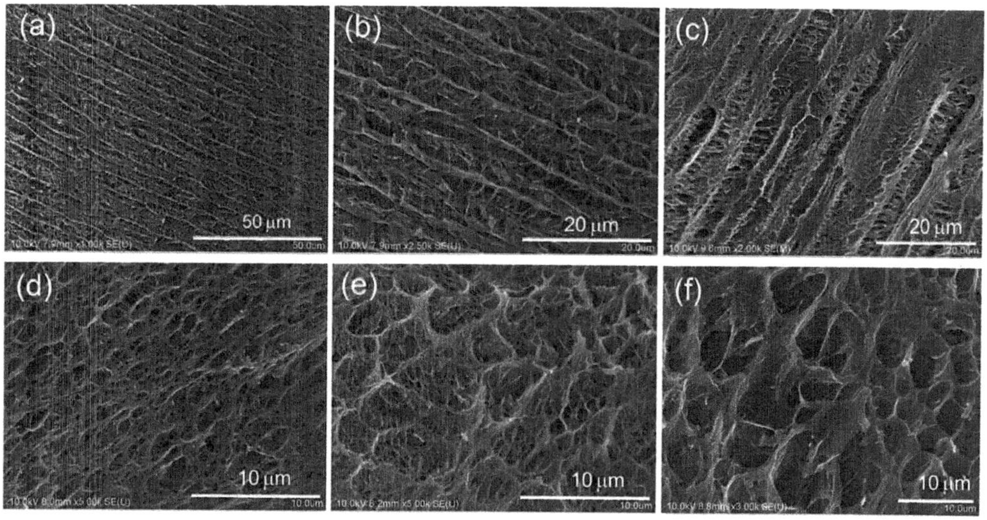

Figure 4.18 SEM micrographs of direction freeze thraw (DFT) PVA hydrogels investigated from the directions parallel (a)–(c) and perpendicular, (d), and (e), to the freezing direction [157].

are hydrophilic, biocompatible, flexible, nontoxic, and nonimmunogenic. A key factor that has stimulated many research publications relates to the fact that PEG layers are notable for their resistance to protein adsorption and thus can minimize nonspecific binding interactions. The PEG system is very much like PVA in the earlier discussion in relation to advantages and limitations when considering application within wound dressings [159]. The PEG monomer themselves have relatively low toxicity and can be coupled with other chemical species such as peptides or growth factors [30,31,158]. The basic structure is highlighted in Fig. 4.19 and it is clear that backbone is less amendable to modification but it can be derivatized through chemical manipulation of the terminal hydroxyl groups. This can create some issues with attempting to create macromolecular structures based solely on PEG where there is a dearth of chemical functionality that can be exploited. There have however been attempts to formulate hydrogel networks through the formation of cross links—irradiating either linear or branched PEG monomers [160] or through a variety of chemical reactions [161,162]. Acrylate-based PEG hybrid monomers have also been used for photopolymerization [158].

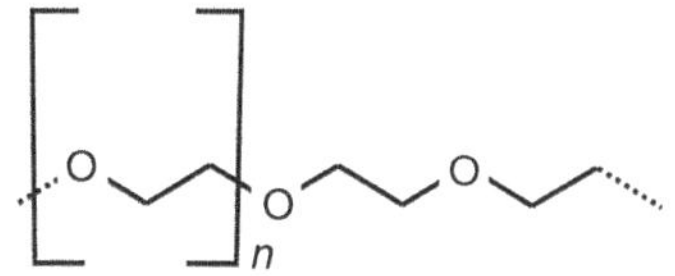

Figure 4.19 ***Basic repeat unit of polyethylene oxide chains.***

A simpler approach has been to blend PEG polymers with other polymer systems to create composite films or networks. Common examples are chitosan, poly(lactic-co-glycolic acid) (PLGA), and poly(propylene fumarate) (PPF). These formulations have been shown to significantly affect solubility, erosion, mechanical and thermal properties, as well as its crystallinity and viscosity [159,163] and thus offer a route through which to specifically tailor the material toward a particular wound application. The use of PEG components within hydrogel formulations has been trialled as a wound dressing [159,164] and has been found to confer several advantages such as improving the proliferation of skin cells, enhanced collagen deposition, and reduced scar formation [165–168]. As with most of the materials discussed within this chapter, those capable of forming a gel have also been used as a slow release matrix in an attempt to impart additional functionality to the dressing, especially where long-term/chronic wounds are concerned. Thus, it is relatively common to find growth factors being loaded to help stimulate faster healing through improved vascularization, enhanced collagen deposition, and maturation and complete reepithelialization [166–168].

4.5.3 Poly(Vinyl Pyrrolidone)

As with the poly(vinyl pyrrolidone) (PVA) and PEG systems, PVP is a hydrophilic and biocompatible material that has been exploited extensively within the pharma industries, but it also has some notable applications in wound healing [169,170]. A major advantage from a commercial perspective for its use in this context relates to the relative ease with which it can be produced and at low cost [159,171]. The polymer is commonly employed as a copolymer with cellulose or PEG to confer some stability, but it can be cross linked with carbodiimides to modify its solubility, delivery and erosion profiles, mechanical properties, softness, and elasticity [159]. One of its common applications is as Povidone in which it is used as a carrier of iodine (Inadine, Aerodine, Betadine), where it is used as an antiseptic [172,173]. The basic structure of PVP and its Povidone-Iodine analogue are shown in Fig. 4.20. The core PVP structure can however be manipulated to carry and dispense other drug or bioactive molecules. One example with particular relevance to DFU treatment relates to an interchain composite in which S-nitrosothiols

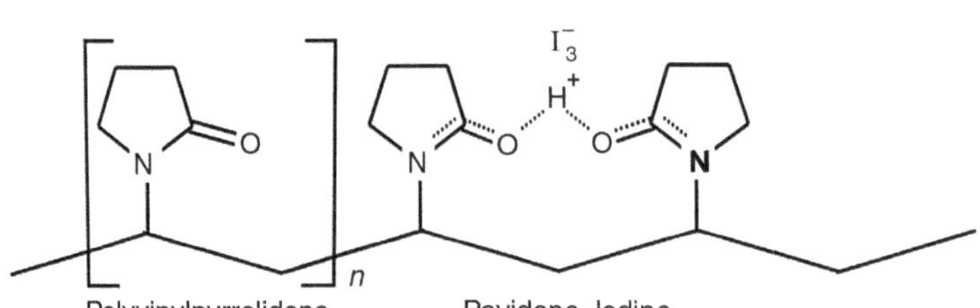

Figure 4.20 ***Basic structure of PVP and Povidone-Iodine.***

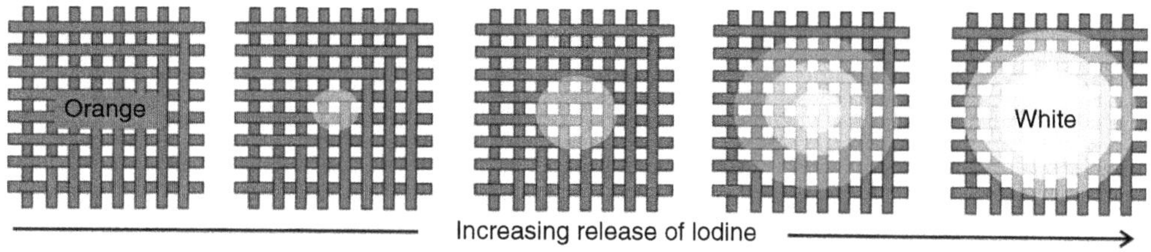

Figure 4.21 ***Inadine dressing release of iodine.***

were grafted onto a poly(vinyl methyl ether co-maleic anhydride) backbone and subsequently formulated along with PVP. The composite was found to enable the controlled release of NO and, when applied in a wound context, was found to accelerate wound closure [174].

One of the advantages of Povidone-iodine as an antiinfective dressing is that it provides a clear indication as to the release/consumption of the iodine as the dressing changes color (Fig. 4.21).

4.5.4 Polyurethanes

Polyurethanes (PUs) are versatile materials that can present different chemical, physical, and biological properties depending on how they are formulated [175]. They are synthesized by condensation and polymerization methods from a wide range of bifunctional or higher-order functional monomers—each can possess and pass on different hydrophilic/hydrophobic characteristics, water sorption, permeation, and degradation profiles to the resulting films. In terms of mechanical and thermal properties, these too can be highly variable depending on the composition of the film and the final film structure, which can be hard, flexible, or elastomeric in nature [176,177]. The films themselves are essentially nontoxic, can be readily sterilized using conventional methods, are nonadherent and nonallergenic [178]. Given the ability to select the monomers, the polymer chains can be cross linked with relative ease or attached to other polymer systems—natural or synthetic and processed into a range of forms such as particles, fibers, films, foams, and hydrogels [179]. The basic reaction scheme involved in the preparation of polyurethane materials is highlighted in Fig. 4.22.

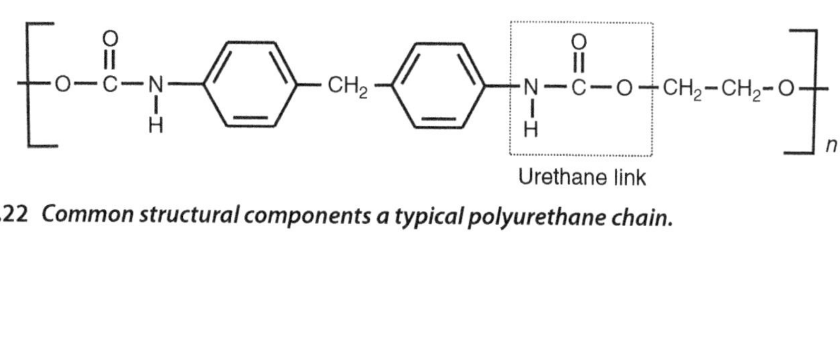

Figure 4.22 ***Common structural components a typical polyurethane chain.***

When used as dressing material, polyurethane nanofibers have been shown to promote wound drainage—which is a key factor in the design of dressing materials [179–181]. There have been a number of studies that have compared the clinical efficacy of polyurethane foam based dressings with conventional systems and found that the former exhibited higher healing capacities [177–181]. The chemical diversity and potential versatility of the polyurethane type materials has meant that there is an extensive literature base available on the material. The inherent capacity of PU-based materials (predominantly as foams) to absorb exudate has effectively established its use in clinical practice. Their implementation however is typically in the form of a hybrid bandage/dressing and is typified by the Meliplex-Ag systems—highlighted previously in Fig. 4.3. In this instance, the polyurethane layer is employed as an absorbant foam in combination with a silicone wound contact interface (described later) and a silver impregnated film. The latter is gas permeable but waterproof and acts to maintain the moist wound environment. The target application would be for those patients who are at risk of infection [182].

4.5.5 Poly(hydroxyethylmethacrylate)

Hydrogels based on poly(2-hydroxyethyl methacrylate) have been extensively investigated for a range of biomedical applications [183], but their oxygen permeability and biocompatibility have generated interest as tissue scaffolds [122,183,184]. As with the other systems described here, the native structure (shown in Fig. 4.23) can be radically manipulated through copolymerization and by cross linking [159].

The poly(hydroxyethylmethacrylate) is seldom used is isolation and is normally employed as a copolymer with other systems described in this chapter. The combination of PHEMA and PEG is a particularly pertinent example of its application in wound healing where the resulting framework was modified to carry MMP inhibitors such that, when placed on the wound bed—the activity of proteases within the matrix is reduced and healing can be reactivated. This approach has been successfully patented and is targeted at DFU treatment [185].

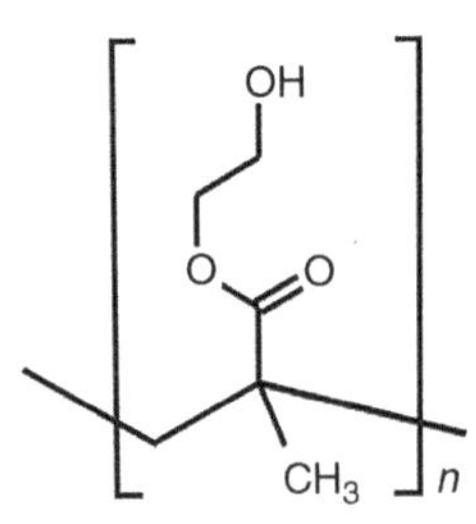

Figure 4.23 ***Basic repeat unit of PHEMA.***

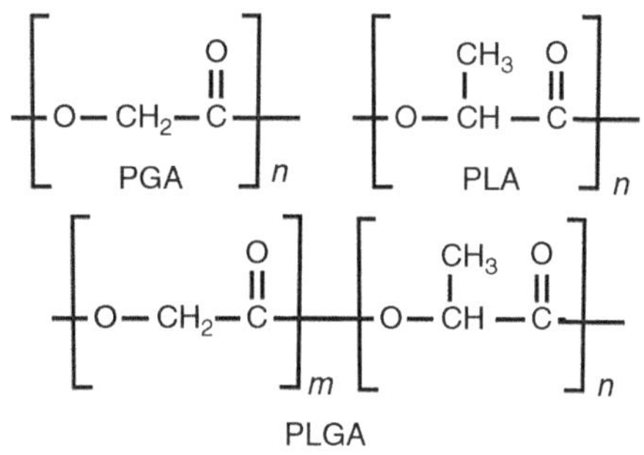

Figure 4.24 ***Repeat units of PGA, PLA and PLGA.***

4.5.6 Poly (α-Esters) (PLA, PGA, PLGA, PCL)

Polyesters have long occupied pivotal roles in biomedical applications but it is relatively recently that engineering polymers such as polylactide (PLA) and polyglycolic acid (PGA) have come to the fore. Polylactide (PLA) is an aliphatic polyester (Fig. 4.24) that is relatively hydrophobic but is biocompatible and biodegradable and is an integral component of drug delivery and tissue engineering applications [186]. The hydrophobicity exhibited by PLA [186–189] contrasts the relatively hydrophyllic nature of polyglycolic acid. The latter is known to degrade faster than PLA and it is little surprise to find that the degradation rate can be tuned through the production of PLA/PGA copolymers—poly(lactic-co-glycolic acid) (PLGA) [188,189]. The PLGA retains the biocompatibility of the homopolymers and it has been shown to be an excellent matrix for facilitating the release of various bioactive substances [190]. PLGA microspheres loaded with rhEGF have been shown to enhance wound healing in diabetic rats through stimulating fibroblast growth. Moreover, the modified dressing was found to be much more effective than applying the rhEGF alone [190,191].

4.5.7 Silicones

Silicone based dressings have a number of diverse functions from low adherent contact layers to absorbent dressings to films for minimizing scarring or keloids. A key advantage is the fact the silicone dressings, when removed from the skin, cause little, if any, damage to the wound or surrounding tissue [192,193]. Most dressings will require the use of some form of top layer film or adhesive tape to maintain their position over the wound site and it is inevitable that frequent dressing changes will cause damage to the skin to which it is adhered [194,195]. This will be especially evident with elderly patients where their skin is liable to be delicate [192]. The degree of damage will depend on the frequency with which the adhesive is applied and removed and the strength of the interaction between it and the skin. In the case of silicone, there is no adhesive as such but there is "tack." The term tack generally relates to the ability of the film to create points of contact between the dressing and skin surface. The greater the ability of the film to conform

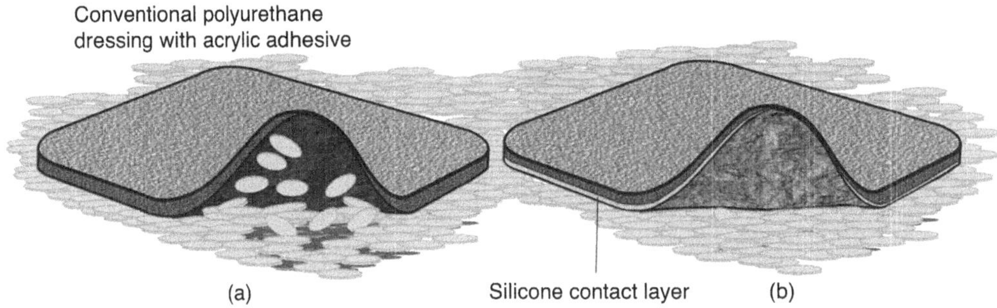

Figure 4.25 Effect of conventional adhesive dressing (a) and Safetac atraumatic silicone layer (b) on skin.

to the surface morphology the greater the number of contact points and the greater the tack. In principle, it should create a tight but easily reversible bond which is still strong enough to prevent the leakage of the wound fluid. In minimizing the exposure of the surrounding tissue to the latter, maceration of the healthy skin is avoided [196]. As there is no adhesive involved, the removal of the film should be relatively harmless (Fig. 4.25).

Comparative studies examining the polyurethane foams with an acrylic adhesive and with silicone contact layers found that the silicone removed less of the stratum corneum [197]. Silicone contact layers are also considered to be "atraumatic" in that they do not cause any damage the wound bed upon removal of the dressing. This is particularly significant on occasions where the absorptive component of the dressing has dried out. In conventional dressings, such as cotton gauze, the dressing will invariably adhere to the new tissue such that when the dressing is removed—so will a significant proportion of new tissue [198,199].

4.6 HONEY

Is honey a wound dressing or an additive to a wound dressing? The use of honey as a wound dressing was introduced in Chapter 3 and its effectiveness has been acknowledged for thousands of years [200,201]. It is only in recent times, however, that clinical evidence has been acquired to substantiate the hitherto old wives tales [202,203]. Once dismissed as a sugar syrup, it is now known to contain a variety of bioactive components that directly influence the biochemical processes at work within the wound. Moreover, the physical structure of honey can perform many of the functions common to those polymers discussed in the previous sections.

It was mentioned in the very beginning of this chapter that a key aim in the design of dressing is to create an environment which is favorable to healing but which discourages the proliferation of bacteria. Honey directly addresses this challenge through its inherent low pH and high osmolarity. The effect of pH is quite stunning, being in the region of pH 3–5, it can stimulate the release of oxygen from haemoglobin, decreases protease activity, and is

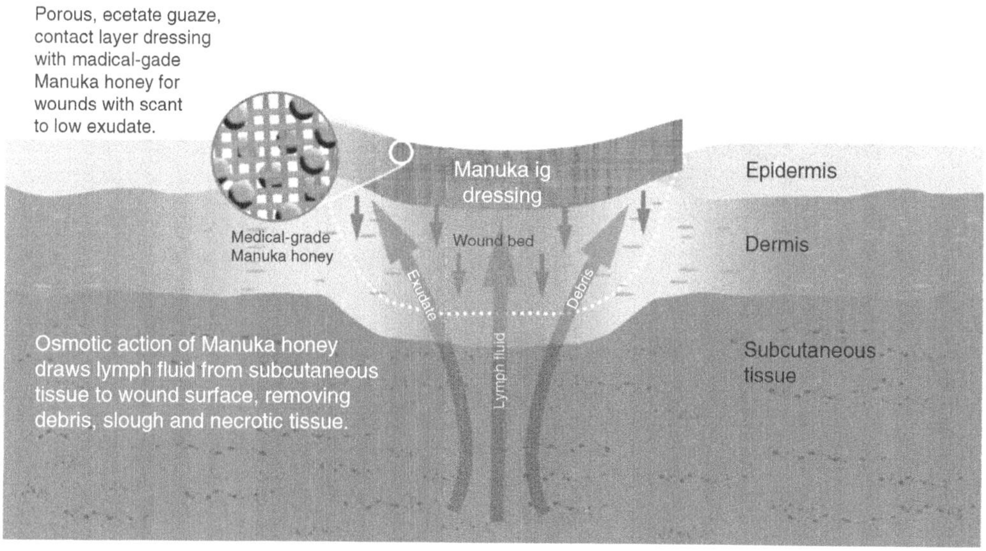

Figure 4.26 ***Modes of action of a honey-based dressing.*** *(Reproduced with permission from Links Medical).*

generally unfavorable for bacteria [204–207]. Moreover, the high osmolarity, generated as a consequence of the high sugar content, effectively draws water from the wound bed as indicated in Fig. 4.26. This can appear counter intuitive as it could be envisaged that this would dehydrate the wound and would run counter to well-established recommendations to keep the wound moist. It is assumed that providing the circulation of blood is sufficient, then the water extracted would be replaced whereby the osmotic effect is simply stimulating an outflow from the lymph [208,209]. In some respects it is akin to negative pressure wound therapy. The osmolarity is also effective against bacteria but the peculiarities of its implementation in that context are discussed in more depth in Chapter 6. It is necessary to keep the honey present at the wound bed interface for these bioactivities to work. This is achieved by the use of primary dressings in which the honey is impregnated in an absorbent material.

4.7 ELECTROSPUN DRESSINGS

The manufacture of the dressing can be achieved using a variety of conventional manufacturing techniques, but electrospinning has garnered considerable interest through its ability to produce finely controlled fibrous meshes [155,210–213]. These materials typically consist of extremely fine fibers with diameters that can be in the low micro to nanometer range and, through careful manipulation of the experimental conditions, provide a high surface area with defined porosity. An example of an electrospun chitosan mesh is shown in Fig. 4.27. The electrospinning approach was first patented by Cooley [214], and although it has been known since 1900, it is only in recent years that

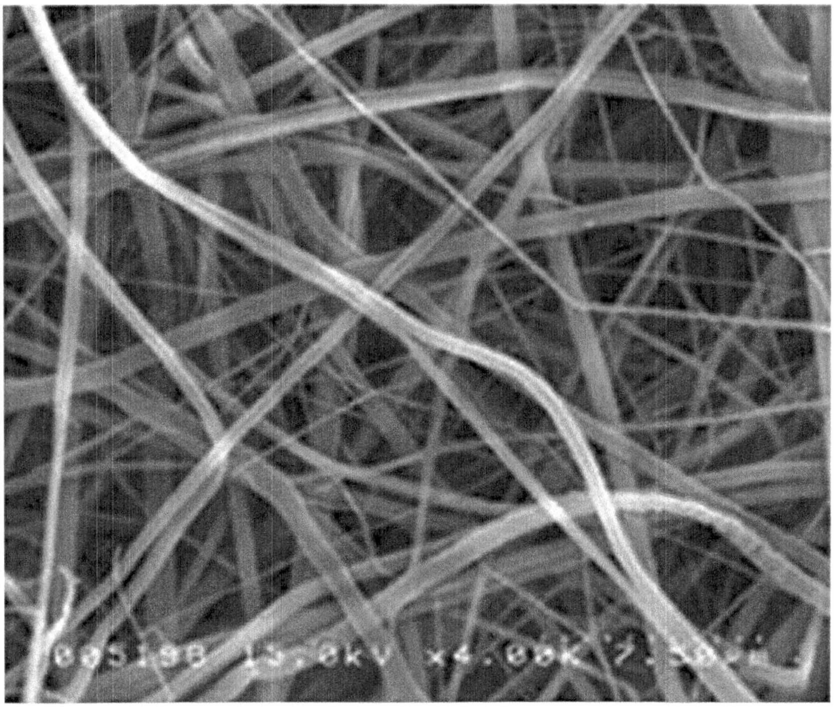

Figure 4.27 ***Electrospun chitosan nanofiber mesh.*** *(Adapated from [234]).*

it has become a highly versatile tool for the fabrication of polymeric scaffolds that cover a diverse range of biomedical applications that includes dressing design and manufacture. As noted earlier in the chapter, it is often useful to combine different polymers to exploit different functionalities that can aid healing. Electrospinning enables different systems to be combined and offers a high degree of control over the final product. The use of electrospinning techniques has been extensively reviewed [210,211] but an overview is given here of the features of direct relevance to wound dressings.

A survey of the literature will reveal that electrospinning of natural polymers is synonymous with tissue engineering and there is now an extensive knowledge base on the creation of electrospun two and three-dimensional polymer scaffolds for this purpose [215]. Many of the properties of these constructs are however directly transferable to the design of dressings where they can serve as a surrogate, or support, to the extracellular matrix within the wound. The latter is chiefly responsible for creating a physical framework and environment through which cells can proliferate and differentiate forming new tissue [216]. Electrospun meshes have been designed to possess many of the physico-chemical properties of the ECM [217,218] and, when implanted into wounds, have been shown to enable fluid absorption and gas permeability which are fundamental to cell respiration and proliferation [219,220]. The high surface area and high degree of interconnected porosity

(60–90%) within the mesh [217] can certainly allow gas permeation but the nanometre pores simultaneously minimize the prospect of moisture loss [221]. Likewise, the small pore dimensions prevent ingress from exogenous microbes while reducing ingrowth of tissue within the actual dressing. The latter is an important consideration where otherwise the removal of the dressing could cause additional trauma to the wound bed [217,221].

4.7.1 Standard Electrospun Processes

The basic procedures involved in the deposition of an electrospun polymer are summarized in Fig. 4.28, whereby a high voltage is applied to a solution (or melt) of the polymer feedstock. Extrusion of the polymer through a syringe equipped with a capillary needle (spinneret) results in the strand being drawn toward a ground collector plate and allows the sustained deposition of a nanostructured/nanofiber mesh [222,223]. A high voltage power supply (~30 kV) is normally used with the potential applied at the tip of the spinneret. The extrusion of a droplet of the feedstock polymer results in the droplet surface becoming charged which induces a transformation into a cone—the Taylor cone. A thin jet emerges from the cone-shaped tip when the electric field force overcomes the surface tension of the feed fluid and moves toward the collector plate during which the solvent evaporates resulting in an ultrafine fiber deposit. Continuation of the process leads to the formation of the randomly aligned nanofibrous mesh [223]. The random nature of the deposition is normally termed a nonwoven mesh but manipulation of the system can enable the production of aligned fiber deposits with uniform dimensions. There are numerous reviews on the manipulation of the extrusion-spinning processes and the effects on the resulting mesh [224,225]. In some cases, polymer blends can be used to create composite mesh structures, especially where there is an advantage to the direct interaction of the two components. In cases where the physical properties of the polymer prevent mixing, or where there is a need for spatially distinct

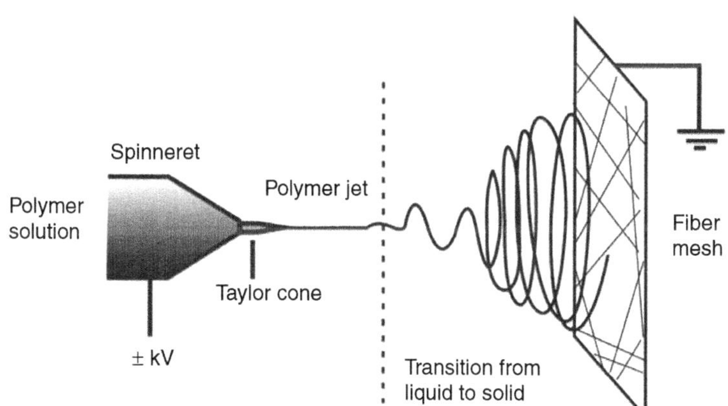

Figure 4.28 ***Electrospun fiber production.***

fibers, multiple spinnerets can be applied to enable codeposition within a single mesh structure [225].

In the previous discussion within this chapter the polymers were divided into two broad categories—natural and synthetic. Electrospinning can be applied to either and also to mixtures (polyblended) depending on the nature of the intended application [226,227]. Among the synthetic pool (Section 4.4), polyurethane [228] and poly(vinyl alcohol) [229] films have been produced and shown to possess high swelling capacity and to be capable of absorbing exudate and maintaining moisture balance. Electrospun hyaluronic acid meshes have also been assessed in vivo and compared favorably to commercial dressings [230]. These have acted in a passive mode but electrospinning can also be used to develop more advanced formulations capable of releasing drugs or other bioactive components into the wound. A conventional approach would have been to entrap the latter within hydrogel systems or to covalently modify the polymeric backbone of a given system to carry the therapeutic agent. Electrospinning can however offer an alternative approach.

4.7.2 Coaxial Electrospinning

This approach is based on a core/shell structure whereby the shell is composed of a suitable polymer that provides structural support, whereas the therapeutic agent is initially retained within the core. The agent can be in the original liquid state being physical/chemically entrapped within a secondary polymer. This requires a slight variation in the nature of the production setup where two feed solutions are used but fed through a single spinneret as indicated in Fig. 4.29. The system involves a single capillary but constructed in such a way so as to have an inner and outer feed channel. The support polymer is fed through the outer channel with the therapeutic feed solution flowing through the inner [231]. The ability to have the therapeutic agent in the liquid or encapsulated

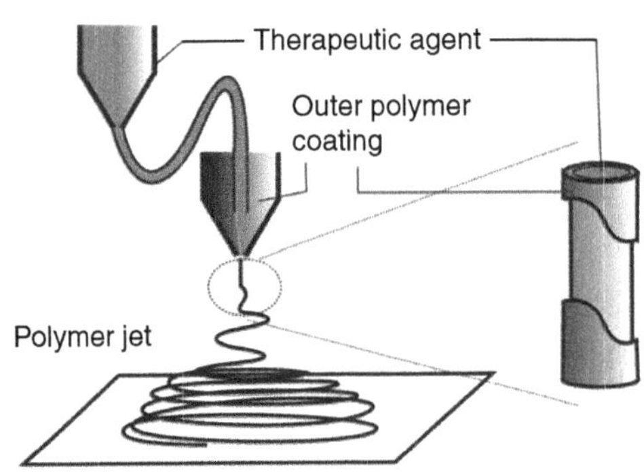

Figure 4.29 ***Coaxial electrospinning for the delivery of therapeutic agents.***

state provides a wealth of flexibility for the controlled release. Moreover, the noncovalent approach enables the delivery of compounds that might be damaged through chemical linkages (ie, growth factors or antimicrobials) and which could otherwise lose their activity. The effectiveness of such approaches needs careful consideration and caution when attempting to transfer from the lab to the wound bed. It has been noted that the release profile can be problematic where there may be a "burst" effect that leads to a higher therapeutic dose being released in the initial stages. While this may be advantageous from the perspective of combating infection, it may prove toxic toward the host's regenerating tissue [155,212]. The approach could, however, prove much more suitable in other situations such as in the delivery of growth factors. There have been studies that have demonstrated the efficacy of such meshes in stimulating the proliferation and differentiation of fibroblasts and keratinocytes [232,233].

The creation of dressings that can effectively mimic the core properties of the extracellular matrix has been a long-held aim as it holds the promise of better cellular responses and, therein, hopefully accelerate the healing process. It was mentioned earlier that simple polymeric nanofiber meshes can go some way to simulating these structures, but it must be noted that the ECM is a heterogeneous matrix consisting of collagens, fibronectin, elastin to name but a few. There is significant diversity of structure and functionality and it can be difficult to imagine one homopolymer fulfilling all the requirements. The ability to electrospin blends (polymer mixtures) is a simple approach that can produce meshes with enhanced functionality that exploit the physico-chemical properties of the blend constituents. Alternatively, the mesh can be built layer by layer. There have been extensive studies examining the cellular interactions with electrospun nanofiber meshes—particularly in relation to fibroblasts. The influence of fiber dimensions (diameter, alignment, and spatial distance) can have a significant effect on cell adhesion, migration [234–237].

Examples of the blend approach have involved mixtures of: keratin and poly(hydroxyl butylate-co-hydroxyvalerate) [238]; polyurethane (PU) and gelatin [239]; collagen, chitosan, and poly(ethylene oxide) (PEO) [240]. Each of these electrospun systems was shown to promote healing. The electrospinning of natural polymers, while clearly possible, can be problematic for much the same reasons as noted earlier in the chapter—particularly the high variability of the feedstock.

Chitosan in particular has generated considerable interest in terms of electrospinning and has the added advantage of combining the ability to aid proliferation while possessing an antibacterial action [240–246]. The electrospinning of chitosan, however, is far from simple and is attributed to the presence of the primary amino groups resulting in polycationic behavior. The latter increases the surface tension of the feed solution and, therefore, a higher potential is needed to force ejection from the droplet. Moreover, it has been noted that hydrogen bonding restricts the degree of movement of the chains during the spinning process [247–249]. The electrospinning performance of chitosan can be improved through treatment with trifluoroacetic acid (TFA) which acts a counter ion and minimizes the influence of the amino groups, but there are issues (expense, toxicity) and, in general, the process has been restricted to low molecular weight variants. Two approaches have been taken to improve the "spinability" of chitosan: blended and prefunctionalized feeds. In the case of blend systems, chitosan has been successfully mixed with a large range of synthetic and natural copolymers: as PEO [250], PVA [247,251,252], PLA [253], nylon-6 [254,255], PCL, [256] silk fibroin [257], collagen [258], and gelatin [259]. The alternative approach is to remove the cationic nature of the polymer prior to electrospinning. This can be done through functionalizing the amino group as a means of improving the solubility and include: N-carboxyethyl [260–262], carboxymethyl [263], galactosylated, [264,265], hexanoyl, [249,266], carboxylation [267], N-[(2-hydroxy-3-trimethylammonium) propyl] chloride [268].

4.7.3 Electroblow-Electrospinning

The addition of an electroblow system to the electrospinning has, however, enabled some of the issues encountered with conventional approaches to be overcome. This technique employs a gas jet (Fig. 4.30) to effectively stretch the fibers creating small diameters and can be used to increase the speed of fiber deposition. The rate at which the fiber mesh is produced is generally limited by the speed at which the polymer feedstock

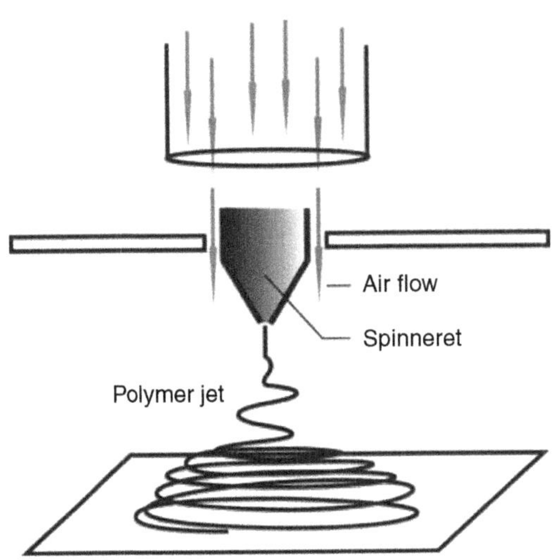

Figure 4.30 ***Schematic of an electroblow—electrospin system.***

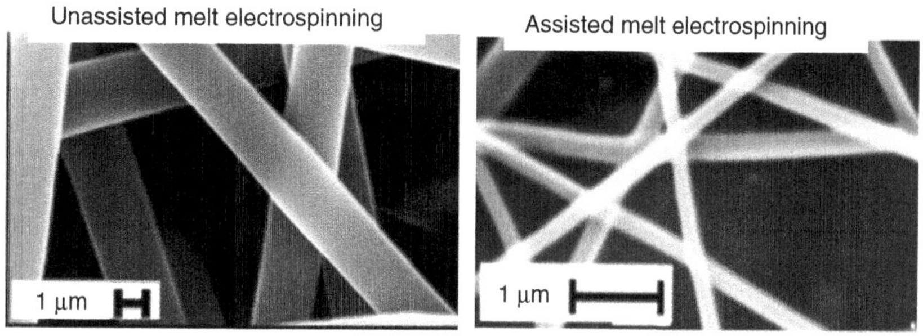

Figure 4.31 ***Comparison of the fiber diameter without (1–2 µm) and with (0.2–0.8 µm) hot air assistance [275].***

is ejected from the spinneret. If the processing speed through the syringe is too high, the polymer can be drip rather than being drawn. The imposition of the additional electroblowing processes allows the flow rate to be increased as the gas jet facilitates the fiber-drawing process. One of the advantages of the combined blowing–spinning approach is that it can improve the morphology of the fibers—producing smooth relatively uniform lengths and minimizing "beads" [269,270].

As mentioned previously, nanofiber meshes formed from hyaluronic acid have shown promising results in wound dressings [260] but, as with chitosan, the production of the material can be problematic due to the high viscosity and surface tension—even in a very dilute solution [269,271]. As with chitosan, there are a variety of options and the experimental conditions that need to be matched to the polymer concerned. The implementation of the electroblow system however can radically transform the production [269,271]. The imposition of an air jet has been shown to enhance the evaporation of the hyaluronic acid feed solution—producing fibers with a high degree of uniformity [272,273]. Heating the air jet can also aid the evaporation process—reducing viscosity and induces greater elongation of the fibers and, as a consequence, reduces the diameter of the fiber [274]. Bubakir [275] have also produced a combination a heated electrospin–electroblow system which deftly separates the heating elements and dispensing units from one another and, using polypropylene as a model system were able to reduce the fiber diameter from a range of 1–2 µm to 0.2–0.8 µm, as shown in Fig. 4.31.

Electrospinning can be scaled and thus, in principle, could be suitable for adaptation to mass production cycles and there are numerous approaches to web formation processes which allow continuous production. One example of such a format is indicated in Fig. 4.32 and highlights the fact that the electrospinning technique is not simply an academic or high speciality curiosity.

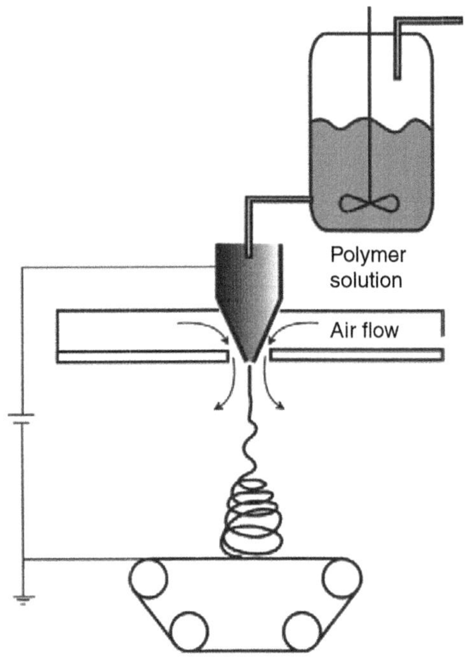

Figure 4.32 ***Schematic of a proposed web-based—electrospin-electroblow fiber manufacture [276].***

4.8 SUMMARY

The qualities of the "ideal" dressing are often quoted but few dressings can achieve all the requirements postulated by Winter. There is a great number of polymer that can be electrospun, but it is clear that rather than use a single polymer composition, hybrid/composite systems are predominantly used where a combination of properties is exploited. In many cases, these embody an asymmetric model in which one layer, the primary, interfaces with the wound site to induce debridement, granulation, and reepithelialization. A secondary layer provides barrier functions, moisture control, gas permeability.

The very first dressings would have contained a variety of components based on myth, folklore, and quite bizarre assumptions; dressings now contain multiple components, but each one is included on the basis of distinct and proven function. There are endless opportunities to vary the composition of the dressing and the science has now progressed to the point where it is possible to tailor the dressing to specific wound types. Chemical functionality has been shown to be a vital component but must be married with advances in a physical form. The latter goes beyond foam/film/gel but must increasingly examine the nanoscale properties as these are critical for interacting with the cellular components within the wound site.

Manufacturing of high specification dressings has also seen tremendous advances and the adoption of electrospinning processes offers a wealth of possibilities. These can be scaled and enable fine control over the fiber composition. The ability to encapsulate therapeutic and bioactive agents (antimicrobials, growth factors, etc) through a number of methods (blending and coaxial coreshell) has captured the imagination of the materials scientists and will undoubtedly continue to expand in the future [277–279].

REFERENCES

[1] Boateng JS, Matthews KH, Stevens NE, Eccleston GM. Wound healing dressings and drug delivery systems: a review. J Pharm Sci 2008;97:2892–923.
[2] Lloyd LL, Kennedy JF, Methacanon P, Paterson M, Knill CJ. Carbohydrate polymers as wound management aids. Carbohydr Polym 1998;37:315–22.
[3] Winter GD. Methods for the biological evaluation of dressings. In: Turner T, KR B, editors. Cardiff: Surgical Dressing Research Unit; 1975.
[4] Schultz GS, Sibbald GR, Falanga V, Yello EEA, Dowsett C, Harding K, Romanelli M, Stacey MC, Teot L, Vanscheidt W. Wound bed preparation, a systemic approach to wound management. Wound Rep Reg 2003;11:1–28.
[5] Osti E, Osti F. Ann Burns Fire Disasters 2004;3:137–41.
[6] Lloyd LL, Kennedy JK, Methacanon P, Paterson M, Knill CJ. Carbohydrate polymers as wound management aids. Carbohydr Polym 1998;37:315–22.
[7] Mulder M. The selection of wound care products for wound bed preparation. Prof Nurs Today 2011;30:15–21.
[8] Parsons D, Bowler PG, Myles V, Jones S. Silver antimicrobial dressings in wound management, a comparison of anti-bacterial physical and chemical characteristics. Wounds 2005;17:222–32.
[9] World Union of Wound Healing Societies. Principles of best practice: Wound exudate and the role of dressings. A consensus document. London: MEP Ltd; 2007.
[10] Barnhart RK. Chambers dictionary of etymology. New York: Chambers Harrap Publishers; 1988.
[11] Kindlen S, Morison M. The physiology of wound healing. In: Morison M, Moffatt CJ, Bridel-Nixon J, Bale S, editors. Nursing management of chronic wounds. 2nd ed. London: Mosby; 1999.
[12] Prompers L, Schaper N, Apelqvist J, et al. Prediction of outcome in individuals with diabetic foot ulcers: focus on the differences between individuals with and without peripheral arterial disease. The EURODIALE Study. Diabetologia 2008;51(5):747–55.
[13] Lavery LA, Armstrong DA, Wunderlich RP, et al. Risk factors for foot infections in individuals with diabetes. Diabetes Care 2006;29(6):1288–93.
[14] Singer AJ, Clark RA. Cutaneous wound healing. N Engl J Med 1999;341:738–46.
[15] Chambers CW, Proctor CM, Kabler PW. Bactericidal effect of low concentrations of silver. J Am Water Works Assoc 1962;54:208–16.
[16] Bowler PG, Davies B. The microbiology of infected and noninfected leg ulcers. Int J Dermatol 1999;38:573–8.
[17] Winter GD. Formation of the scab and the rate of epithelization of superficial wounds in the skin of the young domestic pig. Nature 1962;193:293–4.
[18] Kallaiinen LK, Gordillo GM, Schlanger RK, Sen C. Topical oxygen as adjunct to wound healing, a clinical case series. Pathophysiology 2003;9:208–16.
[19] Boateng JS, Matthews KH, Stevens HN, Eccleston GM. Wound healing dressings and drug delivery systems: a review. J Pharm Sci 2008;97(8):2892–923.
[20] Mayet N, Choonara YE, Kumar P, Tomar LK, Tyagi C, Du Toit LC, Pillay V. A comprehensive review of advanced biopolymeric wound healing systems. J Pharm Sci 2014;103:2211–30.
[21] Dreifke MB, Jayasuriy AA, Jayasuriya AC. Current wound healing procedures and potential care. Mater Sci Eng C 2015;48:651–62.

[22] Wounds International. International best practice guidelines: wound management in diabetic foot ulcers. Available at: www.woundsinternational.com; 2013.
[23] Dowsett C, Blelby A, Searle R. Reconciling increasing wound care demands with available resources. J Wound Care 2014;23:552–62.
[24] Augustin M, Brocatti LK, Rustenbach SJ, Schafer I, Herberger K. Cost-of-illness of leg ulcers in the community. Int Wound J 2014;11:283–92.
[25] Moura LIF, Dias AMA, Carvalho E, de Sousa HC. Recent advances on the development of wound dressings for diabetic foot ulcer treatment—a review. Acta Biomater 2013;9:7093–114.
[26] Hilton JR, Williams DT, Beuker B, Miller DR, Harding KG. Wound dressings in diabetic foot disease. Clin Infect Dis 2004;39(Suppl 2):S100–3.
[27] Fletcher J, Moore Z, Anderson I, Matsuzaki K. Pressure ulcers and hydrocolloids. Wound Int 2011;2:1–6.
[28] Jones V, Grey JE, Harding KG. ABC of wound healing—wound dressings. BMJ 2006;332:777–80.
[29] Turner TD. Hospital usage of absorbent dressings. Pharm J 1979;222:421–4.
[30] Slaughter BV, Shahana SK, Fisher OZ, Khademhosseini A, Peppas NA. Hydrogels in regenerative medicine. Adv Mater 2009;21:3307–29.
[31] Hoffman AS. Adv Drug Deliv Rev 2012;64:18–23.
[32] Rosiak JM, Yoshii F. Hydrogels and their medical applications. Nucl Instrum Meth B 1999;151:56–64.
[33] Caló E, Khutoryanskiy VV. Biomedical applications of hydrogels: a review of patents and commercial products. Eur Polym J 2015;65:252–67.
[34] Fonder MA, Lazarus GS, Cowan DA, Aronson-Cook B, Kohli AR, Mamelak AJ. Treating the chronic wound: a practical approach to the care of nonhealing wounds and wound care dressings. J Am Acad Dermatol 2008;58:185–206.
[35] Dumville JC, Soares MO, O'Meara S, Cullum N. Systematic review and mixed treatment comparison: dressings to heal diabetic foot ulcers. Diabetologia 2012;55:1902–10.
[36] Edwards J, Stapley S. Debridment of diabetic foot ulcers. Cochrane Database Syst Rev 2010;20:1–44.
[37] Murphy PS, Evans GRD. Advances in wound healing: a review of current wound healing products. Plast Surg Int 2012;2012:1–8.
[38] Stashak TS. Update on wound dressings: Indications and best use. Clin Tech Equine Pract 2004;3:148–63.
[39] Skorkowska-Telichowska K, Czemplik M, Kulma A, Szopa J. The local treatment and available dressings for chronic wounds. J Am Acad Dermatol 2011;5:1–11.
[40] Weller C, Sussman G. Wound dressings update. J Pharm Pract Res 2006;36:318–24.
[41] Jeffcoate WJ, Price P, Harding KG. Wound healing and treatments for people with diabetic foot ulcers. Diabetes Metab Res Rev 2004;20(Suppl 1):S78–89.
[42] Meaume S, Van De Looverbosch D, Heyman H, et al. A study to compare a new self-adherent soft silicone dressing with a self-adherent polymer dressing in stage II pressure ulcers. Ostomy Wound Manage 2003;49(9):44–51.
[43] Cunningham D. Treating venous insufficiency ulcers with soft silicone dressing. Ostomy Wound Manage 2005;51(11A Suppl):19–20.
[44] Matthews KH, Stevens HNE, Auffret AD, Humphrey MJ, Eccleston GM. Lyophillised wafers as a drug delivery system for wound healing containing methylcellulose as a viscosity enhancer. Int J Pharm 2005;289:51–62.
[45] Gao D, Heimann RB. Structural and mechanical properties of superabsorbent poly (acrylamide) montmorrilonite composite hydrogels. Polym Gel Netw 1993;1:225–46.
[46] Lansown ABG, Jensen K, Jensen MQ. Contreet foam and contreet hydrocolloid, an insight into two new silver-containing dressings. J Wound Care 2003;12:205–10.
[47] Queen D, Orsted H, Sanada H, Sussman G. A dressing history. Int Wound J 2004;1:59–77.
[48] Harding KG, Jones V, Price P. Topical treatment: which dressing to choose. Diabetes Metab Res Rev 2000;16(Suppl 1):S47–50.
[49] Czaja W, Krystynowicz A, Bielecki S, Brown RM Jr. Microbial cellulose—the natural power to heal wounds. Biomaterials 2006;27:145–51.
[50] Ferreira LM, Sobral CS, Blanes L, Ipolito MZ, Horibe EK. Proliferation of fibroblasts cultured on a hemi-cellulose dressing. J Plast Reconstr Aesthet Surg 2009;5:865–9.

[51] Espinoza-Herrera N, Pedrosas-Islas R, Martin-Martinez ES, Cruz-Orea A, Tomes SA. Thermal, mechanical and microstructures properties of cellulose derivatives films: a comparative study. Food Biophys 2011;6:106–14.
[52] Zoher K, Kolli ME, Riahi F, Doufnoune R. Preparation and characterization of hydrocolloid biopolymer-based films for dressings application. Int J Polym Mater 2009;58:665–80.
[53] Boateng JS, Matthews KH, Stevens HN, Eccleston GM. Wound healing dressings and drug delivery systems: a review. J Pharm Sci 2008;97:2892–923.
[54] Zahedi P, Rezaeian I, Ranaei-Siadat S, Jafari S, Supaphol P. A review on wound dressings with an emphasis on electrospun nanofibrous polymeric bandages. Polym Adv Technol 2010;21:77–95.
[55] Tabata Y. Biomaterial technology for tissue engineering applications. J Roy Soc Interface 2009;S311–24.
[56] Samal SK, Dash M, Van Vlierberghe S, Kaplan DL, Chiellini E, van Blitterswijk C, Moronid L, Dubruel P. Cationic polymers and their therapeutic potential. Chem Soc Rev 2012;41:7147–94.
[57] Sell SA, Wolfe PS, Garg K, McCool JM, Rodriguez IA, Bowlin GL. The use of natural polymers in tissue engineering: a focus on electrospun extracellular matrix analogues. Polym Adv Technol 2010;2:522–53.
[58] Huang S, Fu X. Naturally derived materials-based cell and drug delivery systems in skin regeneration. J Control Release 2010;142:149–59.
[59] Jayakumar R, Prabaharan M, Sudheesh Kumar PT, Nair SV, Tamura H. Biomaterials based on chitin and chitosan in wound dressing applications. Biotechnol Adv 2011;29:322–37.
[60] Tessmar JK, Gopferich AM. Matrices and scaffolds for protein delivery in tissue engineering. Adv Drug Deliv Rev 2007;58:274–91.
[61] Dai T, Tanaka M, Huang YY, Hamblin MR. Chitosan preparations for wounds and burns: antimicrobial and wound-healing effects. Expert Rev Anti Infect Ther 2011;9:857–79.
[62] Khoushab F, Yamabhai M. Chitin research revisited. Mar Drugs 2010;8:1988–2012.
[63] Madihally SV. Processing chitosan for tissue regeneration. Curr Trends Polym Sci 2011;15:83–8.
[64] Koide SS. Chitin-chitosan: properties, benefits and risks. Nutr Res 1998;13:1091–101.
[65] Kim IY, Seo SJ, Moon HS, Yoo MK, Park IY, Kim BC, et al. Chitosan and its derivatives for tissue engineering applications. Biotechnol Adv 2008;26:1–21.
[66] Jayakumar R, Prabaharan M, Nair SV, Tamura H. Novel chitin and chitosan nanofibers in biomedical applications. Biotechnol Adv 2010;28:142–50.
[67] Dash M, Chiellini F, Ottenbrite RM, Chiellini E. Chitosan—a versatile semisynthetic polymer in biomedical. Progress Polym Sci 2011;678:981–1014.
[68] Rinaudo M. Chitin and chitosan: properties and applications. Prog Polym Sci 2006;31: 603–32. 112.
[69] Censi R, Di Martino P, Vermonden T, Hennink WE. Hydrogels for protein delivery in tissue engineering. J Control Release 2012;161:680–92.
[70] Muzzarelli RAA, Muzzarelli C. Chitosan chemistry: relevance to the biomedical sciences. Adv Polym Sci 2005;186:151–209.
[71] Kumar MNVR. A review of chitin and chitosan applications. React Funct Polym 2000;46:1–27.
[72] Saranya N, Moorthi A, Saravanan S, Devi MP, Selvamurugan N. Chitosan and its derivatives for gene delivery. Int J Biol Macromol 2011;48:234–8.
[73] Azad AK, Sermsintham N, Chandrkrachang S, Stevens WF. Chitosan membrane as a wound-healing dressing: characterization and clinical application. J Biomed Mater Res B Appl Biomater 2004;69:216–22.
[74] Bhattarai N, Gunn J, Zhang M. Chitosan-based hydrogels for controlled, localized drug delivery. Adv Drug Deliv Rev 2010;62:83–99.
[75] Takei T, Nakahara H, Ijima H, Kawakami K. Synthesis of a chitosan derivative soluble at neutral pH and gellable by freeze-thawing, and its application in wound care. Acta Biomater 2012;8: 686–93.
[76] Patterson J, Martino MM, Hubbell JA. Biomimetic materials in tissue engineering. Mater Today 2010;13:14–22.
[77] Liao YH, Jones SA, Forbes B, Martin GP, Brown MB. Hyaluronan pharmaceutical characterization and drug delivery. Drug Deliv 2005;12:327–42.

[78] Price RD, Berry MG, Navsaria HA. Hyaluronic acid: the scientific and clinical evidence. J Plast Reconstr Aesthet Surg 2007;60:1110–9.

[79] Xu H, Ma L, Shi H, Gao C, Han C. Chitosan-hyaluronic acid hybrid film as a novel wound dressing: in vitro and in vivo studies. Polym Adv Technol 2007;18:869–75. 136.

[80] Galeano M, Polito F, Bitto A, Irrera N, Campo GM, Avenoso A, et al. Systemic administration of high-molecular weight hyaluronan stimulates wound healing in genetically diabetic mice. Biochim Biophys Acta 2011;1812:752–9.

[81] Vazquez JR, Short B, Findlow AH, Nixon BP, Boulton AJM, Armstrong DG. Outcomes of hyaluronan therapy in diabetic foot wounds. Diabetes Res Clin Pract 2003;59:123–7.

[82] Gall Y. Hyaluronic acid: structure, metabolism and implication in cicatrization. Ann Dermatol Venereol 2010;(Suppl 1):S30–9. 137.

[83] Sannino A, Demitri C, Madaghiele M. Biodegradable cellulose-based hydrogels: design and applications. Materials 2009;2:353–73.

[84] Helenius G, Backdahl H, Bodin A, Nannmark U, Gatenholm P, Risberg B. In vivo biocompatibility of bacterial cellulose. J Biomed Mater Res Part A 2006;76A:431–8.

[85] Mano JF, Silva GA, Azevedo HS, Malafaya PB, Sousa RA, Silva SS, et al. Natural origin biodegradable systems in tissue engineering and regenerative medicine: present status and some moving trends. J R Soc Interface 2007;4:999–1030.

[86] Serafica G, Mormino R, Oster GA, Lentz KE, Koehler KP. Microbial cellulose wound dressing for treating chronic, wounds. US7704523 B2 2010.

[87] Cullen MB, Silcock DW, Boyle C. Wound dressing comprising oxidized cellulose and human recombinat collagen. Patent US 20107833790 B2; 2010.

[88] d'Ayala GG, Malinconico M, Laurienzo P. Marine derived polysaccharides for biomedical applications: chemical modification approaches. Molecules 2008;13:2069–106.

[89] Jin ZY, Harvey AM, Mailloux S, Halamek J, Bocharova V, Twiss MR, Katz E. Electrochemically stimulated release of lysozyme from an alginate matrix cross-linked with iron cations. J. Mats Chem 2012;22:19523–8.

[90] Horniblow RD, Dowle M, Iqbal TH, Latunde-Dada GO, Palmer RE, Pikramenou Z, Tselepis C. Alginate-Iron Speciation and Its Effect on In Vitro Cellular Iron Metabolism. PLoS ONE 2015;10. Article Number: e0138240.

[91] Lee KY, Mooney DJ. Hydrogels for tissue engineering. Chem Rev 2001;101:1869–79.

[92] Boanini E, Rubini K, Panzavolta S, Bigi A. Chemico-physical characterization of gelatin films modified with oxidized alginate. Acta Biomater 2010;6:383–8.

[93] Jeon O, Powell C, Solorio LD, Krebs MD, Alsberg E. Affinity-based growth factor delivery using biodegradable, photocrosslinked heparin-alginate hydrogels. J Control Release 2011;154:258–66.

[94] Kim JO, Choi JY, Park JK, Kim JH, Jin SG, Chang SW, et al. Development of clindamycin-loaded wound dressing with polyvinyl alcohol and sodium alginate. Biol Pharm Bull 2008;31: 2277–82.

[95] Han J, Zhou Z, Yin R, Yang D, Nie J. Alginate-chitosan/hydroxyapatite polyelectrolyte complex porous scaffolds: preparation and characterization. Int J Biol Macromol 2010;46:199–205.

[96] Foster AVM, Greenhill MT, Edmonds ME. Comparing two dressings in the treatment of diabetic foot ulcers. J Wound Care 1994;3:224–8.

[97] Tarun K, Gobi N. Calcium alginate/PVA blended nano fibre matrix for wound dressing. Indian J Fibre Text Res 2012;37:127–32.

[98] Lee CH, Singla A, Lee Y. Biomedical applications of collagen. Int J Pharm 2001;221:1–22.

[99] Valenta C, Auner BG. The use of polymers for dermal and transdermal delivery. Eur J Pharm Biopharm 2004;58:279–89.

[100] Arul V, Kartha R, Jayakumar R. A therapeutic approach for diabetic wound healing using biotinylated GHK incorporated collagen matrices. Life Sci 2007;80:275–84.

[101] Cen L, Liu W, Cui L, Zhang W, Cao Y. Collagen tissue engineering: development of novel biomaterials and applications. Pediatr Res 2008;63:492–6.

[102] Parenteau-Bareil R, Gauvin R, Berthod F. Collagen-based biomaterials for tissue engineering applications. Materials 2010;3:1863–87.

[103] Lammers G, Tjabringa GS, Schalkwijk J, Daamen WF, van Kuppevelt TH. A molecularly defined array based on native fibrillar collagen for the assessment of skin tissue engineering biomaterials. Biomaterials 2009;30:6213–20.
[104] Lin Y, Tan F, Marra KC, Jan S, Liu D. Synthesis and characterization of collagen/ hyaluronan/chitosan composite sponges for potential biomedical applications. Acta Biomater 2009;5:2591–600.
[105] Kondo S, Niiyama H, Yu A, Kuroyanagi Y. Evaluation of a wound dressing composed of hyaluronic acid and collagen sponge containing epidermal growth factor in diabetic mice. J Biomater Sci Polym Ed 2012;23:1729–40.
[106] Lee CR, Grodzinsky AJ, Spector M. The effects of cross-linking of collagenglycosaminoglycan scaffolds on compressive stiffness, chondrocytemediated contraction, proliferation and biosynthesis. Biomaterials 2001;22:3145–54.
[107] Chen ZG, Wang PW, Wei B, Mo XM, Cui FZ. Electrospun collagen-chitosan nanofiber: a biomimetic extracellular matrix for endothelial cell and smooth muscle cell. Acta Biomater 2010;6:372–82.
[108] Srinivasan A, Sehgal PK. Characterization of biocompatible collagen fibers—a promising candidate for cardiac patch. Tissue Eng Part C Methods 2010;16:895–903.
[109] Samal SK, Dash M, Van Vlierberghe A, Kaplan DL, Chiellini E, van Blitterswijk C, Moronid L, Dubruel P. Cationic polymers and their therapeutic potential. Chem Soc Rev 2012;41:7147–94.
[110] Gioffrè M, Torricelli P, Panzavolta S, Rubini K, Bigi A. Role of pH on stability and mechanical properties of gelatin films. J Bioact Compat Polym 2012;27:67–77.
[111] Zhong SP, Zhang YZ, Lim CT. Tissue scaffolds for skin wound healing and dermal reconstruction. Nanomed Nanobiotechnol 2010;2:510–25.
[112] Grover CN, Cameron RE, Best SM. Investigating the morphological, mechanical and degradation properties of scaffolds comprising collagen, gelatin and elastin for use in soft tissue engineering. J Mech Behav Biomed Mater 2012;10:62–74.
[113] Farris S, Song J, Huang Q. Alternative reaction mechanism for the cross-linking of gelatin with glutaraldehyde. J Agric Food Chem 2010;58:998–1003.
[114] Rujitanaroj P, Pimpha N, Supaphol P. Wound-dressing materials with antibacterial activity from electrospun gelatin fiber mats containing silver nanoparticles. Polym Degrad Stab 2008;49:4723–32.
[115] Saha N, Saarai A, Roy N, Kitano T, Saha P. Polymeric biomaterial based hydrogels for biomedical applications. J Biomater Nanobiotechnol 2011;2:85–90.
[116] Singh O, Gupta SS, Soni M, Moses S, Shukla S, Mathur RK. Collagen dressing versus conventional dressings in burn and chronic wounds: a retrospective study. J Cutan Aesthet Surg 2011;4:12–6.
[117] Arul V, Masilamoni JG, Jesudason EP, Jaji PJ, Inayathullah M, Dicky John DG, et al. Glucose oxidase incorporated collagen matrices for dermal wound repair in diabetic rat models: a biochemical study. J Biomater Appl 2012;26:917–38.
[118] Adhirajan N, Shanmugasundaram N, Shanmuganathan S, Babu M. Collagen based wound dressing for doxycycline delivery: in-vivo evaluation in an infected excisional wound model in rats. J Pharm Pharmacol 2009;61:1617–23.
[119] Kawai K, Suzuki S, Tabata Y, Nishimura Y. Accelerated wound healing through the incorporation of basic fibroblast growth factor-impregnated gelatin microspheres into artificial dermis using a pressure-induced decubitus ulcer model in genetically diabetic mice. Br J Plast Surg 2005;58:1115–23.
[120] Kanda N, Morimoto N, Ayvazyan AA, Takemoto S, Kawai K, Nakamura Y, et al. Evaluation of a novel collagen-gelatin scaffold for achieving the sustained release of basic fibroblast growth factor in a diabetic mouse model. J Tissue Eng Regenerative Med 2014;8(1):29–40.
[121] Ahmed TAE, Dare EV, Hincke M. Fibrin: a versatile scaffold for tissue engineering applications. Tissue Eng Part B 2008;14:199–245.
[122] Harding K, Innovation wound healing. J Wound Care 2015;24:7–13.
[123] Chen TM, Tsai JC, Burnouf T. A novel technique combining platelet gel, skin graft, and fibrin glue for healing recalcitrant lower extremity ulcers. Dermatol Surg 2010;36:453–60.
[124] Pedroso DC, Tellechea A, Moura L, Fidalgo-Carvalho I, Duarte J, Carvalho E, et al. Improved survival, vascular differentiation and wound healing potential of stem cells co-cultured with endothelial cells. PLoS One 2011;6:1–12.

[125] Muthukumar T, Anbarasu K, Prakash D, Sastry TP. Effect of growth factors and pro-inflammatory cytokines by the collagen biocomposite dressing material containing Macrotyloma uniflorum plant extract-In vivo wound healing. Colloids Surf B 2014;121:178–88.
[126] Mandal BB, Kundu SC. Cell proliferation and migration in silk fibroin 3D scaffolds. Biomaterials 2009;30:2956–65.
[127] Inpanya P, Faikrua A, Ounaroon A, Sittichokechaiwut A, Viyoch J. Effects of the blended fibroin/aloe gel film on wound healing in streptozotocin-induced diabetic rats. Biomed Mater 2012;7:035008.
[128] Du N, Yang Z, Liu XY, Li Y, Xu HY. Structural origin of the strain-hardening of spider silk. Adv Funct Mater 2011;21(4):772–8.
[129] Li SF, McGhie AJ, Tang SL. New internal structure of spider dragline silk revealed by atomic force microscopy. Biophys J 1994;66(4):1209–12.
[130] Oroudjev E, Soares J, Arcdiacono S, Thompson JB, Fossey SA, Hansma HG. Segmented nanofibers of spider dragline silk: atom force microscopy and single-molecule force spectroscopy. Proc Natl Acad Sci USA 2002;99(9 suppl 2):6460–5.
[131] Augsten K, Muehlig P, Hermann C. Glycoproteins and skin-core structure in Nephila clavipes spider silk observed by light and electron microscopy. Scanning 2000;22(1):12–5.
[132] Putthanarat S, Stribeck N, Fossey SA, Eby RK, Adams WW. Investigation of the nanofibrils of silk fibers. Polymer 2000;41(21):7735–47.
[133] Du N, Liu XY, Narayanan J, Li L, Lim MLM, Li D. Design of superior spider silk: from nanostructure to mechanical properties. Biophys J 2006;91(12):4528–35.
[134] Padamwar MN, Pawar AP. Silk sericin and its applications: a review. J Sci Ind Res 2004;63(4):323–9.
[135] Simmons AH, Michal CA, Jelinski LW. Molecular orientation and two-component nature of the crystalline fraction of spider dragline silk. Science 1996;271(5245):84–7.
[136] Termonia Y. Molecular modeling of spider silk elasticity. Macromolecules 1994;27(25):7378–81.
[137] Baldwin AD, Kiick KL. Polysaccharide-modified synthetic polymeric biomaterials. Biopolymers 2010;94:128–40.
[138] Hwang MR, Kim JO, Lee JH, Kim YI, Kim JH, Chang SW, et al. Gentamicin loaded wound dressing with polyvinyl alcohol/dextran hydrogel: gel characterization and in vivo healing evaluation. AAPS PharmSciTech 2010;11:1092–103.
[139] Sun G, Zhang X, Shen Y, Sebastian R, Dickinson LE, Fox-Talbot K, et al. Dextran hydrogel scaffolds enhance angiogenic responses and promote complete skin regeneration during burn wound healing. Proc Natl Acad Sci USA 2011;108:20976–81.
[140] Parulkar BG, Sobti MK, Pardanani DS. Dextranomer dressing in the treatment of infected wounds and cutaneous ulcers. J Postgrad Med 1985;31:28–33.
[141] Koria P, Yagi H, Kitagawa Y, Megeed Z, Nahmias Y, Sheridan R, et al. Self assembling elastin-like peptides growth factor chimeric nanoparticles for the treatment of chronic wounds. Proc Natl Acad Sci USA 2011;108:1034–9.
[142] Vasconcelos A, Gomes AC, Cavaco-Paulo A. Novel silk fibroin/elastin wound dressings. Acta Biomater 2012;8:3049–60.
[143] Daamen WF, Veerkamp JH, van Hest JC, van Kuppevelt TH. Elastin as a biomaterial for tissue engineering. Biomaterials 2007;28:4378–98.
[144] Wise SG, Mithieux SM, Weiss AS. Engineered tropoelastin and elastin-based biomaterials. Adv Protein Chem Struct Biol 2006;78:1–24.
[145] Mithieux SM, Rasko JEJ, Weiss ASAS. Synthetic elastin hydrogels derived from massive elastic assemblies of self-organized human protein monomers. Biomaterials 2004;25:4921–7.
[146] Leach JB, Wolinsky JB, Stone PJ, Wong JY. Crosslinked alpha-elastin biomaterials: toward a processable elastin mimetic scaffold. Acta Biomater 2005;1:155–64.
[147] Mithieux SM, Tu Y, Korkmaz E, Braet F, Weiss AS. In situ polymerization of tropoelastin in the absence of chemical cross-linking. Biomaterials 2009;30:431–5.
[148] Jannesari M, Varshosaz J, Morshed M, Zamani M. Composite poly(vinylalcohol)/poly(vinyl acetate) electrospun nanofibrous mats as a novel wound dressing matrix for controlled release of drugs. Int J Nanomed 2011;6:993–1003.
[149] Bourke SL, Al-Khalili M, Briggs T, Michniak BB, Kohn J, Poole-Warren LA. A photo-crosslinked poly(vinyl alcohol) hydrogel growth factor release vehicle for wound healing applications. AAPS Pharm Sci 2003;5:E33.

[150] Varshney L. Role of natural polysaccharides in radiation formation of PVA-hydrogel wound dressing. Nucl Instrum Methods Phys Res Sect B 2007;255:343–9.
[151] Kim JO, Park JK, Kim JH, Jin SG, Yong CS, Li DX, et al. Development of polyvinyl alcohol-sodium alginate gel-matrix-based wound dressing system containing nitrofurazone. Int J Pharm 2008;359:79–86.
[152] Xia C, Xiao C. Preparation and characterization of dual responsive sodium alginate-g-poly(vinyl alcohol) hydrogel. J Appl Polym Sci 2012;123:2244–9.
[153] de Souza Costa-Junior E, Pereira MM, Mansur HS. Properties and biocompatibility of chitosan films modified by blending with PVA and chemically crosslinked. J Mater Sci Mater Med 2009;20:553–61.
[154] Fathi E, Atyabi N, Imani M, Alinejad Z. Physically crosslinked polyvinylalcohol-dextran blend xerogels: morphology and thermal behavior. Carbohydr Polym 2011;84:145–52.
[155] Agarwal S, Wendorff JH, Greiner A. Use of electrospinning technique for biomedical applications. Polymer 2008;49:5603–21.
[156] Masters KS, Leibovich SJ, Belem P, West JL, Poole-Warren LA. Effects of nitric oxide releasing poly(vinyl alcohol) hydrogel dressings on dermal wound healing in diabetic mice. Wound Rep Reg 2002;10:286–94.
[157] Zhang L, Zhao J, Zhu J, He C, Wang H. Anisotropic tough poly(vinyl alcohol) hydrogels. Soft Matter 2012;8:10439–47.
[158] Zhu J. Biactive modification of poly(ethylene glycol) hydrogels for tissue engineering. Biomaterials 2010;31:4639–56. 218.
[159] Gibas I, Janik H. Review: synthetic polymer hydrogels for biomedical applications. Chem Technol 2010;4:297–304.
[160] Peppas NA, Keys KB, Torres-Lugo M, Lowman AM. Poly(ethylene glycol)- containing hydrogels in drug delivery. J Controlled Release 1999;62:81–7.
[161] Beamish JA, Zhu J, Kottke-Marchant K, Marchant RE. The effects of monoacrylated poly(ethylene glycol) on the properties of poly(ethylene glycol) diacrylate hydrogels used for tissue engineering. J Biomed Mater Res Part A 2010;92:441–50.
[162] Metters A, Hubbell J. Network formation and degradation behavior of hydrogels formed by Michael-type addition reactions. Biomacromolecules 2005;6:290–301.
[163] Sun G, Zhang X, Chu C. Effect of molecular weight of polyethylene glycol (PEG) on the properties of chitosan-PEG-poly (N-isopropylacrymide) hydrogels. J Mater Sci Mater Med 2008;19:2865–72.
[164] Sokolsky-Papkov M, Agashi K, Olaye A, Shakesheff K, Domb AJ. Polymer carriers for drug delivery in tissue engineering. Adv Drug Deliv 2007;59:187–209.
[165] Lee PY, Cobain E, Huard J, Huang L. Thermosensitive hydrogel PEG-PLGA-PEG enhances engraftment of muscle-derived stem cells and promotes healing in diabetic wound. Mol Ther 2007;15: 1189–94.
[166] Yang Y, Xia T, Chen F, Wei W, Liu C, He S, et al. Electrospun fibers with plasmid bFGF polyplex loadings promote skin wound healing in diabetic rats. Mol Pharm 2012;9:48–58.
[167] Huang Z, Lu M, Zhu G, Gao H, Xie L, Zhang X, et al. Acceleration of diabetic wound healing with PEGylated rhaFGF in healing-impaired streptozocin diabetic rats. Wound Rep Reg 2011;19:633–44.
[168] Biazar E, Roveimiab Z, Shahhosseini G, Khataminezhad M, Zafari M, Majdi A. Biocompatibility evaluation of a new hydrogel dressing based on polyvinylpyrrolidone/polyethylene glycol. J Biomed Biotechnol 2012;2012:343989.
[169] Himly N, Darwis D, Hardiningsih L. Poly(n-vinylpyrrolidone) hydrogels: hydrogel composites as wound dressing for tropical environment. Radiat Phys Chem 1993;42:911–4.
[170] Lugão AB, Machado LDB, Miranda LF, Alvarez MR, Rosiak JM. Study of wound dressing structure and hydration/dehydration properties. Radiat Phys Chem 1998;52:319.
[171] Lugão AB, Rogero SO, Malmonge SM. Rheological behaviour of irradiated wound dressing poly(vinyl pyrrolidone) hydrogels. Radiat Phys Chem 2002;63:543–6.
[172] Sebe I, Szabo B, Nagy ZK, Szabo D, Zsidai L, Kocsis B, Zelko R. Polymer structure and antimicrobial activity of polyvinylpyrrolidone-based iodine nanofibers prepared with high-speed rotary spinning technique. Int J Pharmaceutics 2013;458:99–103.
[173] Campbell N, Campbell D. Evaluation of a non-adherent, povidone-iodine dressing in a case series of chronic wounds. J Wound Care 2013;22:401–6.

[174] Li Y, Lee PI. Controlled nitric oxide delivery platform based on S-nitrosothiol conjugated interpolymer complexes for diabetic wound healing. Mol Pharm 2010;7:254–66.
[175] Naira LS, Laurencin CT. Biodegradable polymers as biomaterials. Prog Polym Sci 2007;32:762–98.
[176] Lee J, Cho Y, Lee J, Kim H, Pyun D, Park M, et al. Preparation of wound dressing using hydrogel polyurethane foam. Trends Biomater Artif Organs 2001;15:4–6.
[177] Chen Z, Lu H. Constructing sacrificial bonds and hidden lengths for ductile graphene/polyurethane elastomers with improved strength and toughness. J Mater Chem 2012;22:12479–90.
[178] Varma AK, Bal A, Kumar H, Kesav R, Nair S. Efficacy of polyurethane foam dressing in debrided diabetic lower limb wounds. Wounds 2008;12:5–8.
[179] Shi R, Chen D, Liu Q, Wu Y, Xu X, Zhang L, et al. Recent advances in synthetic bioelastomers. Int J Mol Sci 2009;10:4223–56.
[180] Khil MS, Cha DI, Kim HY, Kim IS, Bhattarai N. Electrospun nanofibrous polyurethane membrane as wound dressing. J Biomed Mater Res B Appl Biomater 2003;67:675–9.
[181] Davis FJ, Mitchell GR. Polyurethane based materials with application in medical devices. Biomater Prototyping Appl Med 2008;3:27–48.
[182] Barrett S. Mepilex Ag: an antimicrobial, absorbent foam dressing with Safetac technology. Br J Nurs 2009;18:S28–36.
[183] adhakumary C, Nandkumar AM, Nair PD. Hyaluronic acid-g-poly(HEMA) copolymer with potential implications for lung tissue engineering. Carbohydr Polym 2011;85:439–45.
[184] Tsou T, Tang S, Huang Y, Wu J, Young J, Wang H. Poly(2-hydroxyethyl methacrylate) wound dressing containing ciprofloxacin and its drug release studies. J Mater Sci Mater Med 2005;16:95–100.
[185] Rayment EA, Dargaville T, Upton Z. Wound repair composition and method. Patent 20100172860 2010.
[186] Wang D, Song YP, Lin L, Wang X, Wang Y. A novel phosphorus-containing poly(lactic acid) toward its flame retardation. Polymer 2011;52:233–8.
[187] Ignatova M, Manolova N, Markova N, Rashkov I. Electrospun non-woven nanofibrous hybrid mats based on chitosan and PLA for wound-dressing applications. Macromol Biosci 2009;9:102–11.
[188] Armentano I, Dottori M, Fortunati E, Mattioli S, Kenny JM. Biodegradable polymer matrix nanocomposites for tissue engineering: a review. Polym Degrad Stab 2010;95:2126–46.
[189] Li S. Hydrolytic degradation characteristics of aliphatic polyesters derived from lactic and glycolic acids. J Biomed Mater Res Part B Appl Biomater 1999;48:342–53.
[190] Dong X, Xu J, Wang W, Luo H, Liang X, Zhang L, et al. Repair effect of diabetic ulcers with recombinant human epidermal growth factor loaded by sustained-release microspheres. Sci China C Life Sci 2008;51:1039–44.
[191] Chu Y, Yu D, Wang P, Xu J, Li D, Ding M. Nanotechnology promotes the full thickness diabetic wound healing effect of recombinant human epidermal growth factor in diabetic rats. Wound Rep Reg 2010;18:499–505.
[192] Thomas S. Atraumatic dressings. WorldWideWounds 2003. Available at: http://www. worldwidewounds.com/2003/january/Thomas/Atraumatic-Dressings.html.
[193] White R. Evidence for atraumatic soft silicone dressing use. Wounds UK 2005;1(3):104–9.
[194] Dykes PJ, Heggie R, Hill SA. Effects of adhesive dressings on the stratum corneum. J Wound Care 2001;10(2):7–10.
[195] Dykes PJ, Heggie R. The link between the peel force of adhesive dressings and subjective discomfort in volunteer subjects. J Wound Care 2003;12(7):260–2.
[196] Rippon M, White R, Davies P. Skin adhesives and their role in wound healing. Wounds UK 2007;3:76–86.
[197] Matsumura H, Imai R, Ahmatjan N. Removal of adhesive wound dressings and its effect on the stratum corneum of the skin. Comparison of eight different adhesive wound dressings. Int Wound J 2012;7. [epub ahead of print].
[198] Dowsett C, Newton H. Wound bed preparation: TIME in practice. Wounds UK 2005;1(3):48–70.
[199] Moffat CJ, Franks PJ, Hollinworth H. Understanding wound pain and trauma. An international perspective. In: European wound management (EWMA) position document. Pain at wound dressing changes. MEP, 2002. Available at: www.woundsinternational.com.
[200] Forrest RD. Early history of wound treatment. J R Soc Med 1982;75(3):198–205.

[201] Majno G. The healing hand. Man and wound in the ancient world. Cambridge, MA: Harvard University Press; 1975.
[202] Molan PC. The evidence supporting the use of honey as a wound dressing. Int J Low Extrem Wounds 2006;5:40–54.
[203] Molan PC. The evidence and the rationale for the use of honey as a wound dressing. Wound Pract Res 2011;19:204–21.
[204] White JW. Composition of honey. In: Crane E, editor. Honey: a comprehensive survey. London: Heinemann; 1975. p. 157–206.
[205] Kaufman T, Eichenlaub EH, Angel MF, Levin M, Futrell JW. Topical acidification promotes healing of experimental deep partial thickness skin burns: a randomised double-blind preliminary study. Burns Incl Therm Inj 1985;12(2):84–90.
[206] Greener B, Hughes AA, Bannister NP, Douglass J. Proteases and pH in chronic wounds. J Wound Care 2005;14(2):59–61.
[207] Biswas A, Bharara M, Hurst C, Gruessner R, Armstrong D, Rilo H. Use of sugar on the healing of diabetic ulcers: a review. J Diabetes Sci Technol 2010;4(5):1139–45.
[208] Chirife J, Scarmato G, Herszage L. Scientific basis for use of granulated sugar in treatment of infected wounds. Lancet 1982;1(8271):560–1.
[209] Topham J. Sugar for wounds. J Tissue Viability 2000;10(3):86–9.
[210] Jian F, Xungai W, Tong L. Nanofibers – production, properties and functional applications (Ed: T. Lin), IInTech, Rijeka, Croatia 2011, Ch. 14, p. 287–326.
[211] Huang ZM, Zhang YZ, Kotaki M, Ramakrishna S. Compos Sci Technol 2003;63:2223.
[212] Sill TJ, von Recum HA. Electro spinning: applications in drug delivery and tissue engineering. Biomaterials 2008;29:1989–2006.
[213] Martins A, Reis RL, Neves NM. Electrospinning: processing technique for tissue engineering scaffolding. Int Mater Rev 2008;53:257–74.
[214] Cooley JF, GB Patent 06385, 1990.
[215] Murugan R, Ramakrishna S. Nano-featured scaffolds for tissue engineering: a review of spinning methodologies. Tissue Eng 2006;12:435–47.
[216] Martins A, Reis RL, Neves N, Araujo J. Electrospun nanostructured scaffolds for tissue engineering applications. Nanomedicine 2007;2:929–42.
[217] Kanani AG, Bahrami SH. Review on electrospun nanofibers scaffold and biomedical applications. Trends Biomater Artif Organs 2010;24:93–115.
[218] Bhattarai N, Edmondson D, Veiseh O, Matsen FA, Zhang M. Electrospun chitosan-based nanofibers and their cellular compatibility. Biomaterials 2005;26:6176–84.
[219] Zhong SP, Zhang YZ, Lim CT. Tissue scaffolds for skin wound healing and dermal reconstruction WIREs. Nanomed Nanobiotechnol 2010;2:510–25.
[220] Kumbar SG, James R, Nukavarapu SP, Laurencin CT. Electrospun nanofiber scaffolds: engineering soft tissues. Biomed Mater 2008;3. Article 034002.
[221] Zhang Y, Lim C, Ramakrishna S, Huang ZM. Recent development of polymer nanofibers for biomedical and biotechnological applications. J Mater Sci Mater M 2005;16:933–46.
[222] Burger C, Hsiao BS, Chu B. Nanofibrous materials and their applications. Ann Rev Mater Res 2006;36:333–68.
[223] Bhardwaj N, Kundu SC. Electrospinning: a fascinating fiber fabrication technique. Biotechnol Adv 2010;28:325–47.
[224] Sahay R, Thavasi V, Ramakrishna S. Design modifications in electrospinning setup for advanced applications. J Nanomater 2011;2011. Article Number: 317673.
[225] Migliaresi C, Ruffo GA, Volpato FZ, Zeni D. Electrospinning for advanced biomedical applications and therapies. In: Neves NM, editor. Smithers Rapra Technology, USA.
[226] Zahedi P, Rezaeian I, Ranaei-Siadat SO, Jafari SH, Supaphol P. A review on wound dressings with an emphasis on electrospun nanofibrous polymeric bandages. Polym Adv Technol 2010;21:77–95.
[227] Gunn J, Zhang M. Polyblend nanofibers for biomedical applications: perspectives and challenges. Trends Biotechnol 2010;28:189–97.

[228] Khil MS, Cha DI, Kim HY, Kim IS, Bhattarai N. Electrospun nanofibrous polyurethane membrane as wound dressing. J Biomed Mater Res B 2003;67:675–9.

[229] Phachamud T, Phiriyawiru M. In vitro cytotoxicity and degradability tests of gallic acid-loaded cellulose acetate electrospun fiber. Res J Pharm Biol Chem Sci 2011;2:85–98.

[230] Uppal R, Ramaswamy GN, Arnold C, Goodband R, Wan Y. Hyaluronic acid nanofiber wound dressing—production, characterization, and in vivo behavior. J Biomed Mater Res B Appl Biomater 2011;97:20–9.

[231] Park J-H, Braun PV. Coaxial electrospinning of self-healing coatings. 2010; 22, 496–499.

[232] Choi JS, Choi SH, Yoo HS. Coaxial electrospun nanofibers for treatment of diabetic ulcers with binary release of multiple growth factors. J Mater Chem 2011;21:5258–67.

[233] Choi JS, Leong KW, Yoo HS. In vivo wound healing of diabetic ulcers using electrospun nanofibers immobilized with human epidermal growth factor (EGF). Biomaterials 2008;29:587–96.

[234] Zhao W, Liu W, Li J, Lin X, Wang Y. Preparation of animal polysaccharides nanofibers by electrospinning and their potential biomedical applications. J Biomed Res 2015;103:807–18.

[235] Sun T, Mai S, Norton D, Haycock JW, Ryan AJ, MacNeil S. Self-organization of skin cells in three-dimensional electrospun polystyrene scaffolds. Tissue Eng 2005;11:1023–33.

[236] Sun T, Norton D, McKean RJ, Haycock JW, Ryan AJ, MacNeil S. Development of a 3D cell culture system for investigating cell interactions with electrospun fibers. Biotechnol Bioeng 2007;97:1318–28.

[237] Nisbet DR, Forsythe JS, Shen W, Finkelstein DI, Horne MK. Review paper: a review of the cellular response on electrospun nanofibers for tissue engineering. J Biomater Appl 2009;24:7–29.

[238] Chu XH, Shi XL, Feng ZQ, Gu JY, Xu HY, Zhang Y, Gu ZZ, Ding YT. In vitro evaluation of a multi-layer radial-flow bioreactor based on galactosylated chitosan nanofiber scaffolds. Biomaterials 2009;30:4533–8.

[239] Kim SE, Heo DN, Lee JB, Kim JR, Park SH, Jeon SH, Kwon IK. Electrospun gelatin/polyurethane blended nanofibers for wound healing. Biomed Mater 2009;4:044106.

[240] Chen JP, Chang GY, Chen JK. Electrospun collagen/chitosan nanofibrous membrane as wound dressing. Colloids Surf A 2008;313–4. 183–188.

[241] Charernsriwilaiwat N, Opanasopit P, Rojanarata T, Ngawhirunpat T. Electrospun chitosan/polyvinyl alcohol nanofibre mats for wound healing. Int Wound J 2014;11(2):215–22.

[242] Yajing L, Fan C, Jun N, Dongzhi Y. Carbohydr Polym 2012;90:1445.

[243] Duan B, Yuan X, Zhu Y, Zhang Y, Li X, Zhang Y, Yao K. A nanofibrous composite membrane of PLGA-chitosan/PVA prepared by electrospinning. Eur Polym J 2006;42:2013–22.

[244] Zhou Y, Yang D, Chen X, Xu Q, Lu F, Nie J. Electrospun water-soluble carboxyethyl chitosan/poly(vinyl alcohol) nanofibrous membrane as potential wound dressing for skin regeneration. Biomacromolecules 2007;9:349–54.

[245] Spasova M, Paneva D, Manolova N, Radenkov P, Rashkov I. Electrospun chitosan-coated fibers of poly(L-lactide) and poly(L-lactide)/poly(ethylene glycol): preparation and characterization. Macromol Biosci 2008;8:153–62.

[246] Ignatova M, Manolova N, Rashkov I. Electrospun antibacterial chitosan-based fibers. Macromol Biosci 2013;13:860–72.

[247] Ohkawa K, Cha DI, Kim H, Nishida A, Yamamoto H. Electrospinning of chitosan. Macromol Rapid Commun 2004;25:1600–5.

[248] Geng X, Kwon OH, Jang J. Electrospinning of chitosan dissolved in concentrated acetic acid solution. Biomaterials 2005;26:5427–32.

[249] Neamnark A, Rujiravanit R, Supaphol P. Electrospinning of hexanoyl chitosan. Carbohydr Polym 2006;66:298–305.

[250] Kriegel C, Kit KM, McClements DJ, Weiss J. Electrospinning of chitosan-poly(ethylene oxide) blend nanofibers in the presence of micellar surfactant solutions. Polymer 2009;50:189–200.

[251] Li L, Hsieh YL. Chitosan bicomponent nanofibers and nanoporous fibers. Carbohydr Res 2006;341:374–81.

[252] Zhang YY, Huang XB, Duan B, Wu LL, Li S, Yuan XY. Preparation of electrospun chitosan/poly(vinyl alcohol) membranes. Colloid Polym Sci 2007;285:855–63.

[253] Xu J, Zhang JH, Gao WQ, Liang HW, Wang HY, Li JF. Preparation of chitosan/PLA blend micro/nanofibers by electrospinning. Mater Lett 2009;63:658–60.
[254] Zhang HT, Li SB, White CJB, Ning X, Nie HL, Zhu LM. Studies on electrospun nylon-6/chitosan complex nanofiber interactions. Electrochim Acta 2009;54:5739–45.
[255] Nirmala R, Navamathavan R, Kang HS, El-Newehy MH, Kim HY. Preparation of polyamide-6/chitosan composite nanofibers by a single solvent system via electrospinning for biomedical applications. Colloid Surf B 2011;83:173–8.
[256] Shalumon KT, Anulekha KH, Girish CM, Prasanth R, Nair SV, Jayakumar R. Single step electrospinning of chitosan/poly(caprolactone) nanofibers using formic acid/acetone solvent mixture. Carbohydr Polym 2010;80:413–9.
[257] Cai ZX, Mo XM, Zhang KH, Fan LP, Yin AL, He CL, Wang HS. Fabrication of chitosan/silk fibroin composite nanofibers for wounddressing applications. Int J Mol Sci 2010;11:3529–39.
[258] Chen ZG, Wang PW, Wei B, Mo XM, Cui FZ. Electrospun collagen-chitosan nanofiber: a biomimetic extracellular matrix for endothelial cell and smooth muscle cell. Acta Biomater 2010;6:372–82.
[259] Dhandayuthapani B, Krishnan UM, Sethuraman S. Fabrication and characterization of chitosan-gelatin blend nanofibers for skin tissue engineering. J Biomed Mater Res B Appl Biomater 2010;94:264–72.
[260] Mincheva R, Manolova N, Rashkov I. Bicomponent aligned nanofibers of N-carboxyethylchitosan and poly(vinyl alcohol). Eur Polym J 2007;43:2809–18.
[261] Penchev H, Paneva D, Manolova N, Rashkov I. Electrospun hybrid nanofibers based on chitosan or N-carboxyethylchitosan and silver nanoparticles. Macromol Biosci 2009;9:884–94.
[262] Penchev H, Paneva D, Manolova N, Rashkov I. Hybrid nanofibrous yarns based on N-carboxyethylchitosan and silver nanoparticles with antibacterial activity prepared by self-bundling electrospinning. Carbohydr Res 2010;345:2374–80.
[263] Shalumon KT, Binulal NS, Selvamurugan N, Nair SV, Menon D, Furuike T, Tamura H, Jayakumar R. Electrospinning of carboxymethyl chitin/poly(vinyl alcohol) nanofibrous scaffolds for tissue engineering applications. Carbohydr Polym 2009;77:863–9.
[264] Chu XH, Shi XL, Feng ZQ, Gu JY, Xu HY, Zhang Y, Gu ZZ, Ding YT. In vitro evaluation of a multi-layer radial-flow bioreactor based on galactosylated chitosan nanofiber scaffolds. Biomaterials 2009;30:4533–8.
[265] Feng ZQ, Chu XH, Huang NP, Wang T, Wang YC, Shi XL, Ding YT, Gu ZZ. The effect of nanofibrous galactosylated chitosan scaffolds on the formation of rat primary hepatocyte aggregates and the maintenance of liver function. Biomaterials 2009;30:2753–63.
[266] Neamnark A, Sanchavanakit N, Pavasant P, Rujiravanit R, Supaphol P. In vitro biocompatibility of electrospun hexanoyl chitosan fibrous scaffolds toward human keratinocytes and fibroblasts. Eur Polym J 2008;44:2060–7.
[267] Du J, Hsieh YL. Nanofibrous membranes from aqueous electrospinning of carboxymethyl chitosan. Nanotechnology 2008;19:125707.
[268] Alipour SM, Nouri M, Mokhtari J, Bahrami SH. Electrospinning of poly(vinyl alcohol)-water-soluble quaternized chitosan derivative blend. Carbohydr Res 2009;344:2496–501.
[269] UM IC, Fang D, Hsiao BS, Okamoto A, Chu B. Electro-spinning and electro-blowing of hyaluronic acid. Biomacromolecules 2004;5:1428.
[270] Peng M, Sun Q, Ma Q, Li P. Mesoporous silica fibers prepared by electroblowing of a poly(methyl methacrylate)/tetraethoxysilane mixture in N,N-dimethylformamide. Microporous Mesoporous Mater 2008;115:562.
[271] Li JX, He AH, Zheng JF, Han CC. Gelatin and gelatin-hyaluronic acid nanofibrous membranes produced by electrospinning of their aqueous solutions. Biomacromolecules 2006;7:2243–7.
[272] Wang XF, Um IC, Fang DF, Okamoto A, Hsiao BS, Chu B. Formation of water-resistant hyaluronic acid nanofibers by blowing assisted electro-spinning and non-toxic post treatments. Polymer 2005;46:4853–67.
[273] Liu Y, Ma GP, Fang DW, Xu JA, Zhang HW, Nie J. Effects of solution properties and electric field on the electrospinning of hyaluronic acid. Carbohydr Polym 2011;83:1011–5.
[274] Ahmad B, Stride E, Stoyanov S, Pelan E, Edirisinghe M. Electrospinning of ethyl cellulose fibres with a heated needle and heated air using a co-axial needle: a comparison. J Med Bioeng 2012;1:1.

[275] Bubakir MM, Li H, Wu W, Li X, Ma S, Yang W. Applications of web produced by hot air assisted melt differential electrospinning method. IOP Conf Series Mater Sci Eng 2014;64:012052.
[276] Bryner MA, Armantrout JE, Johnson BS Patent US/20110171335.
[277] Lee Y, Chang J, Yang M, Chien C, Lai W. Acceleration of wound dressing in diabetic rats by layered hydrogel dressing. Carbohydr Polym 2012;88:809–19.
[278] Meinel A, Germershaus O, Luhmann T, Merkle HP, Meinel L. Electrospun matrices for localized drug delivery: current technologies and selected biomedical applications. Eur J Pharm Biopharm 2012;81:1–13.
[279] Drury JL, Mooney DJ. Hydrogels for tissue engineering: scaffold design variables and applications. Biomaterials 2003;24:4337–51.

CHAPTER FIVE

Wound Diagnostics and Diagnostic Dressings

J. Davis, A. McLister
School of Engineering, Ulster University, Jordanstown, Northern Ireland, United Kingdom

5.1 INTRODUCTION

Diagnostics play an increasingly important role in the wound management plan for chronic wounds as they can provide valuable insights into why a wound is failing to progress [1–3]. The ability to extract quantitative data on the dynamics of key molecular players rather than relying on gross physical symptoms and visual clues can enable more informed decisions on which treatment route to pursue [3]. As mentioned in Chapter 1, there are a range of standard tests which will be conducted as part of a routine assessment. These can involve checking for the presence of systemic inflammatory markers (ie, C-reactive protein), temperature, or blood pressure, but they may not be specific to the wound, and although they may help to inform the clinician, they do not, by themselves, indicate a particular diagnosis [3]. The development of tests that can provide detailed information on the activity of cellular and molecular species within the wound would clearly be a major benefit to treatment. Such tests however are seldom available to the attending clinician in a convenient point of care format, and usually requires the transport of samples to a central laboratory [1–3]. The time delays in receiving the analysis results will often be of little value as the wound condition may have changed in the intervening days.

One of the key findings in the recent World Union of Wound Healing Societies' report: "Diagnostics and Wounds: A Consensus Document" was that "diagnostic tools need to be moved into the clinic or the patient's home to ensure optimal care is provided for patients with wounds" [3]. The dearth of diagnostic instruments has created a clear opportunity for those involved in biomedical science and engineering to develop system that can be used in the clinic but there is also a need for more autonomous sensing devices [4,5]. The notion of a smart dressing has been introduced in Chapter 1, and, in Chapter 4, it has been shown how material formulations can certainly impart interactivity into modern dressing designs. There is, however, a need to have dressings that can actively monitor the activity of key analytes—particularly where there is the possibility of detecting the early onset of infection. The findings by Dowsett et al. [6] have indicated that the majority of patients with chronic wounds are treated within the community and thus the availability of tests that can be performed in the clinic will limit their influence. The transfer of the tests for use by patients or community nurses is one option, but again it assumes compliance and expertise in the use of the test systems and, given the complexity of the sampling procedures necessary for assessing chemical concentrations, will leave the device subject to potential errors negating its intended use. The application of a smart dressing would, however, effectively take the user (patient and nurse) out of the equation and, it would be hoped, offer more accurate data. There are a lot of assumptions in such proposals and, as a consequence, there are substantial hurdles to be overcome to produce a robust system [1–5]. The science behind the measurement is not the only issue that needs to be addressed: direct integration of the sensor dressing within a conventional bandage also necessitates that it is disposable and cost effective.

5.2 IDEAL PROPERTIES AND KEY CHALLENGES

The significance of the problem of designing sensors for measuring chemical species within biological systems and the translation of the technology toward remote/autonomous sensing for decentralized use has been recognized by many funders including the UK Engineering and Physical Sciences Research Council. Among their Healthcare Grand Challenges call is a raft of objectives with direct relevance to the development of smart bandages and some are highlighted in Table 5.1 [7].

Table 5.1 Healthcare grand challenges

- Design of bioelectronic devices for long-term sensing and control.
- Production of novel, low-cost diagnostic devices, for timely and accurate diagnosis which could ultimately inform appropriate and timely interventions reducing costs improving outcomes.
- Design of novel noninvasive sensing platforms for the capture of real-time health enabling automated intervention—for example, controlled release of a drug—providing better disease control and allowing patients to lead more normal, independent lives.
- Optimizing care through effective diagnosis, patient-specific prediction, and evidence-based intervention. Using real-time information to support self-management of health and well-being, and to facilitate timely interventions.
- Methods for recognizing person-specific abnormal patterns in physiological time course data, providing early warning of deterioration to patients, carers, and healthcare professionals.
- Decision support dashboards and tools for healthcare professionals, supporting safe and effective management in the community of patients with long-term conditions or following early discharge.
- Individually adaptive data collection, interaction with healthcare professionals, and self-reporting requests, to support effective care while minimizing intrusion.
- Technologies for promoting well-being by providing timely, personalized feedback, and exploiting social networking to influence health behaviors.

Source: Adapted from EPSRC Priorities [7].

It is easy to idealize a smart device encompassing all (or most) of the above and, were the device made real, it could provide tremendous benefits for the patient and healthcare administrators. The above list is, of course, a "wish list" but there have been substantial gains in technology in recent years across the main objectives. It could be that one of the "Grand Challenges" will be to unite the advances into a single application.

The aim of this chapter is to provide an overview of the technologies that are seeking to address the key objectives mentioned above and give some insights into the methodologies being applied and the relative merits and limitations of the various approach. The prime focus of this chapter is on electronic devices that can provide telemetry of the wound condition and are capable of being integrated within a bandage of some description.

5.3 WOUND FLUID

The journey toward developing a sensor for measuring chemical species whether for point care application or incorporation within a dressing will require some indication as to what to actually detect. Before that can be accomplished, it is necessary to briefly consider the issue of samples and sampling [8–11]. The latter will be necessary for any diagnostic as the sensor will ultimately work on a discrete portion of wound component, be immersed in it or placed in direct contact with it. The two most common types of sample will be either tissue biopsy or the fluid which bathes the actual wound site [8,9]. There is no consensus regarding which is the better option or, whether one or the other is a truer reflection of the chronic wound and, the choice will also depend on the nature of the device (and wound type) and its intended operation.

In either case, it can be extremely difficult to obtain meaningful data as a consequence of the highly variable nature of both the wound and the sample itself. Wound fluid may, on first consideration, appear to be the more accessible and this is supported by the fact that majority of studies tackling the characterization of chronic wounds take this approach. There are however many concerns over the reliability/reproducibility and representative nature of the results as a consequence of the inherent variability of the sample collection step and subsequent standardization [8–11]. Short and long-term storage are pressing issues, especially in regard to the fact that the fluid is a dynamic matrix where even minor manipulation or short-time delays between collection and analysis can affect composition [8,9].

The fluid bathing the wound originates from a variety of sources and comprises a highly heterogeneous mixture and its composition is assumed to reflect the clinical condition of the wound at the time of sampling [8,9]. The composition of the fluid will vary considerably over the course of the healing process as a consequence of changes in the microenvironment as cell migration and tissue remodeling progresses and, knowing what stage the wound is presently at, is one of the driving forces behind the development of wound-monitoring technologies. Underlying conditions (ie, diabetes, neuropathy) can also influence the nature of the fluid [8,9]. Exogenous factors such as bacterial load, treatments applied (either systemic or topical), and the nature of the wound dressing will also contribute to and affect the milieu [9] and again, the ability to assess the changes in the wound environment through simple diagnostics test could revolutionize treatment [8].

In chronic ulcers, wound fluid is normally defined as an exudate with a high viscosity and protein content that exceeds 30 mg/mL [12]. Temporal issues are critical when considering the fluid under examination as it was found by Jones et al. [13] that immediately following surgery, there can be significant contamination from material being transported directly from the blood stream—accounting for some 30% of the proteinaceous material found with the wound fluid. It is important to consider the etiologies involved in the samples under consideration (ie, comparing acute to chronic wounds), whereby the concentrations of target biomarkers in one particular sample may not correlate to the actual bioactivity in another.

The need for temporal caution in sampling has been highlighted in a number of studies investigating the influence of different sampling periods on the analysis of various biomarkers. Early studies by Jalkanen et al. [14] on the effects of exudates from experimental granulation tissue demonstrated that wound fluid, obtained 4 days (after implantation), initiated the proliferation of fibroblasts, whereas, in contrast, exudates sampled at 10 and 14 days inhibited the process. It has been postulated that, while it is very possible to measure high concentrations of mitogenic cytokines and growth factors in a wound, their effects may be offset by similarly high concentrations of protease enzymes which degrade the former before they have any opportunity to influence the wound progression. A series of experiments by Zillmer et al. [15] on the concentration of interleukins (IL-1a, IL-1b, and IL-8) within wound exudate found similar trends to that of Jalkanen, whereby early sampling (within the first hour) stimulated fibroblast activity but subsequent sampling (at 8-hour intervals) was found to elicit little response. The concentration of the IL markers was found to have increased markedly after the initial sampling, but despite the accumulation there was no significant increase in bioactivity. The concentration of matrix metalloprotease (MMP-9) was assayed throughout and found to remain relatively constant and, would appear to counter the argument that degradation of promoting factors was the principal contributory element. It must be appreciated that such studies are hampered by the complexity of the wound fluid and that there can be a multitude of inhibitory factors which can impact the healing progression.

Wound fluid can be collected using a variety of methods but the selection of the appropriate technique will depend on the nature of the wound, the volume available, and the purpose for which the sample is required. Irrespective of end-use, obtaining reproducible samples, however, is widely regarded as a considerable challenge, and it must be noted from the outset that the sampling procedure may, in all likelihood, induce alterations in the sample itself. The standard approach pioneered by Varghese et al. [16] has been to use occlusive dressings in which the wound fluid accumulates and can be easily sampled by aspiration with a micropipette, syringe, needles, or vaccutainers. A variety of modifications to the general approach have been investigated, but the basic methodology has effectively remained the same since its first inception. There are however issues with the approach with the time through which the dressing is applied and the degree of wound bed preparation and local treatments applied prior to placement being among the more common [8]. It must also be noted that the heterogeneous nature of the wound itself will be a significant factor and will inevitably influence the amount of and nature of the fluid obtained. Direct extraction by pipette can be problematic if there is little fluid available, in which case, passive trapping using absorption into an occlusive dressing may be a more viable option [8]. The provision of control fluids is a highly contentious issue where the appropriateness of alternative biofluids such as serum, plasma, acute wound fluid, and surgical fluid have all been debated and, Broadbent et al. [9] have proposed the use of patient-matched serum/plasma taken at the time of the wound fluid collection. It should be expected that tissues, as with their corresponding wound fluid, will be rich in wound-related molecules. Tissue is surgically removed or obtained by punch biopsy under local anaesthetic and then frozen or immediately preserved prior to analysis. The sampling sites are usually selected from around the wound margins and may also involve intact epidermis to serve as controls [9].

5.4 POTENTIAL BIOMARKERS

There are a large number of biochemical species within the wound fluid and each will have some part to play in the wound dynamics and healing processes. As discussed previously, there is no ideal sample for biomarker discovery, but it could be assumed that a noninvasive approach is the preferred option—both in terms of patient comfort but through lessening the possibility of artefacts arising from the actual sampling process. One issue that may arise relates to the sensitivity of the technique when considering wound fluid where a high volume can unduly dilute the target and hinder discovery. In such cases, an argument can be made for the sampling of tissue, but it creates a dilemma in that there will be a need for a patient-matched control sample from healthy tissue which could initiate a secondary wound. There are also concerns that the concentration of protein biomarkers can vary significantly from one tissue site to another [9].

At present, there is a tremendous effort to elucidate the significance of each of these players and to identify those most likely to be diagnostically useful in the clinical management of chronic wounds. Monitoring markers that can provide key warnings toward the complications, particularly infection, is the critical challenge that faces the development of the next generation of smart dressings. Clinical investigations of wound fluids, exudates, and tissues have provided considerable insights and there have been a number of attempts to classify the main protagonists involved in the healing progression of the wound. Broadbent et al. [9] have detailed over 150 proteins (highlighted in Table 5.2)

Table 5.2 Potential wound biomarkers

α-1-antitrypsin	Haemopexin
α-1-acid glycoprotein	Hepatocyte growth factor
α-1-globulin	Haptoglobin
α-2-macroglobulin	Heparin binding protein
Alanine aminotransferase	IgA
Albumin	IgG
Alkaline phosphatase	Insulin-like growth factor-1
Angiostatin	Insulin-like growth factor binding protein-2
Antichymotrypsin	Insulin-like growth factor binding protein 3
Apolipoprotein A-1	Inter-α-inhibitor
Asparate	Interferon-inducible protein-10
Aminotransferase	Interleukin-1, 1a, 1b, 6, 8, 10
β-1-globulin	Interleukin-1 receptor antagonist protein
β-globulin	Keratin 6
β-2-glycoprotein-1	H, L-Kininogens
Basic fibroblast growth factor	Lactate dehydrogenase
Calgranulin A and B	Macrophage inflammatory protein 1a, 1b
Cathepsin G	Matrix metalloproteinases-1, 2, 8, 9
Ceruloplasmin	Monocyte chemoattractant protein 1
Collagen I and III	Nucleosome assembly protein 2
Complement C3 and C4	Neutrophil cathepsin-D
C-reactive protein	Orosomucoid 1
Creatine kinase	p55, p75
Cytokeratin-1	Plasmin
Elafin	Plasminogen
Elastase	Plasminogen activator
Elastase (Neutrophil)	Plasminogen activator inhibitor
Endostatin	Platelet-derived growth factors AA, AB
Epithelial growth factor	Platelet factor-4
Epithelial neutrophil activating peptide – 78	Tenascin-C
Factor B	Tetranectin
Fibrinogen-α, b gA chains	Tissue inhibitor of metal proteinases-1 and 2
Fibronectin	Tumor necrosis factor-α
Ferritin	Transferrin
γ-globulin	Transforming growth factor-β, B1
γ-glutamyltranspeptidase	Urokinase plasminogen activator
Glypican-1	Vascular endothelial growth factor
Granulocyte macrophage colony stimulating factor	Vitamin D binding protein
Growth regulated oncogene-α	Vitronectin

Source: Adapted from Broadbent et al. [9].

Table 5.3 Common wound diagnostic markers

Bacterial metabolites	**Inflammatory mediators**
Pyocanin*	Cytokines
Nitrite*	Interleukins
Hydrogen sulfide*	Nitric oxide
Enzymes	Reactive oxygen species
Matrix metalloproteinases	**Nutritional factors**
Plasmin	Zinc
Collagenase	Glutamine
Growth factors/hormones	Glucose
Platelet-derived growth factor (PDGF)	Ascorbic acid
Sex steroids (andmgens/oestrogens)	Glutathione
Thyroid hormones	**Physico-chemical parameters**
Immunohistochemical markers	Wound fluid pH*
Integrins	Water loss*
Chemokine receptors	Temperature*
Transforming growth factor Beta II receptors	Oxyegen
	Carbon dioxide

whose concentrations are influenced by the cellular/tissue remodeling and associated inflammatory responses. The upregulation of proteases and growth factor dysregulation have been identified as offering considerable therapeutic and prognostic value [17,18]. As mentioned previously, the ability to control the activation of such species has been shown to aid the healing process, but such interventions clearly require the provision of analytical tools through which their concentration/activity can be speedily and easily measured at the time of consultation [3].

Despite the extensive candidate list indicated in Table 5.2, the diagnostic community has tended to focus on a more limited group and an overview of the chemical components which are presently being investigated is highlighted in Table 5.3 [3]. These follow much the same pattern as that outlined by Harding and can be separated into two groupings reflecting the size of the target biomarker [3]. It must be noted however that although significant strides have been made in terms of characterizing the biochemical fluxes that can occur within a chronic wound environment—the diagnostic community has tended to focus on a much more limited group and that, despite such narrowing, there is, as yet, no set of definitive markers.

5.5 CONVENTIONAL DIAGNOSTICS

There is an increasing effort to design and develop new approaches to the construction of decentralized tests and sensors for use in biomedical applications [1,2,4,5]. The core rationale behind these analytical devices is that they can perform a rapid

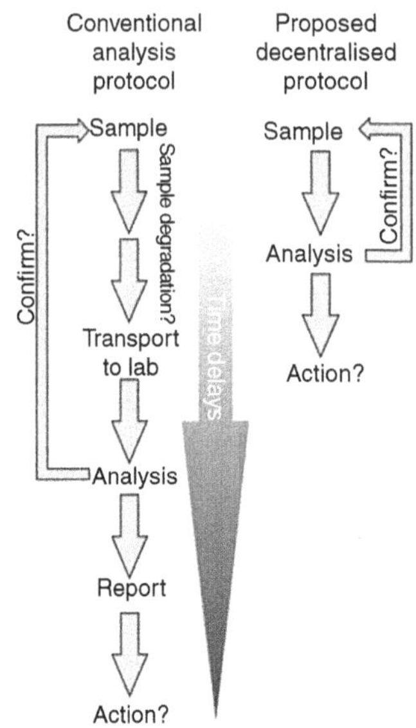

Figure 5.1 ***Central lab versuss point of care analysis.***

analysis of a given sample and provide the user with immediate feedback on a particular physical parameter (ie, temperature) or a chemical concentration(glucose) or enzyme activity (ie, proteases). The term decentralized refers to the fact that the devices can be used outside the normal laboratory environment and by users with varying scientific background. The intention would be for implementation within the clinic, by a community healthcare provider or even by the patients themselves. As such, they should be portable, robust and provide a quick and simple measurement that does not require any sample manipulation by the user. These criteria embody the guidelines proffered by Harding and colleagues [3]. The principal benefit is that they avoid the time delays associated with conventional lab-based analysis (indicated in Fig. 5.1). In the context of wound management, rapid analysis and reporting should, in principle, enable a much speedier intervention and inform the selection of dressings (Chapter 4), which, it is hoped, would restart the healing processes and improve the outcome. This is especially vital in clinical practice where time delays between diagnosis and treatment can have considerable consequences [19].

Any analytical device which is capable of being used outside a normal bioanalytical laboratory, irrespective of the application context, falls under the general heading of a "decentralized test." Those designed for biomedical applications are normally classified as "point of care" or "near patient test" and common examples include thermometers, blood pressure meters, urine dip tests, protease activities, etc [20]. There is often a degree of overlap between the sensors designed for different applications as advances in the underlying technology of one area can often be translated or adapted to fit within the other. For example, advances in industrial gas sensing technology could lead to the development of electronic nose systems for the detection of volatile compounds emitted from infected wounds.

5.5.1 Core Methodologies

The main complication lies in attempting to make a device sensitive and selective to one particular analyte in a particular application context without the need for extensive sample manipulation. It is unreasonable to expect the clinician (or patient) to undertake the sampling of the wound and then have to perform a series of chemical manipulations before the results can be obtained. This is not simply an issue of time but, rather of the possible errors that can be introduced with each step. Any test must therefore be as simple as possible and require a minimum of manipulation and, in a practical sense, should only involve the sampling of the wound fluid [3]. This places a huge responsibility on the underlying technology to process the sample and pick out the target analyte. This is a considerable challenge given the compositional complexity of wound fluid [8,9]. The basic rationale behind the test systems, irrespective of actual application context, is shown in Fig. 5.2. The sample considerations can be different depending on the nature of the wound—a wound that has lots of slough will present a radically different challenge than a wound that has been freshly debrided. It may be necessary to add in additional layers of procedure (such as debridement) or instrumentational sophistication (ie, permselective barriers) to address the demands of a particular sample.

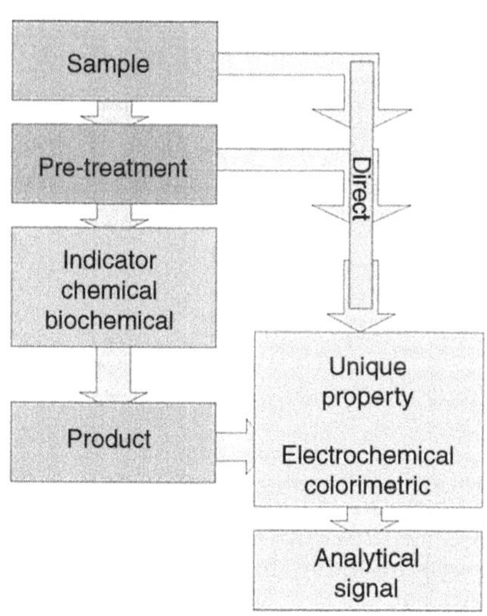

Figure 5.2 ***Assay/device development methodology.***

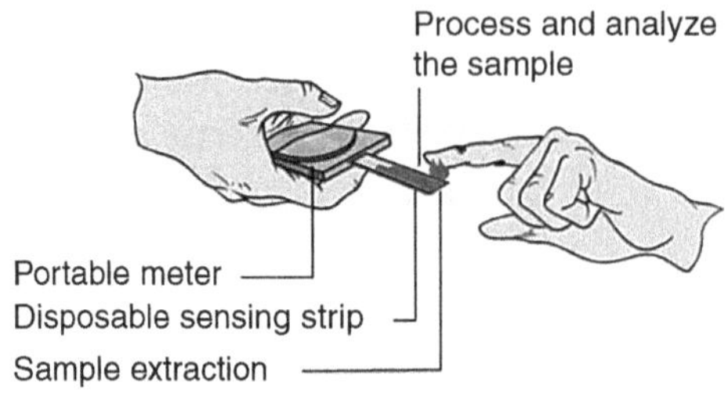

Figure 5.3 ***Conventional blood glucose sensor.***

Identifying the analyte from all the other species that may be present within the sample matrix is however the central issue—without selectivity the test is useless [20]. Much research is targeted at developing the chemistry so that the analyte is selectively transformed into something else which has a "unique and measurable" property with little or no interference from the other components as indicated in Fig. 5.2. In many cases, this requires the design of a chemical indicator that will readily and selectively react with the analyte or the use of a biological agent (enzyme or antibody) that can selectively act upon that particular substrate. As noted previously, it is important that the labeling is done with minimal sample preparation and hence little interaction by the user beyond simply adding the sample. The classic example is the use of glucose test strips, whereby the patient is only required to conduct a finger prick test to release a few microliters of blood (Fig. 5.3) which can be delivered to a test strip. The strips are designed with an enzyme (typically glucose oxidase) which will selectively react with glucose in the sample while ignoring a plethora of other sugar molecules. The sample is conducted in whole blood with no sample manipulation.

In some cases it is also possible to design devices that act directly upon the analyte—avoiding the need for any additional reactions. This approach is less common and usually exploits the inherent differences in electrochemical or spectroscopic properties of the molecules present within the sample and is usually reserved for very simple samples. The optimization of the chemistry on the sensing surface of the proposed device to enhance the detection properties is another area of high interest to both the bioanalytical and materials science communities [1,2].

5.5.2 Dipstick Tests

The earliest and simplest POCT designs were based on simple color changes [20]. Direct measurement by colorimetric approaches can be much more complex due to the "broadness" of the spectra and the inevitable overlap of different species creating a highly

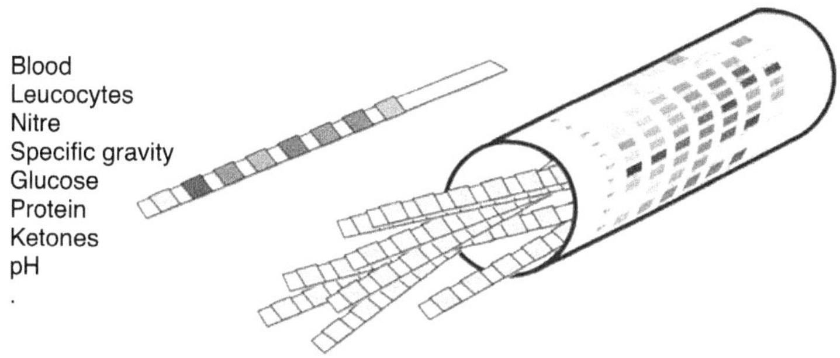

Figure 5.4 ***Conventional urinanalysis test strip.***

ambiguous signal. As such, spectroscopic analysis tends to be used in conjunction with indicator systems to generate a "unique property." This typically results in a reaction that leads to the production of a wholly new absorption band in a region of the spectrum where there is no existing process and hence can be measured without interference. There is a wealth of colorimetric autoanalyser assays which operate on the basis of enzymic transformations resulting in a colored product (typically λ_{max} ~560 nm), but there is often a requirement for the sample to be plasma or serum which will have no native components in that particular region of the spectrum.

Test strips with an indicating reagent immobilized within an absorbent pad was the next step in the evolution of spot tests, the most common example being the urinanalysis dipstick test (Fig. 5.4) that is performed in GP surgeries [20]. A drop of the aqueous sample is added to the strip and the color allowed to develop and can be used to test for a range of analytes such as glucose, leukocytes, nitrite, pH, protein, etc.

This has a number of procedural advantages (operational simplicity and reagent-less nature of the test being the more important), but the interpretation and quantification issues remain. The systems are typically designed/selected to obey Beers Law but there are a number of problems associated with this approach [20]:

1. color variability of the actual sample (background color)
2. chemical variability of the sample (pH)
3. availability of the analyte (complexation or covalent binding)
4. presence of interferences (false positives)
5. perception of the color on the band and its relation to the calibration chart.

The simple dipstick technologies are seldom used for complex samples such as wound fluid as they rely on fairly simple chemical reactions. The selective detection of target proteins, such as matrix metalloproteases, requires far greater degree of sophistication,

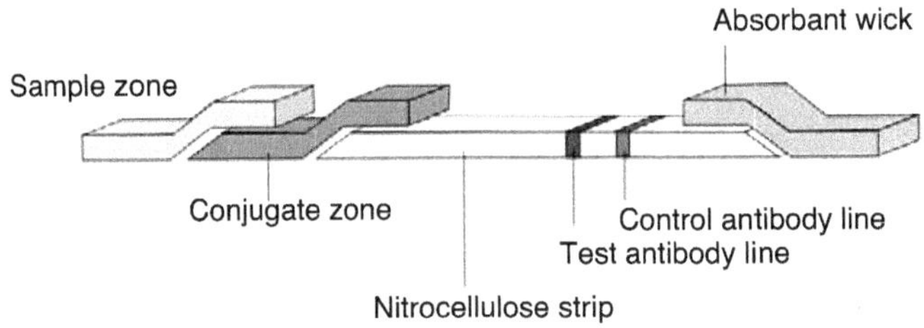

Figure 5.5 ***Basic components of an immunochromatographic (lateral flow) test strip.***

but there have been considerable strides made in the development of alternative approaches to the traditional dip stick test.

5.5.3 Lateral Flow Diagnostics

Lateral flow systems embody immobilized antibodies using a capillary flow system to separate out the target analytes from the other components. These have been used for a large range of target analytes and have been extensively commercialized as point of care devices across a number of biomedical contexts. The design and operation of the devices are relatively generic (Fig. 5.5) and differ mainly in the identity and selectivity of the conjugate and capture antibodies [21].

The conjugate antibodies are freely diffusing species which are solubilized upon passage of the sample solution along the capillary membrane and are responsible for the initial binding event with the target analyte. The conjugate antibodies are normally labeled with a chromophore of some description (commonly gold nanoparticles giving a red indication or latex providing a blue line) [21,22]. As they move along the nitrocellulose strip, the primary antigen–antibody complexes encounter a line of immobilized antibody which will be selective toward a different epitope of the target analyte. Thus, in the presence of the target, the conjugate antibodies bind, are transported to the "test" line, and are captured with the nanoparticle label providing a visual indication of the presence of the analyte (positive result). In the absence of the target analyte—there will be no secondary binding event and the conjugate-labeled antibody will pass through into the absorbant pad and hence no visual indication (negative result) will be apparent. The basic operation is highlighted in Fig. 5.6.

In most lateral flow designs, a "control" line is added to ensure that the device has functioned properly. This involves an additional antibody capture system which will have a similar label to that of the conjugate antibody. In this case, however, the control antibody (IgG in Fig. 5.6) takes no part in the conjugation process but is simply transported along with the flow and, upon reaching the capture zone, is caught by the secondary antibody. Providing the sample has progressed along the nitrocellulose

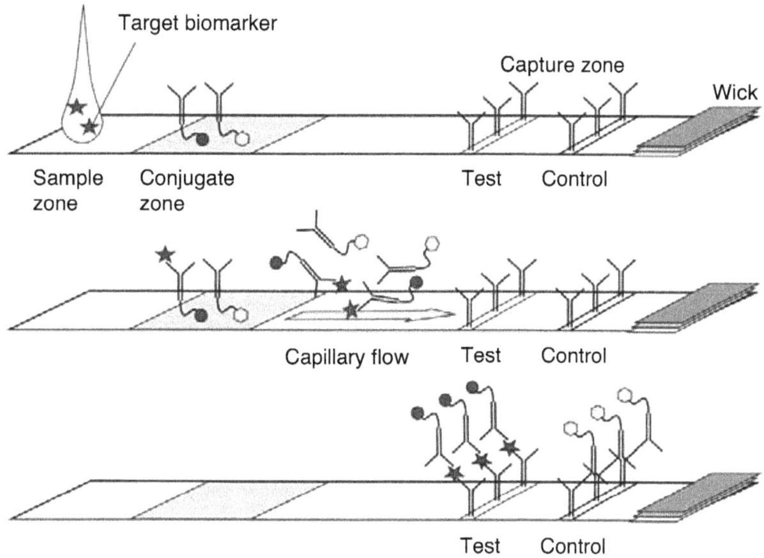

Figure 5.6 ***Typical operation of a lateral flow test strip.***

strip, the capture of the labeled control antibody will give a visual signal similar to that of the test line. If the "control" line is not visible, it would imply that the sample has not been transported (ie, high viscosity or blockage of the permselective screen) and the test has failed. The latter is a failsafe against the reporting of false negatives [21,22].

In terms of wound diagnostics, Table 5.2 indicates there is an extensive list of candidate targets that could be of value in building a picture of the wound condition, and it could be envisaged that through substituting the relevant antibody system, the technology advocated in Figs. 5.5 and 5.6 could be adapted. As yet, the only target to have emerged within the commercial sector is a screening tool for the presence of matrix metalloproteases. The WoundChek system (Fig. 5.7) is a simple lateral flow test designed for use by the clinician to gauge the activity (over activity) of MMPs.

The simple lateral flow systems would typically provide a yes/no response and would be designed around a particular threshold value. In the case of the protease detection system, there will be a natural background of protease activity, and thus the threshold can be manipulated to provide a positive result when excessive levels have been reached. The simple strip type systems are inherently semiqualitative, but there is an increasing move toward the introduction of electronic readers that can provide a quantitative evaluation of concentration/activity through assessing the intensity of the chromophore on the test line [21–24].

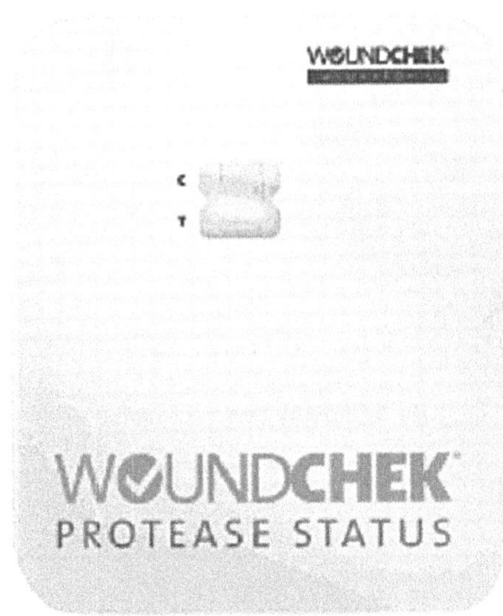

Figure 5.7 ***Woundcheck™ lateral flow system for detecting high MMP activity.***

5.6 MOVING TOWARD SMART DRESSINGS

The provision of a digital "readout" of the analysis result removes the ambiguity of ascribing a color to a given chart is a large component of the uncertainty of the measurement [20] and the numerical value provided by the electronic systems can be considered a significant step forward. While there are a large number of systems that could ultimately be applied to wound monitoring [1,2,4,5], the present overview has focused predominantly on those targeting pH and endogenous wound biomarkers. Biomarkers arising from the immune response to bacterial infection and the release of bacterial metabolites are considered in more depth in Chapter 6. Many of approaches have been investigated with the intention of implementation within a clinic setting, but acquiring sufficient selectivity with minimal sample preparation is a severe challenge, especially when considering the limited time available during a patient consultation.

5.7 MONITORING WOUND pH

The pH of wound exudate is known to vary depending on the stage of healing (Fig. 5.8), and it is widely recognized that the prevailing pH plays a key role in the multitude of biochemical reactions taking place. Although the normal pH of the skin will vary from one person to another, it tends to fluctuate within a relatively narrow acidic range

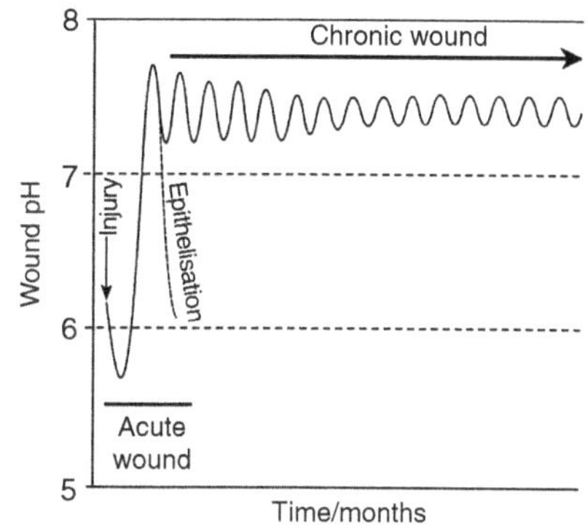

Figure 5.8 ***Typical pH profiles observed for acute and chronic wounds.*** *(Adapted from Scheinder et al. [25]).*

between pH 4 and pH 6. In maintaining the surface pH at this level, bacterial proliferation is impeded and acts as an aid in minimizing infection. A cutaneous wound, however, exposes the underlying tissue which, being homeostatically regulated at the higher pH of 7.4, can encourage bacterial growth and increase the susceptibility to infection. Acute wounds tend to follow a predictable trajectory whereby the pH returns to the normal acidic skin regime as the wound heals [25].

The pH of the chronic wound is known to oscillate within a narrow, weakly alkaline range and this can have the effect of increasing the susceptibility of the patient to infection. It has been postulated that bacteria increase the pH of the local wound fluid to create an environment that is more accommodating for their continued growth [25,26]. The increase in pH could therefore be exploited as a simple diagnostic handle or screening tool through which to identify the onset of infection [27] or, at the very least, raise an alarm for particular vigilance. It must be acknowledged that this is a rather simplistic model, as there have yet to be conclusive studies that demonstrate a definitive change in pH upon infection, let alone provide confirmation that all bacteria influence the wound in the same manner. It may therefore be more useful to use the oscillation in pH as a baseline and any significant and sustained deviation from the regular pattern being a sufficient cause to raise an alarm. There has been a considerable effort to develop disposable sensors and modified dressings that could be applied to monitoring wound pH using a range of analytical methodologies.

5.8 COLORIMETRIC pH SYSTEMS

5.8.1 Visual pH Devices

Mohr and coworkers have pioneered the use of chromophore and fluorophore-modified textiles to produce smart fabrics that respond to changes in pH [28]. Their work has significant ramifications across a range of medical applications and

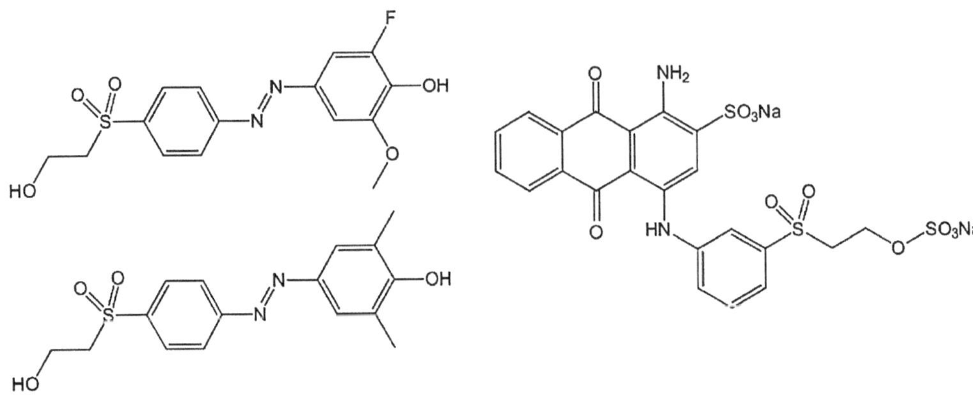

Figure 5.9 ***Structures of the dye components used by Mohr to provide a "traffic light system" indicator [28].***

is particularly valuable in that the indicator system employs an innovative use of the well-recognized "traffic light" warning sequence to alert the healthcare worker to possible issues [29,30]. Mohr's team have successfully incorporated specific combination of dyes (Fig. 5.9) directly onto the polymer backbone to provide a green-to-red transition with increasing pH and are universally associated with the change from "good" to "bad." The significance of their work relates to the fact that there is no single indicator capable of providing the desired color change and thus the need for a specific formulation.

The approach has been used in the design of smart textiles designed to monitor the pH of the skin, but the technology has also been proposed as a smart swab through which to assess the pH of chronic wounds (Fig. 5.10). The covalent immobilization of the dyes onto the cotton fiber of the swab serves to minimize the possibility of leaching [28]. There are obvious issues with this system, as noted, there is considerable debate as to the value of swabbing [8,10,11] and it necessitates that there is sufficient wound fluid available. It also assumes that high pH is a true indication of infection which has yet to be proven and, therefore, while the green–red transition provides a clear visual indicator, there is a possibility of false negatives arising.

Trupp and colleagues have proposed an alternative to the swab system in which the colorimetric indicators are loaded onto an actual dressing complete with transparent protective film as indicated in Fig. 5.11. The rationale is similar to that demonstrated by Mohr, albeit without the traffic light sequence, but it can be envisaged that it will encounter much the same issues.

Both approaches by Mohr and Trupp rely on visual inspection, which has the advantage of easing issues of cost and manufacturing, but they are nevertheless dependent upon the subjective color perception of the person conducting the test/inspection.

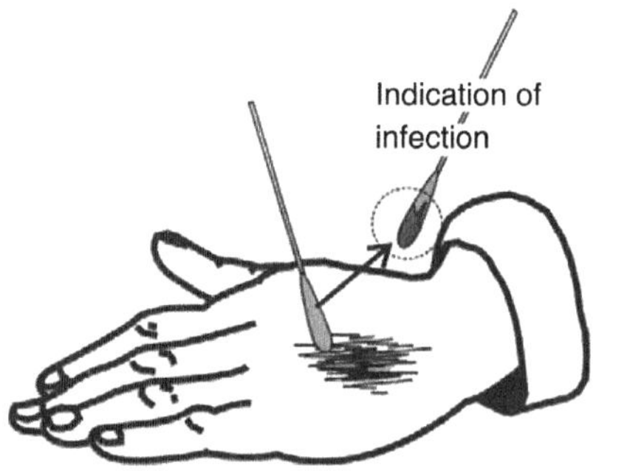

Figure 5.10 ***Proposed implementation of the "traffic light" pH swab.***

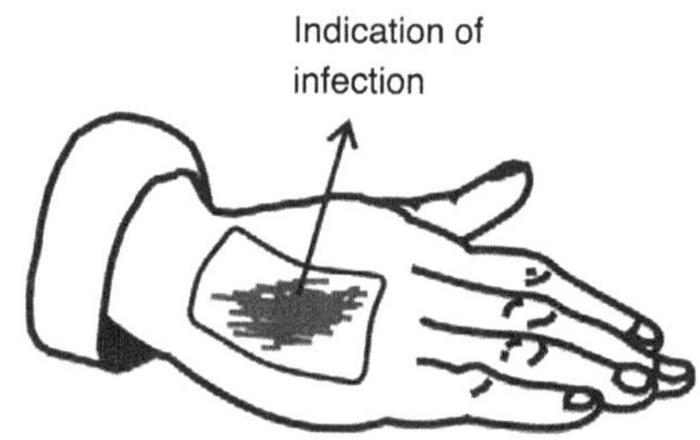

Figure 5.11 ***Proposed pH-sensitive bandage by Trupp and coworkers.***

5.8.2 Quantitative Wound pH Imaging

In contrast, Schreml and coworkers took a more quantitative approach through employing a luminescent detection technique to obtain two-dimensional images of oxygen and pH distributions across the wound bed [31]. Palladium(II)-meso-tetraphenyltetrabenzoporphyrin was deployed within poly(styrene-co-acrylonitrile) microparticles as the oxygen probe [32–34] with fluorescein–isothiocyanate covalently immobilized on aminoethylcellulose microparticles as the pH-dependent system. The microparticles sensing elements were then embedded in a polyurethane hydrogel layer with a transparent poly(vinylidenechloride) (PVdC) interface layer to provide mechanical support and prevent leaching of the components into the wound bed itself. The basic structure of the approach is highlighted in Fig. 5.12.

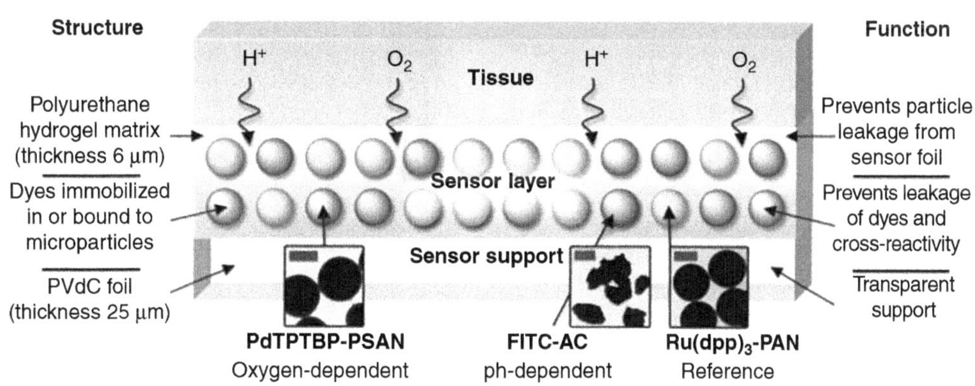

Figure 5.12 ***Modified dressing for measuring pH and pO_2 [31].***

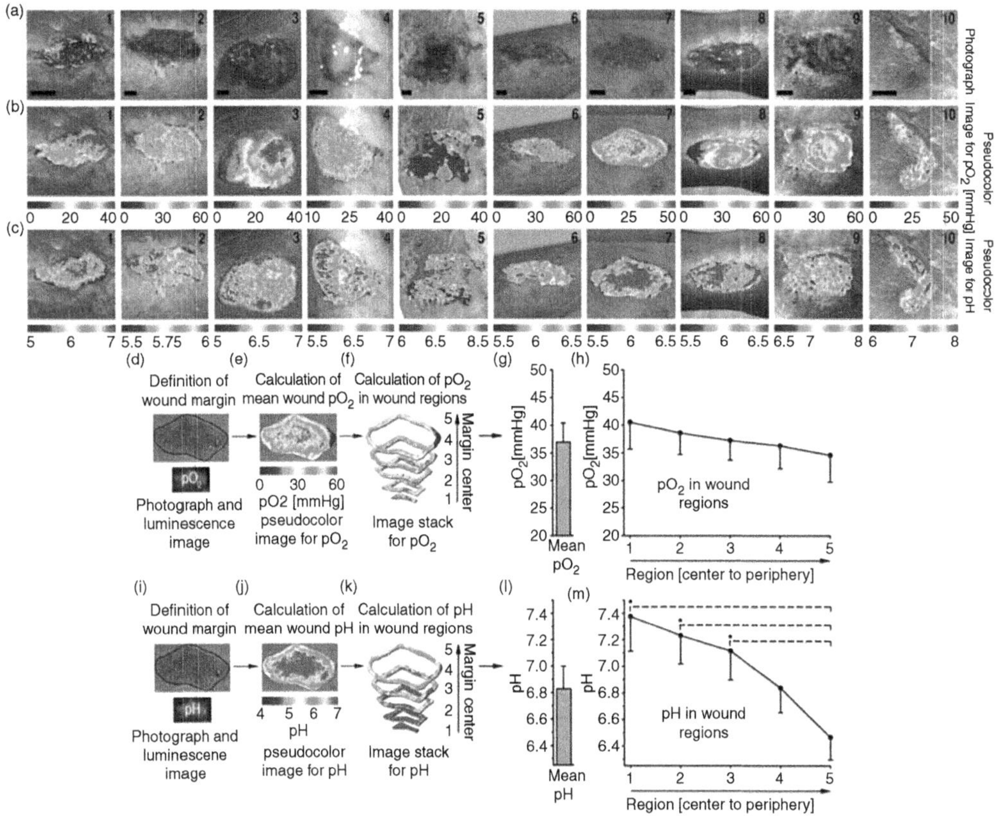

Figure 5.13 ***Spatial patterns of*** pO_2 ***and pHe on chronic wound surfaces.*** (a) Photographs of chronic venous ulcers on the lower legs of patients. Scale bars, 1 cm. (b, c) Distribution of pHe and pO_2 in chronic wounds. pO_2 values range from 0 up to 60 mmHg with high spatial variability. pHe values range from ~5 up to ~8 with high interindividual variability. In large areas, pHe increased from the wound peripheries toward the wound centers. (d, i) After defining the wound margins, mean pO_2/pHe for the entire wound surface was calculated (e,j,g,l). (f, k) Self-programmed computerized macros (Materials and Methods, Macro S1) served to obtain pO_2/pHe-data for the different wound regions. (g, l) Mean pO_2 mounted to ~37 mmHg for the entire wound surface, and mean pHe was ~6.8. (h) A relatively homogenous distribution of pO_2 values was found when analyzing data from all wound regions. (m) There were significant differences in pHe values between the wound periphery and regions in the wound center. A pHe gradient was found, starting with high mean pHe in the wound center (~7.4) and decreasing to low pHe near the wound margins (~6.5). n = 10, mean ± s.e.m., one-way ANOVA $p < 0.001$, $*p < 0.05$ in post-hoc Tukey tests [31].

The luminescence was detected using a charge-coupled device (CCD) camera and the signal separated by optical filters. Sample data collected using the sensing foil is highlighted in Fig. 5.13. The sensing layer needs to be applied with a degree of caution to avoid the entrapment of air bubbles which will compromise the oxygen and proton measurements, but the polymeric membrane has been found to be sufficiently flexible so as to conform to the wound enabling surface wetting and subsequent adherence to the wound contours [31]. The sensing foil is photoexcited with an appropriate LED and the time gated luminescence signals acquired and pseudo-colour maps of the respective oxygen and pH levels rendered as shown in Fig. 5.13. The system is a highly sophisticated tool which may be more applicable to investigation into wound dynamics than routine diagnostics. Schreml et al. [31] demonstrated the presence of extracellular pH gradients that were found to negatively influence keratinocyte viability, proliferation, and migration at the wound periphery. This can have significant implications for wound closure where decreasing pH within the wound center inhibits keratinocyte recruitment. The acquisition of such information is clearly of diagnostic benefit and may offer the possibility of more targeted/spatial therapeutic interventions, but there is a considerable expertise and equipment overhead in its application. While extensive information can be obtained, its application will be more suitable for use within a clinic setting.

An alternative approach to the use of CCDs was proposed by Sawada, Hizawa and colleagues [35,36]. Rather than employing a luminescent indicator system, their strategy employed a solid state membrane based on silicon nitride (Si_3N_4) to serve as a pH-sensitive layer which is scanned by an integrated analysis system to provide a two-dimensional pH image of the wound. The system is built on a CMOS fabrication system as outlined in Fig. 5.14. The prototype system is based on a 10 by 10 pixel array covering a size of 5.1 x 5.1 mm [36]. The system has been shown to provide a sensitivity (50.9 mv/pH) which is consistent with most ion-selective electrochemical systems (discussed in the next section). Although the device heralds a considerable achievement in terms of the underlying engineering, there are considerable limitations to its implementation. The cost of the device, especially if considering disposability, will be a major impediment. Moreover, the limited resolution, positioning within irregular wounds, and conformity to the wound are all issues that would need to be overcome.

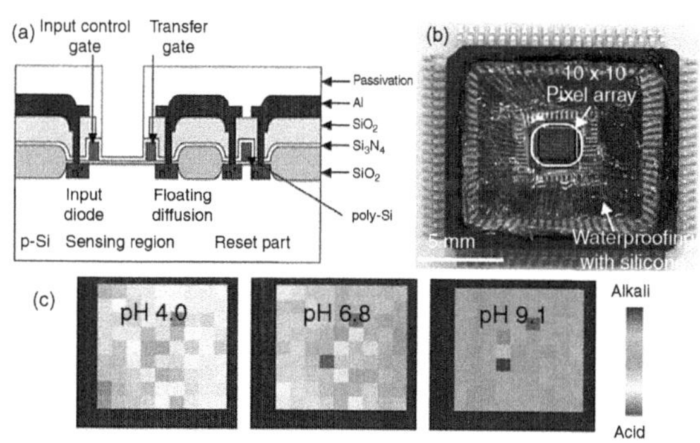

Figure 5.14 ***Silicon nitride CCD pH imaging [36].***

5.8.3 Radiofrequency Identification Optical Sensors

There have been many developments in the use of wireless protocols (Bluetooth, Zigbee, etc.) for sensing applications [37–39] and many of these are discussed in detail within Chapter 7. Radiofrequency identification (RFID) was originally intended for product identification applications that could be scanned over a very short range (typically less than 2 m) [39,40]. It has however received considerable interest as potential adjunct to chemical sensors [38–40] and could be ideally suited toward wound monitoring. Given its present use as a label for consumer goods, the production of economically viable sensors could, in principle, be exploited for use in wounds that need frequent replacement. Steinberg and Steinberg have developed a contactless, battery-free, optical sensor based on an RFID protocol [40]. The sensing layer involves the encapsulation of a pH-sensitive dye (Bromocresol Green) within a sol-gel film. The sol-gel approach to chemical sensors is well established [41], but few have been applied to a wound context and there are some disadvantages to the approach—leaching of the dye and the relative inflexibility of the matrix with the encapsulated indicator dye to probe across the wound fluid.

A schematic outlining the basis of the approach is highlighted in Fig. 5.15 [40]. The RFID-based sensor does not possess a battery but is powered by a vicinity-integrated circuit card (VICC) that passively harvests energy from an electromagnetic field generated

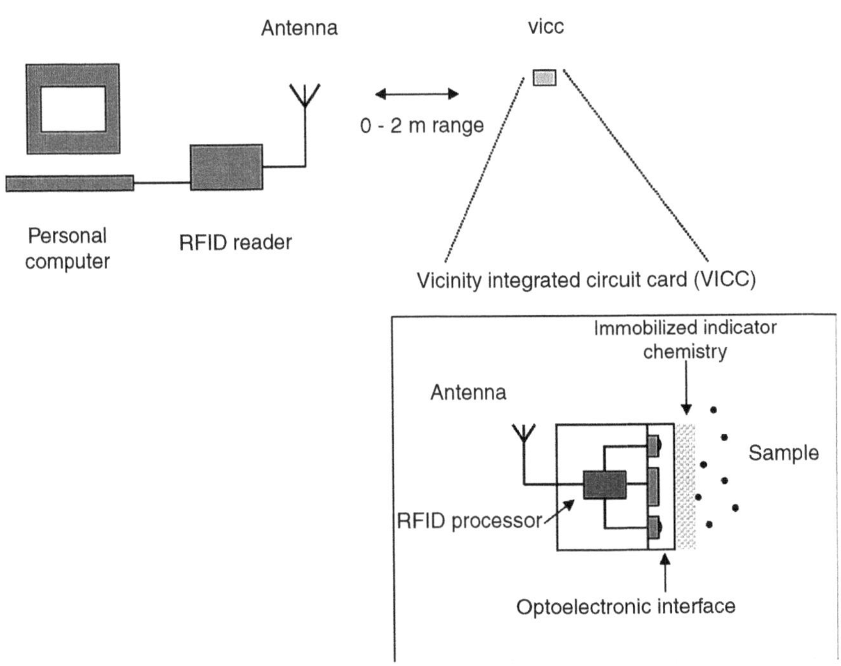

Figure 5.15 ***RFID pH detection methodology [40].***

by a suitable reader [40]. The prototype sensor consists of the antenna, the RFID processor, the optoelectronic interface, and sol-gel/indicator interface.

The detection methodology is based on the differential absorbance of light measured at two wavelengths: 435 nm and 619 nm capturing λ_{max} for the protonated and deprotonated forms of bromocresol green respectively [40]. The two LEDs on the VICC tag were tuned to 505 nm (the isobestic point used as a reference) and 619 nm with the intensity from each measured by a photodiode and allowed a measurement range of pH 5.2–pH 8.3 which covers the majority of pH transitions expected within a chronic wound [25]. The RFID sensor has yet to be tested on complex matrices, and it is likely that there could be substantial interference given the wavelengths being used, but while the applicability of sensing component may be questionable, the underlying technology clearly has considerable promise.

5.9 ELECTROCHEMICAL pH SYSTEMS

There are a large number of commercial electrochemical probes for monitoring pH but the majority are based on the traditional glass bulb electrode and designed predominantly for use within a bioanalytical laboratory. The fragility of the glass membrane renders these conventional systems almost unusable for direct monitoring of wound pH, but there have been significant advances in the design methodologies employed in recent years. These have arisen largely in response to the limitations of the traditional glass potentiometric systems [1,2,43], but it must be noted not all are designed specifically for biomedical contexts, nor can they all be readily applied to the latter. The introduction of electrochemical sensor systems within wound-monitoring contexts gives rise to numerous concerns such as probe size and disposability and is hampered by situations where sample volume can be limited (ie, dry wounds or those with low exudate). A number of approaches have been pursued in an effort to address these issues and both potentiometric [42–55] and voltammetric [56–67] methodologies have been investigated. To confer selectivity, a functional material containing a pH-sensitive component is normally applied to the surface of the sensor substrate. A variety of modification methods and designs have been assessed that include adsorption of monolayers [50,59], polymer films [37,54], printed inks [36,39,41,48], covalent binding [47,48], or the use of electrodeposited layers [33,34,38,43–45,53]. A summary of the surface modification and associated sensitivities is presented in Table 5.4.

The need to modify the surface of the sensor is acceptable from the perspective of designing a point of care sensor, but there are clear issues over electrode fouling, biocompatibility, and the possibility of the pH-sensitive component leaching into the biological matrix. As such, the majority of the approaches can become limiting when considering the integration of the sensor within a dressing designed to be worn by the patient.

Table 5.4 Comparison of electrochemical pH sensors

Electrode modifier	Method	mV/pH	Error (mV)
Iridium oxide	P	69	1
Polyglycine	P	52	NS
Ion-selective membrane	P	61	1.7
Metalloporphyrins	P	54	NS
CeO_2	P	51	NS
Carbon nanotubes	P	43	NS
TiO_2 nanotubes	P	54	NS
Co/AI hydroxides	P	76	0.6
Nitroso-phenyl/Ferrocene	V	60	2
Ferrocene/dyad	V	52	NS
Anthraquinone/diphenylphenylenediamine	V	114	NS
Polyplumbagin	V	51	3
Nafion/Benzoquinone	V	59	NS
Uric acid	V	62	NS
Ferrocene/phenathraquinone	V	97	3

Where P = potentiometric; V= voltammetric; NS = not specified.

5.9.1 Screen-Printed Potentiometric Smart Dressings

Wang and co-workers exploited the use of a polyaniline-modified screen-printed sensor to monitor changes in wound pH [68]. Their approach encompasses the concept of a smart bandage with the sensor incorporated on the gauze dressing and encased in an adhesive polymer bandage. The various components are indicated in Fig. 5.16.

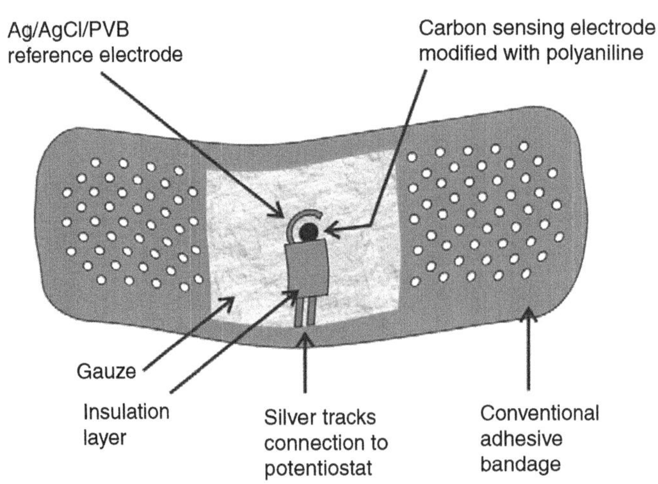

Figure 5.16 ***Smart bandage based on screen printed sensors with a polyaniline (PANI) sensing layer [68].***

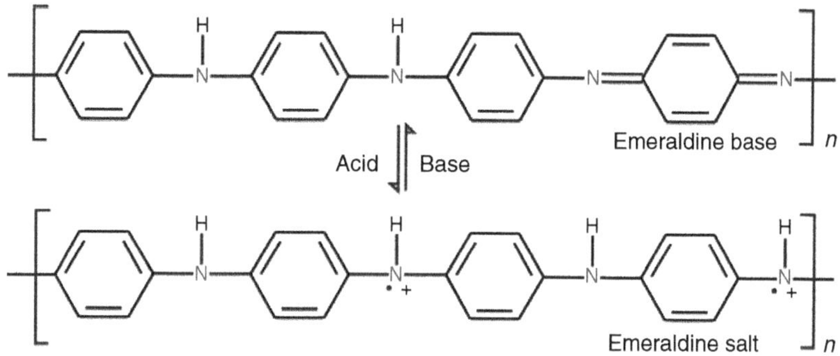

Figure 5.17 ***pH transition of the emeraldine salt and bases within polyaniline.***

The analytical signal arises from measuring the potential difference between the working (sensing) electrode and the PVB/silver–silver chloride reference. The carbon layer is modified with polyaniline and the system exploits the transition between the emeraldine salt and emeraldine base moieties within the polymer backbone [69–71], as indicated in Fig. 5.17. The strategy deftly combines the manufacturing simplicity/reproducibility of screen printing with solid state potentiometry and the devices have been shown to exhibit a conventional Nernstian behavior over pH 4-pH 8 as indicated in Fig. 5.18.

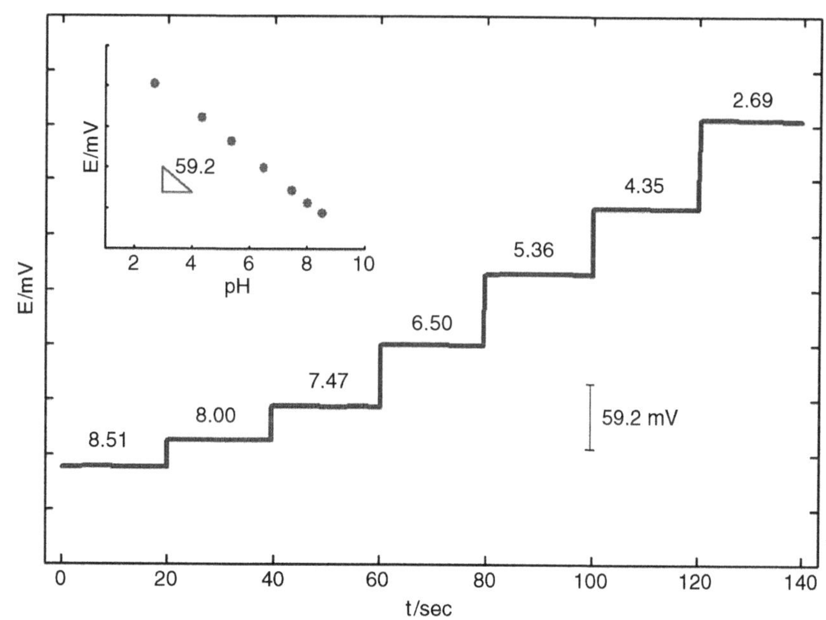

Figure 5.18 ***Potentiometric response to varying pH at the polyaniline smart bandage [68].***

The system offers several advantages in terms of the simplicity of its operation, but there are a number of limitations—particularly the need to modify the surface with an exogenous component.

5.9.2 Carbon Fiber pH Sensors

One innovative approach to counter this issue was proposed by Anderson et al. [72] whereby carbon fiber was used to probe pH. Carbon fiber, more commonly associated with high specification structural engineering applications, is particularly interesting in the present context as it is mechanically flexible, conductive, and relatively inexpensive. The electroanalytical performance of the unmodified fiber is, however, relatively poor and initial studies found a distinct lack of selectivity toward changes in pH from either potentiometric or voltammetric methodologies. Rather than add exogenous groups onto the surface, Anderson's team exploited the redox chemistry endogenous to the carbon surface itself as a means of enhancing the pH response through a voltammetric approach. In contrast to the more passive potentiometric system utilized by Wang, voltammetry examines the current response as a function of potential. Different electroactive species can give rise to different voltammetric profiles as indicated in Fig. 5.19.

A complete description of the underlying principles of the techniques and different waveforms employed is beyond the scope of this book, but there are a substantial number of resources available [73–75]. In essence, the technique examines the oxidation-reduction characteristics of a particular target analyte such that upon applying a sufficient potential at the electrode surface, transfer of electrons occurs and can give rise to a peak-like profile as indicated in Fig. 5.19. The position of the peak can give some indication as to the identity of the analyte and the magnitude of the current is proportional to the concentration within the sample. The principal issue with voltammetry of complex matrices (particularly biofluids) relates to the fact that there will be a large number of candidate molecules that can be oxidized or reduced and this can lead to overlapping signals which obscure the response of the target biomarker (Fig. 5.19). The challenge is to obtain a clear, unambiguous signal from one particular target without interference from the milieu. Voltammetry has been extensively used for electroanalytical purposes, and, in most cases, the surface of the electrode is modified to confer selectivity toward a given analyte [76] but it is only recently that it has employed for the measurement of pH. The approach taken has generally been to exploit the pH dependence of a redox couple—typically quinone-hydroquinone (Q/H_2Q) systems. The analytical signal is extracted by measuring the peak position of the oxidation processes associated with the hydroquinone moiety. As the system involves a transfer of protons, there is an inherent pH dependence, and thus the position of the oxidation peak can be related to the pH of the sample in accordance with the well-established Nernst relationship of 0.059 m/n V/pH (m/n is the ratio of protons to electrons). In this case, the quinoid forms are present as an integral component of the carbon surface as indicated in Fig. 5.20.

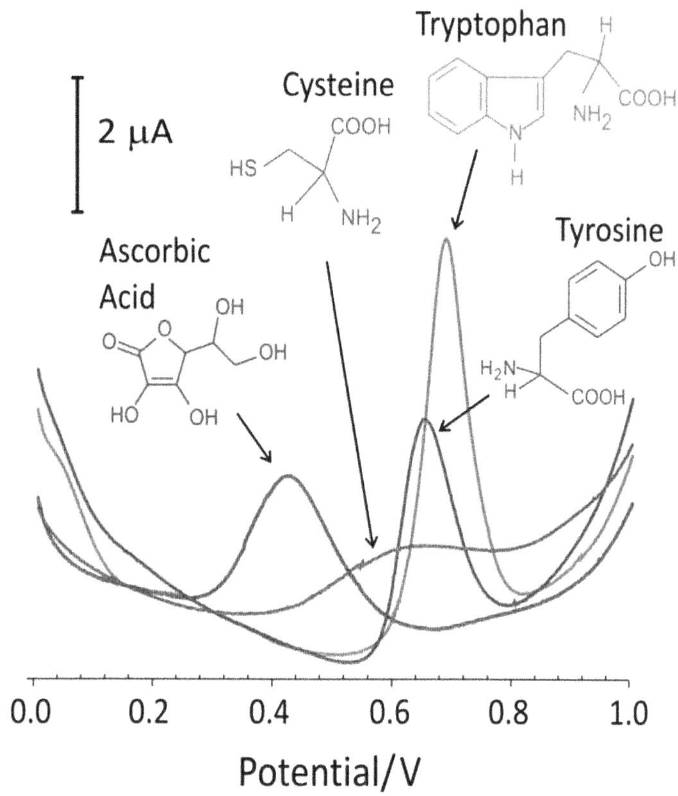

Figure 5.19 ***Square wave voltammograms of common electroactive species liable to be encountered within a wound sample.***

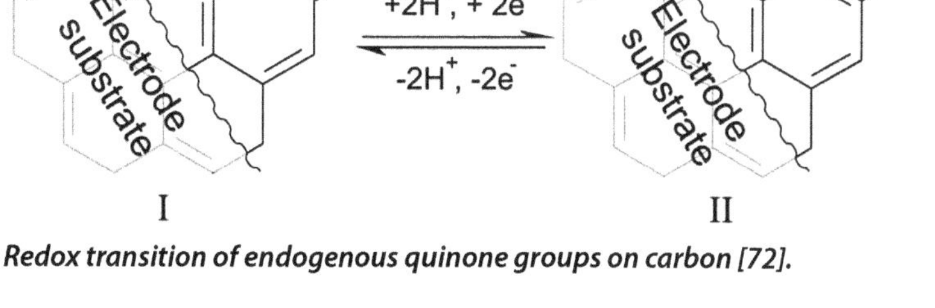

Figure 5.20 ***Redox transition of endogenous quinone groups on carbon [72].***

The endogenous population of quinone groups on conventional, unprocessed carbon fiber is relatively low and hence the failure of initial experiments to establish a relationship between the electrode response and pH. The surface of the carbon electrode can, however, be manipulated to increase the proportion of redox groups through a variety of processes such as laser ablation, plasma treatment, or electrochemical oxidation. Anderson's approach was to utilize the latter to modify the electrode behavior. This technique has been widely used to enhance electrode performance for a large range of analytes as it fractures the underlying carbon and results in a marked increase in edge plane sites [66,67]. It could be anticipated that quinoid functionality would be similarly increased and that this would lead to a more identifiable redox peak process from which to indirectly determine pH. Examination of carbon fiber before and after electrochemical anodization was conducted using X-ray photoelectrospectroscopy (XPS) to identify changes in the surface profile and two examples are compared in Fig. 5.21 [72].

It can be seen that there is a marked change in the chemical functionality at the electrode surface and corresponds to the exfoliation of the carbon—partially destroying the sp^2 character but dramatically increasing the proportion of quinoid groups (as indicated by the C = O peak in Fig. 5.21). Square wave voltammograms comparing the response of the carbon fiber before and after electrochemical anodization are shown in Fig. 5.22a. The response of the anodized fiber to varying pH is indicated in Fig. 5.22b.

The integration of the carbon figure as a working, standalone sensor has been demonstrated through its encapsulation within a novel laminate manufacturing process outlined in Fig. 5.23. The design strategy involves encasing conductive carbon fiber filaments (10 μm diameter) within a laminate layer (2 mm wide) which served as the sensing electrode. A second sheath containing a chloridized silver wire (50 μm diameter, 10 mm length exposed) served as the combined reference-counter electrode. The approach offers numerous advantages over conventional colorimetric swabs through offering a quantitative analysis, yet retaining the disposability and inexpense associated with carbon fiber. A major advantage however is the small dimensions of the assembled probe which could enable the rapid analysis of ultrasmall samples of wound fluid. The design outlined in Fig. 5.23 highlights the adaptation of the system for use within a point of care context, but it could be extrapolated for use as sensor within a conventional dressing.

5.9.3 Screen-Printed Voltammetric Sensors

The techniques listed in Table 5.4 have the potential for transfer to a wound context, but their applicability has yet to be tested and most focus on the underpinning science rather than providing a critical examination of their clinical use/accessibility. There are

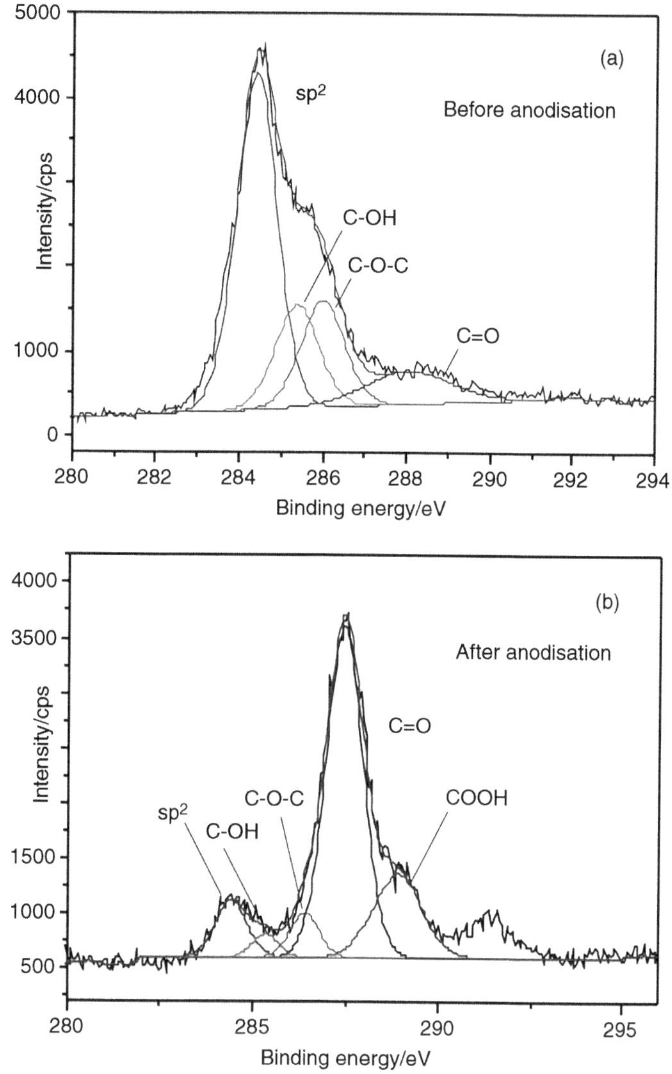

Figure 5.21 ***XPS profiles of carbon fiber before and after electrochemical anodization [72].***

however a number of important exceptions. Phair et al. [67] proposed a screen-printed sensor specifically designed for assessing wound pH based on the voltammetric determination of uric acid and the various components used in its construction are shown in Fig. 5.24.

In contrast to many of the approaches listed in Table 5.4, the sensor does not rely on the modification of the electrode substrate with an exogenous pH-sensitive

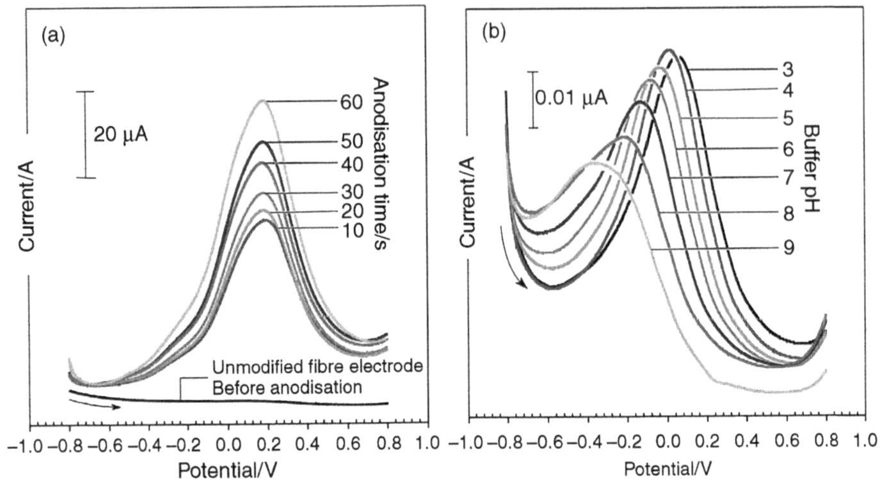

Figure 5.22 (a) Voltammograms highlighting the creation of quinoid groups on the carbon surface. (b) Influence of pH on the redox behavior of the endogenous quinones [72].

indicator. In this case, the sensor relies on the oxidation of urate which will be present within the wound fluid to provide an indirect measure of the pH. Uric acid is ubiquitous within biofluids as a consequence of the catabolism of purines and is relatively easy to detect at a conventional, unmodified, electrode [77]—in most electroanalytical applications it is considered to be a rather pernicious interference precisely due to these characteristics [76,77]. The oxidation of urate involves protons (Fig. 5.25) and thus the peak position of the associated electrode process will be dependent upon the prevailing pH within the solution (or wound fluid). This is analogous to the approach taken by Anderson but in this case the oxidation peak is due to a diffusing solution based species rather than quinone groups anchored within the carbon substrate [67]. Square wave voltammograms detailing the response to urate under different pH regimes are compared in Fig. 5.26 where it can be seen that there is a distinct shift in the peak position.

The shift in the position of the oxidation peak can be used as the basis of a calibration graph from which the pH of an unknown sample could be determined. The single disposability of the system does not adequately meet the objectives of the Harding Consensus document as it still requires the use of the device by the healthcare provider [3]. It does, however, offer a much more direct route to manufacture that the laminate system proffered by Anderson and it could be envisaged that the printing of sensors through large-scale web processes akin to that used in glucose strip manufacture could be possible.

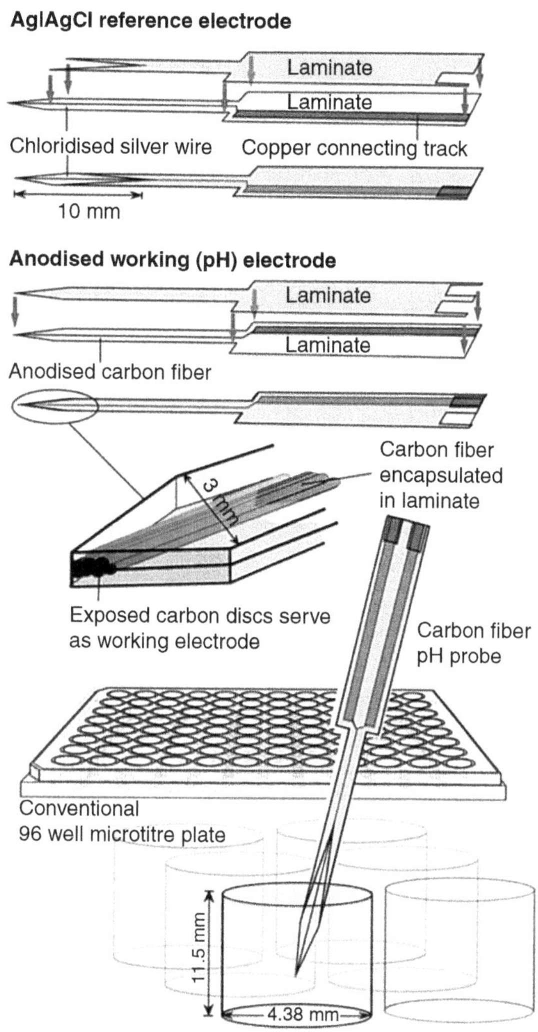

Figure 5.23 ***Probe design specifications [72].***

It could be argued that it could be exploited much in the same way as glucose meters and effectively used by the patients themselves to monitor the condition of the wound but, in reality, compliance will be a major issue [78,79]. The ideal approach, as advocated in Chapter 1, would center on the development of a system that periodically monitors the pH—providing telemetry of the wound condition which can be viewed by the healthcare professional. This requires the integration of the device within the dressing itself.

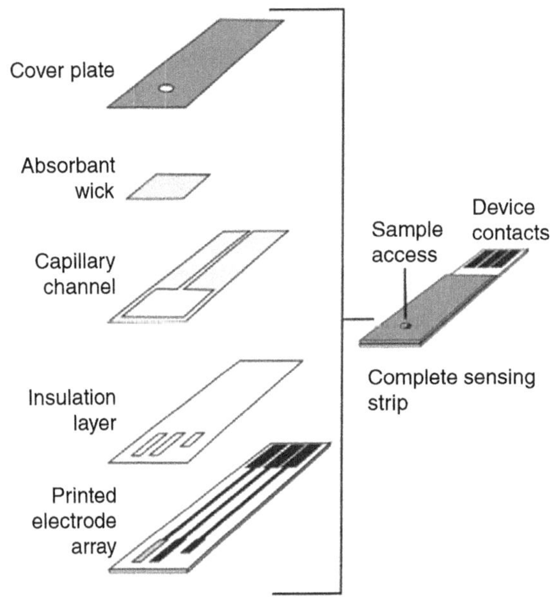

Figure 5.24 ***Fabrication of the screen printed urate pH sensor [67].***

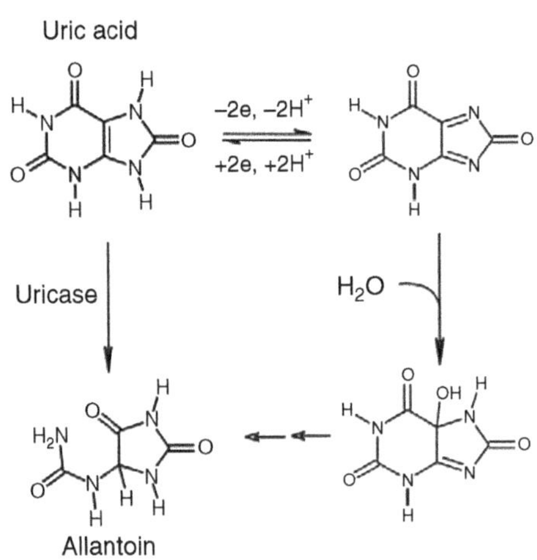

Figure 5.25 ***Electrochemical oxidation of urate.***

5.9.4 Carbon Fiber Weave Dressings

Dowsett et al. [6] conducted a survey to elucidate the key factor involved in the treatment of wounds within the United Kingdom and while many of the results have already been discussed in the previous chapters, the issue of dressing changes needs to be highlighted here. It was reported that the average number of dressing changes was X per week [6]. This has significant ramifications for the development of a smart dressing in

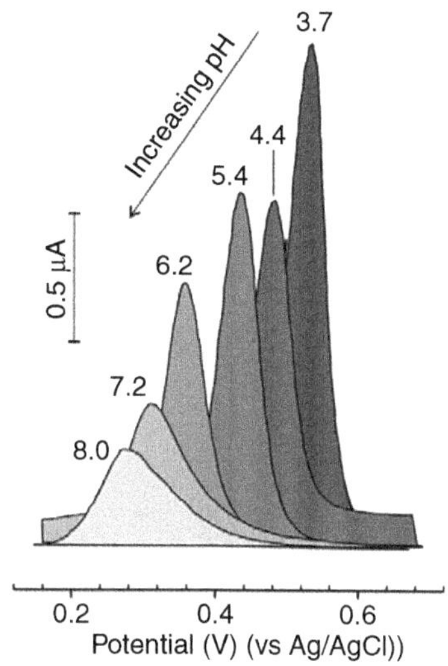

Figure 5.26 ***Influence of pH on the voltammetric response to urate at a screen-printed sensor [67].***

that the technology being employed must be inherently disposable and therefore come at a low cost. The ability to produce large numbers of sensors through the screen printing technique could go some way to addressing such concerns. One issue with the use of a single, discrete probe would relate to the positioning within the dressing to ensure that the sensing element was active. This requires that the sensor is in contact with the wound fluid such that a measurement can be obtained. It also assumes that the measurement is representative of the wound fluid in general and is not due to an isolated pocket of fluid, disconnected from the main wound bed.

One innovative approach to overcome this issue employed aspects of both carbon fiber and urate analysis as the core detection rationale. The carbon fiber weave is sufficiently flexible to follow the contours of wounds that can present a highly variable surface morphology and can be manufactured in the volumes necessary to enable the mass production of dressing at relatively low cost [80]. It was envisaged that the carbon component would provide the framework for electrochemical transduction enabling quantitative information on key biomarkers associated with wound healing to be extracted through an appropriate electronic monitor—worn either by the patient or connected at the time of consultation. As indicated in the work by Anderson, the structure of the carbon can be readily modified to enhance the electrochemical performance—either using endogenous quinone groups [72] or exploiting the presence of uric acid [67]. It could be envisaged that the carbon fiber weave (Fig. 5.27a) could be directly inserted between the dressing layers as indicated in Fig. 5.27b.

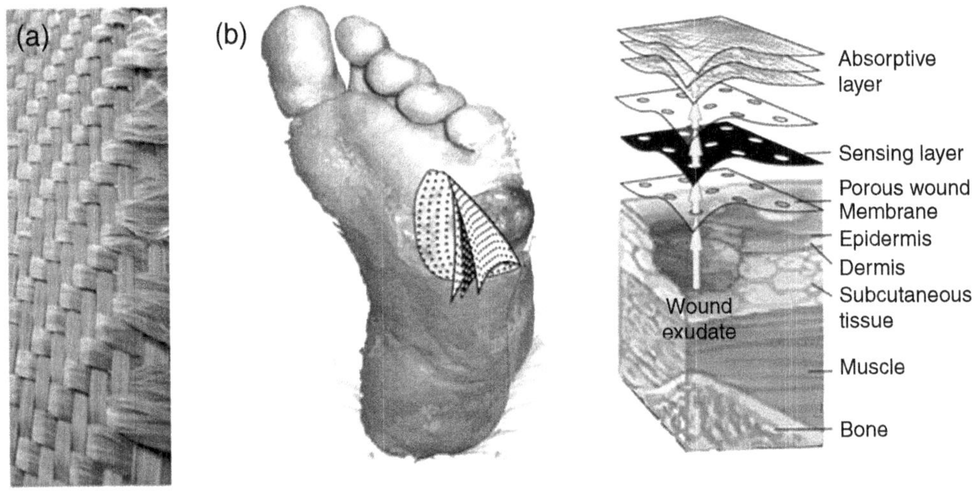

Figure 5.27 (a) Structure of the carbon fiber weave and (b) proposed implementation.

5.9.5 Carbon Composite Film Dressings

Carbon fiber can present some additional issues in that, although generally flexible, the fracturing of individual fibers could contaminate the wound with fragments that could exacerbate the irritation and lead to a prolonging of inflammation. An alternative has been proffered in which a carbon composite polymer based on polyethylene doped with carbon particles that could be integrated within a conventional wound dressing [81,82]. The core rationale is similar to that outlined in Fig. 5.27 but with the polymer film replacing the carbon fiber weave. This would be a more viable solution given the inherent mechanical flexibility of the composite film—a prerequisite given the high degree of morphological variability encountered with chronic wounds. This approach also stands in marked contrast to the brittleness associated with the carbon fiber matting [80] previously investigated and offers the critical advantage of component simplicity (requiring only carbon and polyethylene) which could be manufactured using conventional bulk polymer processing techniques and not dissimilar to those used for the manufacture of film-based dressings [81,82].

The carbon-polymer approach has clear advantages but it also has some significant drawbacks in that the effective electrode area through which to analyze the sample is relatively small. Despite the film being large—it must be remembered that the composite effectively consists of carbon particles (nm-micron diameter) encapulsated within a sea of polymer as highlighted in Fig. 5.28.

The electrode is only active where the carbon particles breach the film and interact with the wound fluid. This is highlighted in Fig. 5.29 where scanning electron micrographs of a carbon–polyethylene film before and after the electrodeposition of silver are

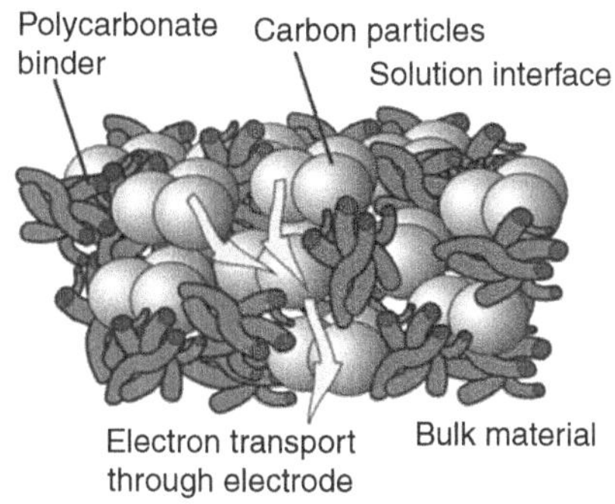

Figure 5.28 ***Schematic highlighting the composite nature of the carbon-loaded films.***

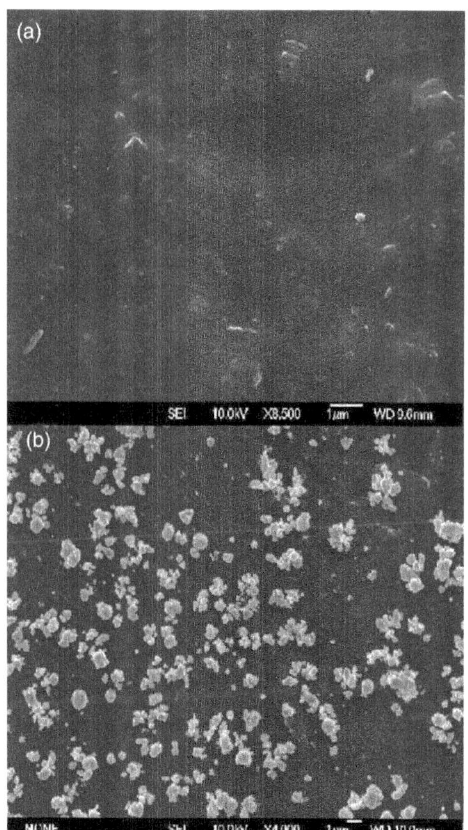

Figure 5.29 ***Scanning electron micrographs detailing the surface of the carbon-loaded polyethylene–carbon electrode before and after the electrodeposition of silver [81].***

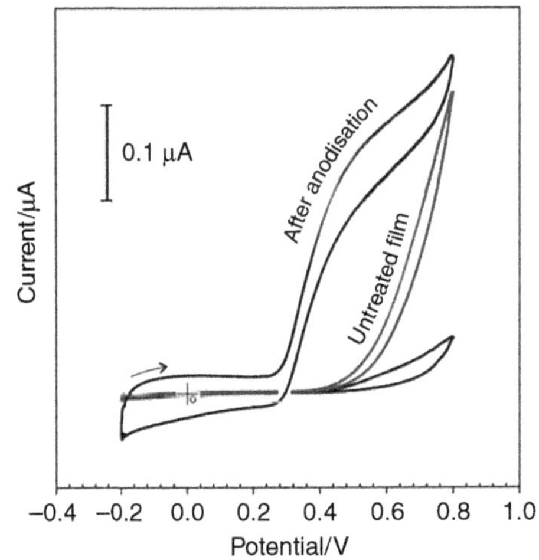

Figure 5.30 ***Cyclic voltammograms detailing the response of the untreated and anodized polyethylene electrode toward 0.244 mM urate (pH 7). Scan rate: 50 mV/s [81].***

compared [81]. It can be seen that the silver deposits appear as microcrystals randomly distributed across the surface of the film and can be attributed to those areas where the carbon particles are exposed and hence capable of facilitating the electro-reduction of silver ion from the solution.

The electroanalytical performance of the film was found to be relatively poor and can be attributed to the fact that the predominant form of the carbon encapsulated within the polymer is a basal plane. It has long been recognized that faster electron transfer and hence improved analytical performance can be obtained at edge plane carbon sites. The latter can be created in situ through the use of electrochemical anodization (as discussed previously in the case of Anderson's carbon fiber probe [72]). Cyclic voltammograms detailing the responses of the film before and after electrochemical anodization toward urate (0.244 mM, pH 7) are shown in Fig. 5.30. As expected, the unmodified film displays very little response to urate and has no diagnostic capability and is similar to the responses observed with the untreated carbon fiber. Electrochemical anodization of the film however had a significant impact on the response, resulting in a sigmoidal profile which is a characteristic of microelectrode behavior and further emphasizes the fact that the interfacial carbon is distributed across the film as isolated islands. It was postulated that the microelectrode behavior arises as a consequence of the relative spatial isolation of the carbon particles at the interface [81].

The polymer film indicated in Fig. 5.29 is impermeable to gases and moisture and therefore would form an occlusive membrane which would be less than ideal as noted in Chapter 4. A key advantage of the film approach lies in the fact that the substrate can easily be manipulated through a variety of processing techniques and patterned to suit

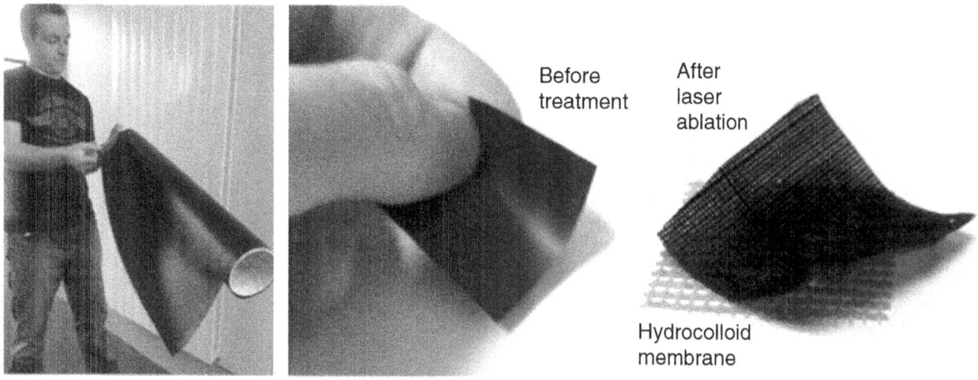

Figure 5.31 ***Carbon-loaded polyethylene before and after laser treatment.***

a given application. Therefore, it is possible to create pores (from the nano-to the milli scale) that can enable the transport of gases and exudate. In the case of the carbon-loaded polyethylene, Phair et al. [81,82] demonstrated the use of laser ablation as a means of creating a mesh within micron size pores (Fig. 5.31), but which, as a consequence of the processing, activated the electroanalytical properties of the resulting film.

Rastering the laser across the film to create trenches in the film had the effect of creating a pore where the laser paths crossed, but it was noted that the laser effectively removed the polymer resulting in more of the carbon being exposed. This can be seen in the electron micrographs in Fig. 5.32 where there is an increase in the surface roughness where the laser has passed.

The laser-etched film can be employed as indicated in Fig. 5.27 as an additional layer within a conventional dressing assembly with the mesh structure enabling the transport of exudates through the film to an overlying gauze or foam absorbant. In doing so, the fluid contacts the sensing surfaces and a pH measurement can be made on the basis of uric acid oxidation—analogous to the methodology employed in the screen print sensor shown in Fig. 5.26. The key advantage is that it avoids errors associated with spatial positioning with the mesh covering the entire wound surface.

5.9.6 Peptide Redox Wires for pH Sensing

An alternative approach to pH measurement within wounds was proposed by McLister and co-workers where tryptophan was used as an indirect indicator of pH [83,84]. In contrast to the use of uric acid, McLister employed a homo polypeptide of tryptophan which effectively immobilized the electroactive moieties at the electrode surface [83,84]. The core rationale relates to the electrochemical generation of quinoid functional groups on the indole substituent of the tryptophan which is propagated along the length of the peptide chain and effectively creates a redox wire [84]. The reaction mechanism is highlighted in Fig. 5.33.

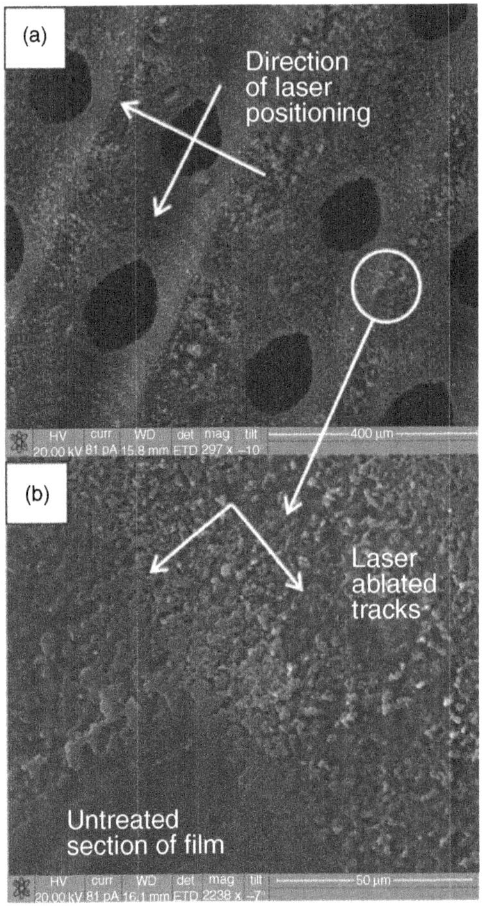

Figure 5.32 ***Scanning electron micrographs of the carbon-loaded polyethylene after laser ablation.*** (a) Effect of x-y rastering on the creation of pores and (b) the ablation of the polymer to leave behind carbon particles [81].

The main rationale behind using poly-L-tryptophan was on the basis that the peak positions of the electrogenerated quinoid functionalities would be pH responsive. This was postulated on the fact that there is a 2 electron, 2 proton transition between the oxidized and reduced components. Therefore, it could be envisaged that the peak potential will shift by −0.059 V per pH unit in accordance with previously published voltammetric pH sensor data [46–58,72]. The voltammograms shown in Fig. 5.34 certainly shift with pH; however, the relationship is sub-Nernstian (Epa (V) = −0.051 pH + 0.462; n = 6; R2 = 0.993) over pH 3 to pH 8. This can be ascribed in part to the slight broadening of the peak at higher pH [84].

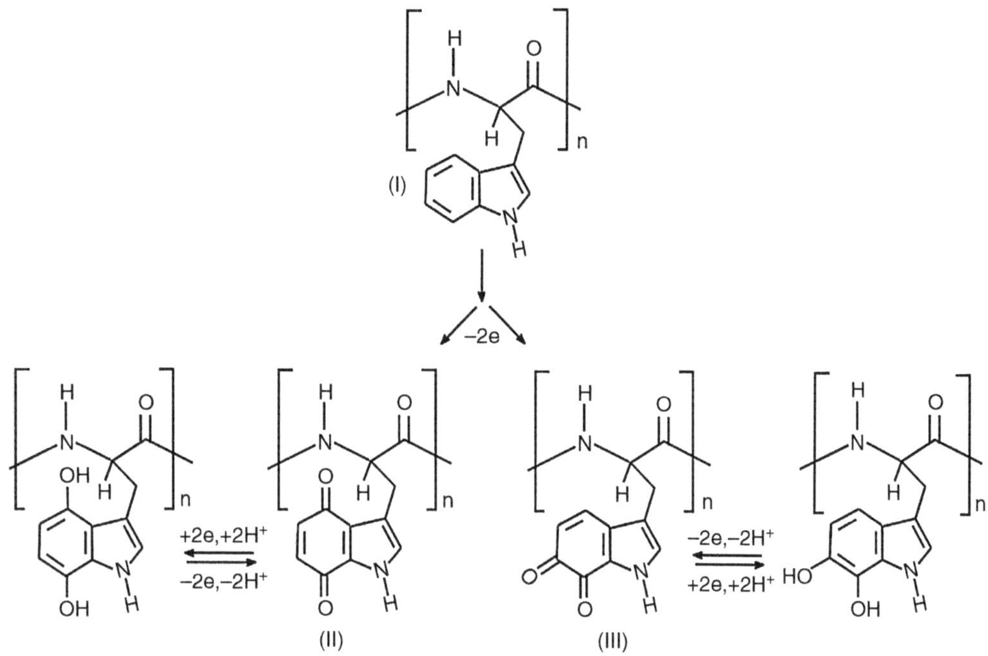

Figure 5.33 ***Electrochemical oxidation of polymer bound tryptophan to the corresponding quinone systems and their corresponding hydroquinone redox system [84].***

5.9.7 Reference Electrode Issues

In both cases, a silver–silver chloride reference was used, but there is an implicit assumption that the chloride concentration will remain constant. This is of concern as while it can be anticipated that the chloride concentration within the blood will be tightly regulated, the dynamics of the wound could be more variable, depending on the injury.

This calibration issue has been addressed, in principle, by measuring the potential difference between two redox peaks to determine the pH. The method employs the use of a pH-sensitive redox indicator such as hydroquinone alkylthiol, anthracene, or nitrophenyl group together with a pH-insensitive redox species such as alkylferrocene [56–61]. Lawrence and coworkers have pioneered a number of these types of systems and an example is highlighted in Fig. 5.35 where the electrode substrate is modified with an anthraquinone–ferrocene conjugate [62].

This molecule has two distinct voltammetric functional groups that differ markedly in redox potential and dependence on pH. The anthraquinone is sensitive to pH whereas the ferrocene is unaffected. This is highlighted in Fig. 5.36 where the voltammetric signature for the anthraquinone moiety moves toward more positive potentials with pH and the ferrocene oxidation remains fixed at +0.4 V [62].

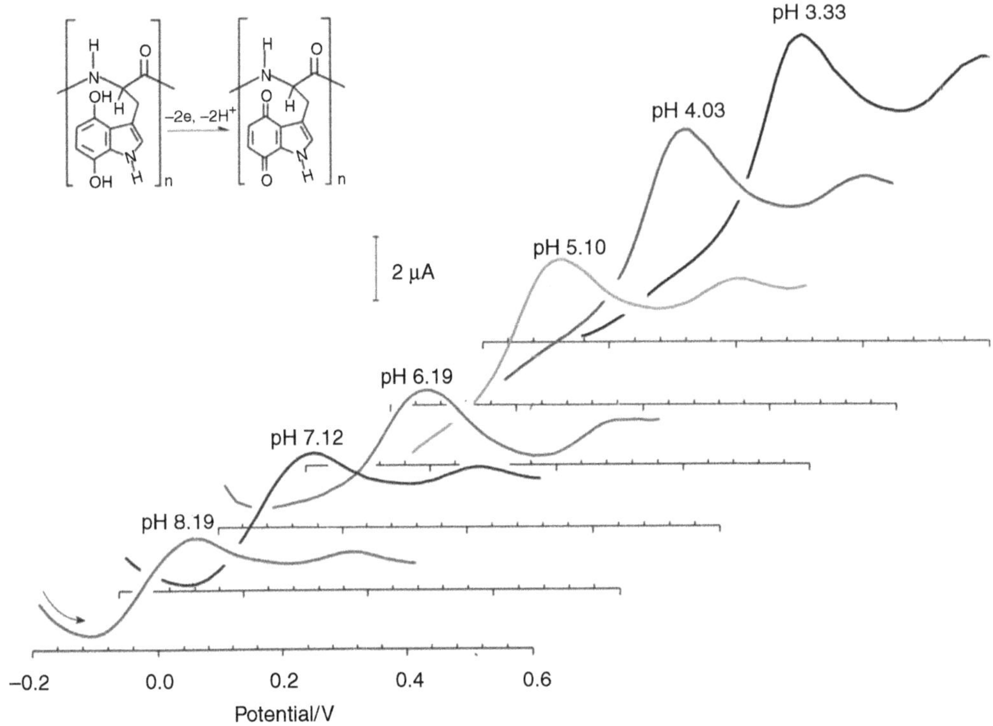

Figure 5.34 ***Square wave voltammograms detailing the influence of solution pH on the response of the poly-tryptophan—carbon fiber composite electrode [84].***

A number of these systems have been investigated with disposable SPE platforms [58] and although the stability of the systems toward pH within control/model solutions is not in question, they have yet to be trialled within a complex matrix like wound fluid. It is also important to assess the influence of other electroactive constituents within the wound fluid and nonspecific absorption of protein absorption onto the surface.

5.10 HYDROGEL SENSORS

An alternative electronic approach to pH measurement which avoids the issues with the reference electrode was proposed by Sridhar and Takahata [85]. Their design was based on the dimensional changes of a hydrogel layer (poly(vinyl alcohol)–poly(acrylic acid) brought about through changes in pH. A schematic of the proposed device is detailed in Fig. 5.37 and the fabrication processes highlighted in Figs. 5.38. The device is based on an inductive transducer (formed from a dual coil sandwich) and which can facilitate wireless reporting. When the hydrogel swells or contracts, there will be change in the inductance which can be measured external to the system [85].

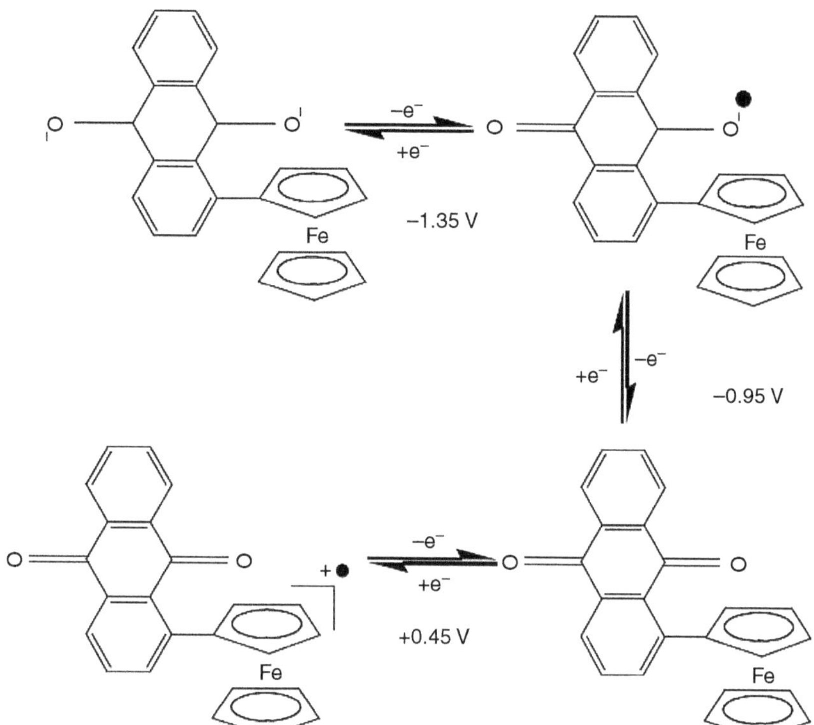

Figure 5.35 ***Structure and redox chemistry of the anthraquinone–ferrocene conjugate [62].***

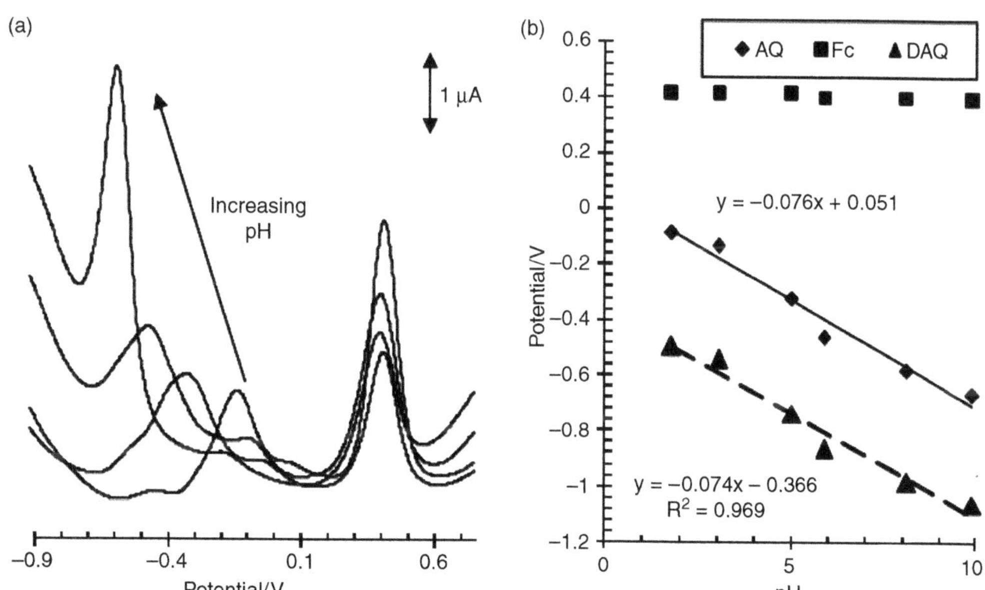

Figure 5.36 (a) Voltammograms detailing the response of the Aq-Fc conjugate to varying pH and (b) corresponding calibration data [62].

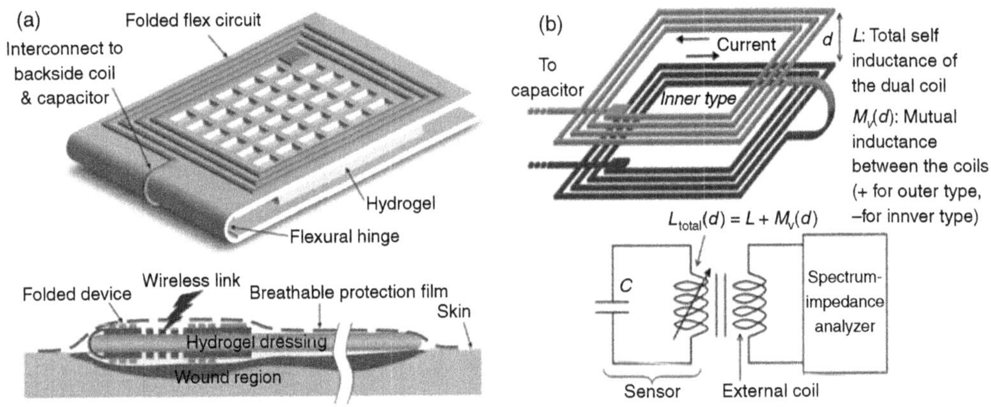

Figure 5.37 ***Inductor coil–sandwich hydrogel system for measuring pH [85].***

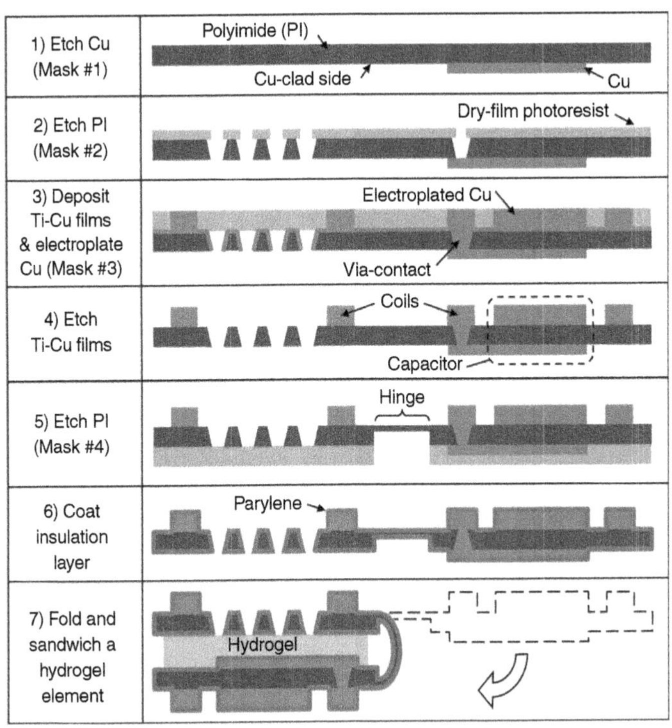

Figure 5.38 ***Fabrication steps in the fabrication of the inductor coil sensor [85].***

In principle, the design provides an elegant option but there are considerable issues over the fabrication and operation of the device. The device is highly dependent upon the hydrogel being mechanically and dimensionally stable under normal condition except in situations where there is a change in pH [85]. This is a large demand and, from the discussion in Chapter 4, will be difficult to fulfil. Hydrogels respond to a host of factors endogenous to the wound but will also be susceptible to external factors (variations in temperature and pressure exerted on the supporting bandage). It may therefore be difficult to acquire a robust measurement in an actual clinical application.

5.11 ENDOGENOUS WOUND BIOMARKERS

The matrix metalloproteinase (MMP) family are key players in the wound-healing process and are responsible for remodeling the extracellular matrix (ECM) through degrading protein matter. Under normal circumstances, they are controlled by their associated tissue inhibiters (TIMPs), but where there is disease or extensive inflammation, the control system can fail, resulting in the over expression of MMPs. The latter has long been recognized as a key factor in chronic wounds, where high MMP activity and low levels of the corresponding TIMPs are used as a critical diagnostic of poor wound healing [86,87]. A number of commercial immunoassays, based on a simple yes/no visual inspection, are available for the detection of MMPs (ie, Systagenix Woundchek discussed in Section 5.5), but a quantitative approach based on an electrochemical assay has been demonstrated by Ciani et al. [88]. The approach involves the immobilization of antibodies for MMP-9 onto gold screen printed electrodes and the use of impedance measurements to quantify the binding events at the electrode. This is effectively a refinement of the lateral flow system outlined earlier and could offer considerable advantages in terms of monitoring more subtle changes in the MMP/TIMPS levels and therein facilitate preemptive treatment. It is however restricted to one shot clinical diagnosis does not possess any capability for transfer to a smart dressing and the requirement for periodic monitoring.

A procedurally simpler approach, involving the measurement of uric acid, has generated considerable interest in recent years as Fernandez et al. [89] have shown that its concentration is elevated as a consequence of tissue remodeling within the wound (Fig. 5.39). The cellular trauma and associated healing processes result in the release of adenosine triphosphate (ATP) into the extracellular wound matrix which is subsequently metabolized into uric acid.

Fernandez and co-workers used a validated chromatographic method to analyze the purine metabolite concentrations in wound fluid collected from 29 patients (total of 70 samples). In addition, the Pressure Ulcer Scale of Healing (PUSH) score for each ulcer was determined to provide a clinical grading of wound severity. The latter is a

Adenosine
Inosine
Hypoxanthine
XO
Xanthine
XO
Uric Acid (UA)
O2−
O2−

Figure 5.39 ***Purine catabolism pathway.***

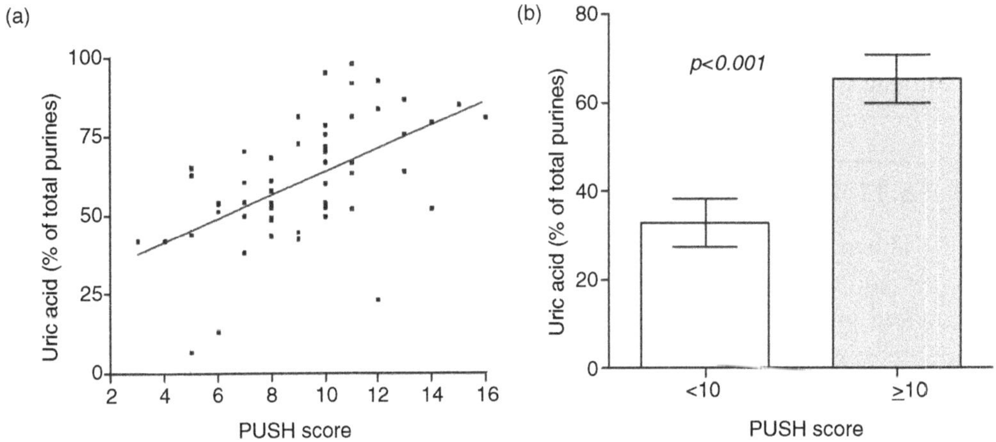

Figure 5.40 (a) Scatter plot of urate expressed as a percentage of total purine versus the PUSH score and (b) Levels expressed as the amount of urate as a percentage of total purines (±SEM) [89].

clinically recognized screening tool (see Chapter 1) which assesses a variety of wound parameters providing a score ranging from 1 to 17—the higher the score the more severe the wound. The amount of urate (as a percentage of the total purines) was plotted against the PUSH score (Fig. 5.40a) and confirmed that urate increases with severity. Further confirmation was obtained through taking one wound sample for each patient and the relative concentrations evaluated against the two PUSH grouping indicated in Fig. 5.40b [89].

As a biomarker, uric acid possesses the prime advantage of being present in relatively high concentrations and there is an extensive amount of literature on its electrochemical detection [76,77]. It is somewhat ironic to note that while the ease with which it can be electrochemically oxidized is often considered to be an interference in electroanalytical methods, it is this same property that has made it attractive as a biomarker in the present context. Thus, the ability to electrochemically monitor its concentration could be useful in determining the extent of inflammation and the subsequent response to treatment—therein providing insights into the healing process [89].

It is possible to directly oxidize urate at the electrode and this has been described in the previous section on pH [77,80–82]. The electrochemical measurement of urate as a means of gauging wound severity was proposed by Joshi and colleagues, whereby a carbon load polyethylene film was modified (in a similar process that was described by Phair et al. [81]). The electrochemical response to a test solution containing urate and tyrosine is highlighted in Fig. 5.41 and highlights the need to obtain voltammetrically distinct signal resolution between the different components.

An issue that is quite often overlooked in the case of electrochemical sensors is how to extract the signal from the wound. A great deal of effort is normally expended on the

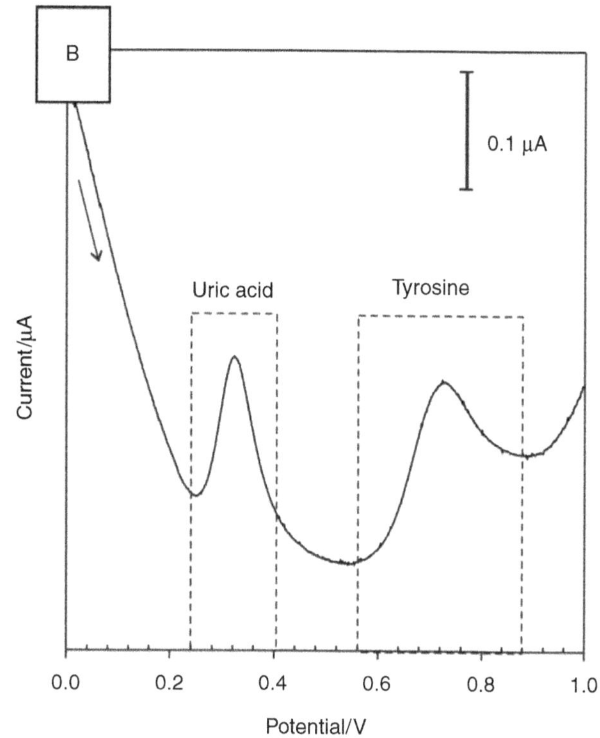

Figure 5.41 ***Volammetric response of the carbon loaded polyethylene film electrode toward uric acid and tyrosine [82].***

materials aspects of the sensor, but the signal acquisition is usually achieved through the use of expensive and cumbersome laboratory-based equipment. Joshi's team developed a small foot print potentiostat that could be used to send the signal to a smart device as indicated in Fig. 5.42 [82].

The major limitation with this approach is the fact that the sensor and controller and data-recording system still requires hard wiring but nevertheless a significant step forward in the path toward a discrete sensor. The system could be minitaurized to a much smaller footprint and highlight the fact that a simple amperometric system could be employed and can relay chemical information that may be useful in wound diagnostics.

An alternative system has been proposed by Wang and coworkers who developed a biosensor approach to the measurement of urate [90]. The voltammograms obtained by Joshi's team (Fig. 5.41) still require a significant positive potential to oxidize urate. This could encounter a level of interference when subjected to complex wound fluid. The enzyme approach advocated by Wang was to use uricase as the detection enzyme as indicated in Fig. 5.43. This would convert the urate into allantoin and in doing so hydrogen peroxide is produced as a by-product. The team exploited the ability of

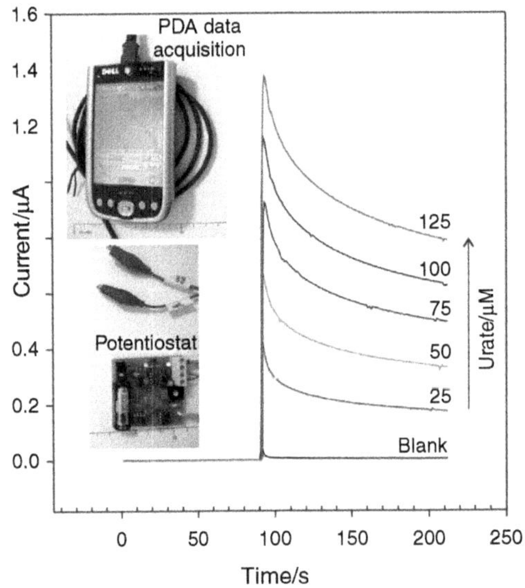

Figure 5.42 ***Amperometric measurement of urate through using a carbon loaded polyethylene film connected to a small foot print potentiostat and smart device [82].***

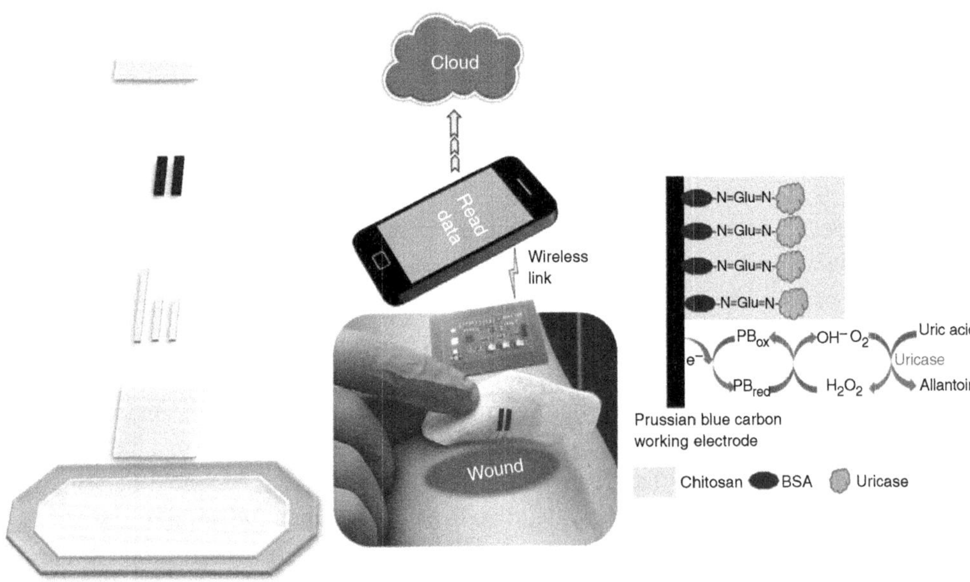

Figure 5.43 ***Fabrication of the urate biosensor and its mode of operation [90].***

Prussian Blue particles to catalyze the reduction of the enzymatically produced peroxide and thus the operating potential can be moved to a potential where there is less likelihood of interference. This is a substantially more complex arrangement but Wang and colleagues have successfully demonstrated the manufacture of screen-printed systems which could open an avenue toward the production of the system. The innovative nature of the approach was further illustrated through the use of wireless signal transduction to a smart device.

It is relatively easy to envisage the translation of the biosensing system from a point of care diagnostic to a smart dressing. The manufacture of the actual sensor can be achieved using conventional screen printing and hence is disposable. The electronics, although nondisposable, could be further miniaturized and adapted for remote/telemonitoring. The key point of interest does not, however, solely rest on the measurement of urate but rather on the generic nature of the methodology itself: uricase is an oxidase enzyme and thus it could be substituted for a range of other enzyme systems and therefore open up the possibility of other analytes being analyzed or multiparametric analysis.

5.12 SUMMARY

There is a wide spectrum of commercially available dressings which have some remarkable properties, and, as outlined in Chapter 4, the variety of form and function can enable the dressings to be tailored to the circumstance of the patient and the needs of the wound. The progression of troublesome wounds toward healing may require several different approaches and therefore there is a need for more information on the chemical dynamics within the wound to inform subsequent interventions. It could be envisaged the development of smart sensors, outlined in this chapter, and which are capable of integration within existing dressing formats, could provide invaluable data on the condition of the wound and thereby facilitate more informed decisions on what type of dressing should be applied to encourage the wound to move between different stages in healing.

Although there are many diagnostic assay and sensing techniques that can be translated from the lab bench to the clinic, the subsequent adaptation for continuous/periodic monitoring that would be required for outpatient monitoring is still some way off. While the transfer of technological solutions to the home, in a way similar to that pioneered by glucose monitors, would be the ideal, the actual implementation of point of care diagnostics remains elusive and problematic. Chronic wounds necessitate that treatment is conducted under aseptic conditions by trained healthcare professionals and, it is likely that were such responsibilities to be devolved to the patient, any drop in the standard of care may compromise the healing progress. This may occur through the mechanical disruption of the wound but also by exposing tissue to possible infection.

A better option, and one where embedded sensors would be of great benefit, can be found in the "Connected Health" model. The direct integration of sensors within the bandage to form a smart dressing would minimize disruption to the wound and remove the ambiguities that can arise through human intervention/measurement. The main requirement is the devices perform periodic monitoring and report back to a central server where the results can be assessed/reviewed by the healthcare team. In many cases, the present impediment to the development process is the robustness of the assays and the need for reagentless sensing. It is unlikely that the demands of the instrumentation will be an issue as RFID technologies are not beginning to emerge and the miniaturization of the electronics continues apace. Designing an economically viable solution will inevitably be a further hurdle but the cost benefits of early treatment, as outlined in Chapter 1, could easily justify the development costs. The latter is especially pertinent considering the current prevalence of chronic wounds and the epidemic predictions for the future.

REFERENCES

[1] Dargaville TR, Farrugia BL, Broadbent JA, Pace S, Upton Z. Sensors and imaging for wound healing: a review. Biosens Bioelectron 2013;41:30–42.

[2] McLister A, Phair J, Cundell J, Davis J. Electrochemical approaches to the development of smart bandages: a mini-review. Electrochem Commun 2014;40:96–9.

[3] World Union of Wound Healing Societies (WUWHS). Principles of best practice: Wound infection in clinical practice. An international consensus. London: MEP Ltd, 2008. Available at: www.mepltd.co.uk.

[4] Mehmood N, Hariz A, Fitridge R, Voelcker NH. Applications of modern sensors and wireless technology in effective wound management. J Biomed Mats Res B 2014;102B:885–95.

[5] Matzeu G, Florea L, Diamond D. Advances in wearable chemical sensor design for monitoring biological fluids. Sens Actuators B 2015;211:403–18.

[6] Dowsett C, Blelby A, Searle R. Reconciling increasing wound care demands with available resources. J Wound Care 2014;23:552–62.

[7] Engineering and Physical Sciences Research Council, United Kingdom. Available at: www.epsrc.ac.uk.

[8] Löffler MW, Schuster H, Bühler S, Beckert S. Wound fluid in diabetic foot ulceration: more than just an undefined soup? Int J Lower Extremity Wounds 2013;12:113–29.

[9] Broadbent J, Walsh T, Upton Z. Proteomics in chronic wound research: potentials in healing and health. Proteomics Clin Appl 2010;4:204–14.

[10] Angel DE, Lloyd P, Carville K, Santamaria N. The clinical efficacy of two semi-quantitative wound-swabbing techniques in identifying the causative organism(s) in infected cutaneous wounds. Int Wound J 2011;8:176–85.

[11] Schmohl M, Beckert S, Joos TO, Königsrainer A, Schneiderhan-Marra N, Loffler MW. Superficial wound swabbing: a novel method of sampling and processing wound fluid for subsequent immunoassay analysis in diabetic foot ulcerations. Diabetes Care 2012;35:2113–20.

[12] Trengove NJ, Langton SR, Stacey MC. Biochemical analysis of wound fluid from nonhealing and healing chronic leg ulcers. Wound Repair Regen 1996;4:234–9.

[13] Jones PW, Taylor DM, Williams DR. Analysis and chemical speciation of copper and zinc in wound fluid. J Inorg Biochem 2000;81:1–10.

[14] Jalkanen M, Haapanen T, Lyytikainen AM, Larjava H. Wound fluids mediate granulation tissue growth phases. Cell Biol Int Rep 1983;7:745–53.

[15] Zillmer R, Trøstrup H, Karlsmark T, Ifversen P, Agren MS. Duration of wound fluid secretion from chronic venous leg ulcers is critical for interleukin-1a, interleukin-1b, interleukin-8 levels and fibroblast activation. Arch Dermatol Res 2011;303:601–6.

[16] Varghese MC, Balin AK, Carter DM, Caldwell D. Local environment of chronic wounds under synthetic dressings. Arch Dermatol 1986;122:52–7.

[17] Cao Y, Croll TI, Rizzi SC, et al. A peptidomimetic inhibitor of matrix metalloproteinases containing a tetherable linker group. J Biomed Mater Res A 2011;96:663–72.

[18] Liu Y, Min D, Bolton T, et al. Increased matrix metalloproteinase-9 predicts poor wound healing in diabetic foot ulcers: response to Muller et al. Diabetes Care 2009;32:e137.

[19] International Best Practice Guidelines: Wound Management in Diabetic Foot Ulcers. Wounds International, 2013. Available at: www.woundsinternational.com.

[20] Kost GJ. Principles and practice of point of care testing. Lippincott Williams and Wilkins, Philadelphia; 2002.
[21] Ngom B, Guo Y, Wang X, Bi D. Development and application of lateral flow test strip technology for detection of infectious agents and chemical contaminants: a review. Anal Bioanal Chem 2010;397:1113–35.
[22] Huang X, Aguilar ZP, Xu H, Lai W, Xiong Y. Membrane-based lateral flow immunochromatographic strip with nanoparticles as reporters for detection: a review. Biosens Bioelectron 2015;75:166–80.
[23] Worsley GJ, Attree SL, Noble JE, Horgan AM. Rapid duplex immunoassay for wound biomarkers at the point-of-care. Biosens Bioelectron 2012;34:215–20.
[24] DETEKT Digital Diagnostic Solutions. Available at: www.idetekt.com.
[25] Schneider LA, Korber A, Grabbe S, Dissemond J. Influence of pH on wound-healing: a new perspective for wound-therapy. Arch Dermatol Res 2007;298:413–20.
[26] Gethin G. The significance of surface pH in chronic wounds. Wounds UK 2007;3:52–6.
[27] Ono S, Imai R, Ida Y, Shibata D, Komiya T, Matsumura H. Increased wound pH as an indicator of local wound infection in second degree burns. Burns 2015;41:820–4.
[28] Mohr GJ, Muller H. Tailoring colour changes of optical sensor materials by combining indicator and inert dyes and their use in sensor layers, textiles and non-wovens. Sens Actuators B 2015;206:788–93.
[29] Evans RC, Douglas P, Williams JAG, Rochester DL. A novel luminescence-based colorimetric oxygen sensor with a Traffic Light response. J Fluoresc 2006;16:201–6.
[30] Wang XD, Chen X, Xie ZX, Wang XR. Reversible optical sensor strip for oxygen. Angew Chem 2008;120:7560–3.
[31] Schreml S, Meier RJ, Kirschbaum M, Kong SC, Gehmert S, Felthaus O, Küchler S, Sharpe JR, Wöltje K, Weiß KT, Albert M, Seidl U, Schröder J, Morsczeck C, Prantl L, Duschl C, Pedersen SF, Gosau M, Berneburg M, Wolfbeis OS, Landthaler M, Babilas P. Luminescent dual sensors reveal extracellular pH-gradients and hypoxia on chronic wounds that disrupt epidermal repair. Theranostics 2014;4:721–35.
[32] Schreml S, Meier RJ, Wolfbeis OS, Landthaler M, Szeimies RM, Babilas P. 2D luminescence imaging of pH in vivo. Proc Natl Acad Sci U S A 2011;108:2432–7.
[33] Schreml S, Meier RJ, Wolfbeis OS, Maisch T, Szeimies RM, Landthaler M. 2D luminescence imaging of physiological wound oxygenation. Exp Dermatol 2011;20:550–4.
[34] Wang XD, Wolfbeis OS. Optical methods for sensing and imaging of oxygen: materials, spectroscopies and applications. Chem Soc Rev 2014;43:3666–761.
[35] Sawada K, Ohshina T, Hizawa T, Takao H, Ishida M. A novel fused sensor for photo- and ion-sensing. Sens Actuators B 2005;106:614–8.
[36] Hizawa T, Sawada K, Takao H, Ishida M. Fabrication of a two dimensional pH image sensor using a charge transfer technique. Sens Actuators B 2006;117:509–15.
[37] Zampolli S, et al. Ultra-low-power components for an RFID Tag with physical and chemical sensors. Microsyst Technol Micro Nanosystems Information Storage Process Syst 2008;14:581–8.
[38] Potyrallo RA, Morris WG. Multianalyte chemical identification and quantitation using a single radio frequency identification sensor. Anal Chem 2007;79:45–51.
[39] Byrne R, Diamond D. Chemo/bio-sensor networks. Nat Mater 2006;5:421–4.
[40] Steinberg IM, Steinberg MD. Radio-frequency tag with optoelectronic interface for distributed wireless chemical and biological sensor applications. Sens Actuators B 2009;138:120–5.
[41] Jeronimo PCA, Araujo AN, Montenegro M. Optical sensors and biosensors based on sol–gel films. Talanta 2007;72:13–27.
[42] Hemmink GJM, Weusten BLAM, Oors J, Bredenoord AJ, Timmer R, Smout AJPM. Ambulatory oesophageal pH monitoring: a comparison between antimony, ISFET, and glass pH electrodes. Eur J Gasteronenterol Hepatol 2010;22:572–7.
[43] Taouil A, Lallemand F, Meolt JM, Husson J, Hihn JY, Lakard B. Effect of polypyrrole modified electrode functionalization on potentiometric pH responses. Synth Met 2010;160:1073–80.
[44] Carrol S, Baldwin RP. Self calibrating microfabricated iridium oxide pH electrode array for remote monitoring. Anal Chem 2010;82:878–85.
[45] Herlem G, Zeggari R, Rauch JY, Monney S, Anzola FT, Guillaume Y, Andre C, Gharbhi T. One-pot electrosynthesis of polyglycine like thin film of platinum electrodes as transducer for solid state pH measurements. Talanta 2010;82. 417–412.

[46] Musa AE, del Campo FJ, Abramova N, Alonso-Lomillo MA, Dominguez-Renedo O, Arcos-Martinez MJ, Brivio M, Snakenborg D, Geschke O, Kutter JP. Disposable miniaturised screen printed pH and reference electrodes for potentiometric systems. Electroanalysis 2011;23:115–21.
[47] Inoue T, Baba T, Yuchi A. Responses of Metalloporphyrin-based ion selective electrodes to pH. Electroanalysis 2011;23:536–42.
[48] Li Q, Li H, Zhang J, Xu Z. A novel pH potentiometric sensor based on electrochemically synthesized polybisphenol A films at an ITO electrode. Sens Actuators B 2011;155:730–6.
[49] Betelu S, Polychronopoulou K, Rebholz C, Ignatiadis I. Novel CeO2 based screen printed potentiometric electrodes for pH monitoring. Talanta 2011;87:126–35.
[50] Lee D, Cui T. Carbon nanotube thin film pH electrode for potentiometric enzymatic acetylcholine biosensing. Microelectron Eng 2012;93:39–42.
[51] Zhuiykov S, Kats E, Kalantar-Zadeh K, Breedon M, Miura N. Influence of thickness of submicron Cu2O doped RuO2 electrode on sensing performance of planar electrochemical pH sensors. Mater Lett 2012;75:165–8.
[52] Kim S, Rim T, Kim K, Lee U, Baek E, Lee H, Baek CK, Meyyappan M, Deen MJ, Lee JS. Silicon nanowire ion sensitive field effect transistor with integrated Ag/AgCl electrode: pH sensing and noise characteristics. Analyst 2011;136:5012–6.
[53] Cherchour N, Deslouis C, Messaoudi B, Pailleret A. pH sensing in aqueous solutions using a MnO2 thin film electrodeposited on a glassy carbon electrode. Electrochim Acta 2011;56:9746–55.
[54] Zhao R, Xu M, Wang J, Chen G. A pH sensor based on TiO2 nanotube array modified Ti electrode. Electrochim Acta 2010;55:5647–51.
[55] Mignani A, Corticelli C, Tonelli D, Scavetta E. A new pH sensor based on a glassy carbon electrode coated with a Co/Al layered double hydroxide. Electroanalysis 2011;23:1745–51.
[56] Hickman JJ, Ofer D, Laibinis PE, Whitesides GM, Wrighton MS. Molecular self assembly of 2-terminal voltammetric microsensors with internal references. Science 1991;252:688–91.
[57] Makos A, Omiatek DM, Ewing AG, Heien ML. Development and characterisation of a voltammetric carbon fiber microelectrode pH sensor. Langmuir 2010;26:10386–91.
[58] Xiong L, Batchelor-McAuley C, Compton RG. Calibrationless pH sensors based on nitrosophenyl and ferrocenyl co-modified screen printed electrodes. Sens Actuators B 2011;159:251–5.
[59] Park W, Kim S. Triggerable single component two electrode voltammetric pH sensors using dyad molecules. Electrochem Commun 2013;26:109–12.
[60] Streeter I, Leventis HC, Wildgoose GG, Pandurangappa M, Lawrence NS, Jiang L, Jones TG, Compton RG. A sensitive reagentless pH probe with a ca. 120 mV/pH unit response. J Solid State Electrochem 2004;8:718–21.
[61] Heald CGR, Wildgoose GG, Jiang L, Jones TGJ, Compton RG. Chemical derivatisation of multiwalled carbon nanotubes using diazonium salts. Chemphyschem 2004;5:1794–9.
[62] Lafitte VGH, Wang WX, Yashina AS, Lawrence NS. Anthraquinone-ferrocene film electrodes: utility in pH and oxygen sensing. Electrochem Commun 2008;12:1831–4.
[63] Davis J, Molina MT, Leach CP, Cardosi MF. Plasma-polyplumbagin modified microfiber probes: a functional material approach to monitoring vascular access line contamination. ACS 2013;8:9367–71.
[64] Webster RA, Xia F, Pan M, Mu S, Dale SEC, Tsang SC, Hammett FW, Bowen CR, Marken F. Voltammetric probing of pH at carbon nanofiber-Nafion-Carbon nanofiber membrane electrode assemblies. Electrochim Acta 2012;62. 197–102.
[65] Fierro S, Mitani N, Comninellis C, Einaga Y. pH sensing using boron doped diamond electrodes. Phys Chem Chem Phys 2011;13:16795–9.
[66] Li M, Phair J, Cardosi MF, Davis J. Nanostructuring carbon fiber probes for use in central venous catheters. Anal Chim Acta 2014;812:1–5.
[67] Phair J, Newton L, McCormac C, Cardosi MF, Leslie R, Davis J. A disposable sensor for point of care wound pH monitoring. Analyst 2011;136:4692–5.
[68] Guinovart T, Valdes-Ramerez G, Windmiller JR, Andrade FR, Wang J. Bandage-based wearable potentiometric sensor for monitoring wound pH. Electroanalysis 2014;26:1345–53.
[69] Kaempgen M, Roth S. Transparent and flexible carbon nanotube/polyaniline pH sensors. J Electroanal Chem 2006;586:72–6.

[70] Lindfors T, Ervela S, Ivaska A. Polyaniline as pH-sensitive component in plasticized PVC membranes. J Electroanal Chem 2003;560:69–78.
[71] Zhang X, Ogorevc B, Wang J. Solid-state pH nanoelectrode based on polyaniline thin film electrodeposited onto ion-beam etched carbon fiber. Anal Chim Acta 2002;452:1–10.
[72] Anderson A, Phair J, Benson J, Meenan BJ, Davis J. Investigating the use of endogenous quinoid moieties on carbon fiber as means of developing micro pH sensors. Mater Sci Eng C-Mater Biol Appl 2014;43:533–7.
[73] Compton R, Banks CE. Understanding voltammetry. Singapore: World Scientific Publishing; 2009.
[74] Monk PMS. Fundamentals of electroanalytical chemistry. New York: Wiley; 2001.
[75] Sholtz F. Electroanalytical methods: guide to experiments and applications. Berlin: Springer; 2014.
[76] Lawrence NS, Beckett EL, Davis J, Compton RG. Advances in the voltammetric analysis of small biologically relevant compounds. Anal Biochem 2002;303:1–16.
[77] Dutt JSN, Cardosi MF, Livingstone C, Davis J. Diagnostic implications of uric acid in electroanalytical measurements. Electroanalysis 2005;17:1233–43.
[78] Bloom C, Hart LK. The relationship between the health belief model and compliance of persons with diabetes mellitus. Diabetes Care 1980;3:594–8.
[79] Jin J, et al. Factors affecting therapeutic compliance: a review from the patient's perspective. Therapeut Clin Risk Manage 2008;4(1). 269–86.
[80] Phair J, Leach CP, Cardosi MF, Davis J. Atmospheric pressure plasma treated carbon fiber weave: a flexible approach to wound monitoring. Electrochem Commun 2013;33:99–101.
[81] Phair J, Benson J, McCormac C, Cundell J, Gracheva S, Wilkinson D, Forsythe S, Davis J. Butyl grafted polyethylene films doped with carbon black: a foundation for the development of smart bandages. Sens Actuators B 2014;193. 764–7.
[82] Phair J, Joshi M, Benson J, McDonald D, Davis J. Laser patterned carbon-polyethylene mesh electrodes for wound diagnostics. Mater Chem Phys 2014;143:991–5.
[83] McLister A, Davis J. Molecular wiring in smart dressings: opening a new route to monitoring wound pH. Healthcare 2015;3:466–77.
[84] McLister A, Lowry N, Anderson A, McHugh J, Davis J. Novel pH sensing redox wire based on a polyamide homopolymer of L-tryptophan. Fibers Polym 2015;16:2294–7.
[85] Sridhar V, Takahata K. A hydrogel-based passive wireless sensor using a flex-circuit inductive transducer. Sens Actuators A 2009;155:58–65.
[86] Lobmann R, Zemlin C, Motzkau M, Reschke K, Lehnert H. Expression of matrix metalloproteinases and growth factors in diabetic foot wounds treated with a protease absorbent dressing. Diabetes Complications 2006;20:329.
[87] Liu Y, Min D, Bolton T, Nube V, Twigg SM, Yue DK, McLennan SV. Increased matrix metalloproteinase-9 predicts poor wound healing in diabetic foot ulcers. Diabetes Care 2009;32:117.
[88] Ciani I, Schulze H, Corrigan DK, Henihan G, Giraud G, Terry JG, Walton AJ, Pethig R, Ghazal P, Crain J, Campbell CJ, Bachmann TT, Mount AR. Development of immunosensors for direct detection of three wound infection biomarkers at point of care using electrochemical impedance spectroscopy. Biosens Bioelectron 2012;31:413.
[89] Fernandez ML, Upton Z, Edwards H, Finlayson K, Shooter GK. Elevated uric acid correlates with wound severity. Int Wound J 2012;9:139–49.
[90] Kassal P, Kim J, Kumar R, de Araujo WR, Steinberg IM, Steinberg M, Wang J. Smart bandage with wireless connectivity for uric acid biosensing as an indicator of wound status. Electrochem Commun 2015;56:6–10.

CHAPTER SIX

Sensors for Detecting and Combating Wound Infection

J. Davis, A. McLister
School of Engineering, Ulster University, Jordanstown, Northern Ireland, United Kingdom

6.1 INTRODUCTION

Wound infection is a particular hazard for those managing a chronic wound as the inevitable delays render the patient more susceptible to complications [1–3]. The consequences are considerable and range from increased healing time to life-threatening events. There is also an added economic burden through hospital admission and subsequent treatment. While the risk of infection is a clear issue, there are considerable concerns over the diagnosis of the condition. A recent survey conducted by Dowsett et al. [4] found that some 74% of wounds are treated in the community which can place the onus of early diagnosis on the visiting healthcare worker and the patient. Delays in responding to an infection could lead to a wound becoming irretrievably damaged and runs a risk of amputation being necessary [2,5,6]. Richards et al. [6] reported that in the French OPIDIA study, nearly half of the patients admitted to a DFU clinic with infection were subsequently found to require lower-limb amputation. Identifying when a wound is infected is far from straightforward and, in the Dowsett survey, 8% of clinicians when asked if the wound was infected responded with a "don't know" [4]. A variety of guidelines have been issued in an attempt to clarify the presence of infection, but visual inspection remains a poor substitute for a quantitative diagnosis [7,8]. The standard approach will be to request a microbial culture of the wound, but this can be far from ideal as variations in swab technique are a contentious issue in itself but further complicated by the interpretation of the results. Wounds will be host to a variety of organisms and, in many circumstances, can heal without being unduly perturbed by their presence. The use of "stages" such as contamination, colonization, critical colonization, and infection are widely known but require expertise to determine within which category a particular wound resides [1,2]. The aim of this chapter is to provide a brief overview of the present approaches to the assessment of wound infection and to highlight the technologies that are emerging in the development of smart materials that can remove some of the limitations associated with visual inspection and improve treatment.

6.2 CLASSICAL SIGNS OF WOUND INFECTION

The classic sign of infection is the formation and release of exudate (pus) from the wound, and it is likely that most readers will have experienced some form of this in their journey through life. The release of purulent exudate only arises as a consequence of the action of white blood cells in combating the invading organisms. This is, of course, a fairly clear indicator of infection but a host of inflammatory signs will arise in advance of this stage and include erythema, edema, heat, and pain [7]. There are however 12 indicators of infection (Table 6.1), but these are less familiar to a lay audience and are associated with secondary wound processes [9]. In the context of chronic wounds, clinical signs can be ambiguous as the characteristics can be affected by underlying complications such as neuropathy, vascular disease, venous disease, and impaired leukocyte function and their use as a diagnostic test for infection has been questioned [10].

The Infectious Disease Society of America guidelines for the diagnosis of infection within diabetic patients proposed using only the classic signs of infection [12] and the release of purulent exudates in particular. As an alternative, two or more classic signs appearing in combination could also be used as a diagnostic tool, but given that diabetic patients commonly have a diminished inflammatory response, the application of such criteria is contentious [13]. Gardner et al. [11] proposed using the seven signs specific to secondary wounds as indicators of wound bioburden and found that the composite predictor provides a moderate level of discrimination that is superior to the Infectious Disease Society of America approach and may be suitable for clinical use.

Table 6.1 Adapted from Gardener et al. [11]

Primary	Eyrthema
	Edema
	Heat
	Pain
	Purulent exudate
Secondary	Serous exudate
	Delayed healing
	Friable granulation tissue
	Discolored granulation tissue
	Foul odor
	Pocketing of wound base
	Wound breakdown

6.3 MICROBIAL CULTURE

It is clear that obtaining a rapid diagnosis of the early onset of infection and the identity of the causative agents is pivotal to the management of the wound to ensure that the healing processes are restored and the associated morbidity and mortality is reduced [14]. It is commonplace for an open wound to be contaminated by bacteria, and despite the presence of the latter, many wounds will continue to heal [14–16]. There can be a huge number of contaminating species and the challenge is to identify those that are liable to give rise to complications in the healing process. Both aerobic and anaerobic organisms will contaminate and colonize wound surfaces and the diversity of species has been illustrated by Bowler and Davies who extracted some 367 isolates from 61 acute and 45 chronic wound samples [17]. It is, however, the nature of the bacterial species present and not necessarily the number of organisms that is important when assessing the propensity toward infection [18] as it has been shown by Wright et al. [19] that surgical wounds would singularly fail to heal when haemolytic Streptococcus pyogenes is present in the tissue. In the case of infected acute wounds, it has been noted that gram-positive organisms are usually the predominant species with *Staphylococcus aureus* being the most common [21–25]. Chronic wounds, partly as a consequence of their extended healing period, are polymicrobial with gram-positive, gram-negative, and anaerobes all liable to be present [18]. In such cases, *S. aureus*, *P. Aeruginosa*, and beta haemolytic streptococci are among the more common protagonists in infection and delayed healing [26–35]. The physiological response to the presence of such pathogens can be incredibly varied irrespective of the wound state, and it must be stressed that the interactions between the host tissues and bacteria will often be the key to determining the influence of the invading organism on the healing processes.

It can be expected that upon suspicion of infection, microbiological culture would be requested to identify the causative agent and to enable the collation of an antibiogram to guide antimicrobial treatment [36,37]. Sampling can be obtained using either tissue biopsy, wound fluid aspirate or through swabbing of the wound surface. The use of tissue biopsy is rather contentious as it risks inflicting further injury to the patient but it is considered the "gold standard" for providing information on the species which have penetrated the soft tissues [38–45]. There are a number of other issues: the expertise of the practitioner taking the sample, the representative nature of the sample, and as both its extraction and subsequent handling are labor intensive, the cost. These factors usually mitigate against its use in routine practice [46]. In contrast, the use of swabbing is much more accessible, noninvasive, easily performed and has become standard for most clinical investigations [47]. There are, however, many drawbacks to this approach as there is no generally accepted method through which the swab should be taken. Given the diversity of wounds, there will always be a wide variation in the approach taken and it is little surprise to find that there is considerable debate as to best practice [36,47–50].

Should the swab be taken from isolated positions or randomly wiped across the surface of the wound bed? Should the wound be cleaned beforehand? These are key questions and it is possible for a wound swab to provide misleading information on the infective agents present. It is possible that a superficial sampling may fail to identify those agents that are responsible for penetrating the soft tissue and which will be responsible for the subsequent infection. The risk of a false positive could have a dramatic effect on the patient outcome [47].

6.4 BIOFILM FORMATION AND COMPLICATIONS

As mentioned, chronic wounds are host to high numbers of multiple bacterial species and it has been established that most of these will be organized into a biofilm of some form. The planktonic (free floating) state is normally surrendered for aggregations on the surface of the wound where they surround themselves with a protective film of extracellular polymeric substances (EPS) [51–53]. The steps involved in the formation of a biofilm are highlighted in Fig. 6.1. The EPS matrix is typically composed of a mixture of polysaccharide, protein, and lipids [54,55]. The protective shroud of the EPS confers numerous advantages to the bacterial communities such as increased resistance to attack from: the host's innate defences, exogenous antimicrobials, and mechanical and chemical debridement [56–58]. The resulting biofilm also results in an alteration of gene transcription as an increased proximity of the bacteria to another also results in the quorum sensing (discussed in later sections) which can influence the expression of virulence factors [59,60].

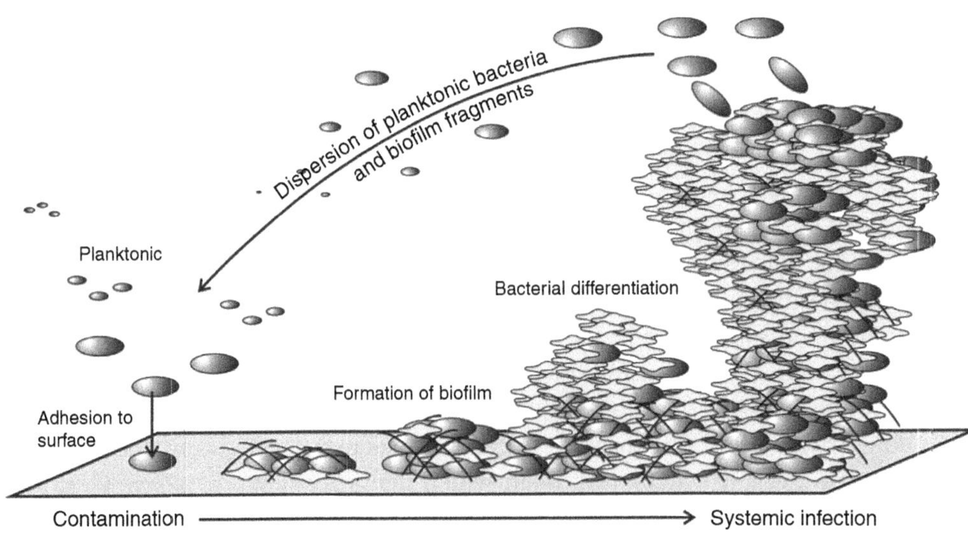

Figure 6.1 ***Stages in the formation of a biofilm.***

Estimates of the prevalence of biofilms within wounds can vary, but it is generally accepted that most, if not all, chronic wounds will have some form of biofilm within the wound bed. The major complication for the management of the wound relates to the fact that the wound bed can appear perfectly healthy despite the presence of a biofilm adhered to the exposed extracellular matrix [61]. The presence of the biofilm can prolong the healing and are typified by a persistent infection that develops slowly. The protective barrier provided by the EPS means that the infection is seldom resolved by the immune response [48] and can require aggressive antimicrobial therapy [15,49,50,62–65].

The biofilm can also be a staging post for the release of planktonic species that can expand the film or create new colonies within the wound bed. This can lead to progressive damage being inflicted on the extracellular matrix, thereby inhibiting the processes necessary to support wound closure. Moreover, it will ultimately lead to local infection [66–68]. The presence of the biofilm will induce an inflammatory response which will involve the release of neutrophils and macrophages to combat the film. These cells secrete a potent cocktail of proteases (discussed in detail in later sections) along with reactive oxygen species in an attempt to dislodge and dissolve the biofilm. This can be a considered "nuclear option" in that there will inevitably be a high degree of indiscriminate damage to the surrounding wound tissue and structures previously constructed to aid healing. Ironically, it has been proposed that the host inflammatory response is actually beneficial to the biofilm communities as the resulting chemical milieu from the attack serves to increase the local nutrition supply to the bacteria [22]. It has also been suggested that *P. aeruginosa* may actively stimulate the inflammation processes through the production of rhamnolipids that protects the communities from phagocytosis [34,35].

Despite the exemplary work by Bolwer and Davies [17], it is likely that the variety of microbe species recovered from a chronic wound is liable to be a gross underestimate [15,16]. It is easy to appreciate that wound swabbing alone can be ineffective in providing a robust picture of the bacterial communities within the wound and compounded by the failure to penetrate the mechanical barrier of the biofilm. The use of debrided tissue as a culture sample, however, can be informative as it can be combined with biomolecular analysis to identify viable but potentially nonculturable microbes [23]. Moreover, histological staining and microscopic analysis of the tissue has been used to excellent effect to identify cluster communities indicative of biofilms. A more recent discovery is that anaerobic species (Bacteroides sp., Fusobacterium sp., Peptostreptococcus sp., and Clostridium sp.) can reside with the deeper tissues and would be completely unreachable using conventional swab techniques [18–22].

Much of the cost associated with the treatment of chronic wounds has been attributed to the complications that arise as a consequence of biofilms [69]. Given their ubiquity, it is evident that being able to identify the bacteria in question could enable more targeted treatments and therein improve outcomes. The development of personalized medicine will be a growth area in the future, provided the technology becomes accessible. For example, Cooper and colleagues applied molecular diagnostics to a patient cohort presenting with chronic wounds and enabled treatment with personalized topical antimicrobial gels that accelerate the healing [48].

6.5 INSTRUMENTAL ANALYSIS TECHNIQUES

Providing detailed analysis of the bacterial bioburden within the wound can be particularly challenging from the perspectives of sampling and instrumental analysis. There have been substantial advances in lab-based techniques in recent years with sequencing technologies offering considerable gains in microbe identification. These are, however, complex and require substantial investment in both staff and equipment [70,71]. Denaturing gradient gel electrophoresis is a relatively common and versatile technique that has been used in a number of research investigations targeting chronic wounds [19,22,27]. The sequence library can be a limitation and will, invariably, be biased toward common pathogens and, as such, many of the denaturing gradient gel electrophoresis profiles can represent previously unsequenced species [16,22,32]. Kirketerp-Moller and coworkers utilized acid–fluorescence in situ hybridization (PNA-FISH) to aid bacterial identification in samples taken from chronic wounds. Although *S. aureus* was the main isolate, there was a discrepancy in the detection *P. aeruginosa* between the PNA-FISH technique and conventional culture with the latter significantly underestimating the prevalence of the microbe in most samples [25,33]. Bacterial tag encoded FLX amplicon pyrosequencing has been utilized by Dowd and colleagues to assess Diabetic Foot Ulcers and revealed a high prevalence of anaerobes which would otherwise have gone undetected by conventional culture methods [72].

A significant issue relates to the speed at which the analysis can be achieved, as the clinician will almost certainly be in a race against time to combat the onset of infection before healing is irreparably compromised. One innovative approach which would appear to go some way to addressing such issues relates to the work by Wolcott and Dowd where *P. aeruginosa* was identified from sample to result within 2 h through the use of quantitative polymerase chain reaction (PCR). This stands in marked contrast to the 24 h required for conventional culture techniques [73]. Wound panel molecular diagnostics are now becoming available as a clinical tool, but as with the conventional lab-based techniques the range of analytes is typically limited to the usual suspects but do offer rapid screening [67,72].

Mass spectroscopy has been a mainstay of analytical techniques designed to identify biochemicals, and while the technique has been used successfully for the detection of proteins, it is now finding increasing application as a versatile diagnostic tool for microbe detection. In contrast to microbial culture, it can offer rapid screening of swab/

biopsy samples and is used as a frontline technique in many hospitals. Matrix-assisted laser desorption ionization time-of-flight mass spectrometry has quickly become an established technique offering a relatively economical and fast turnaround that can effectively compete with conventional phenotype identification techniques [74–78]. The technique has the prime advantage of requiring minimal sample preparation, whereby the sample is fixed/crystallized within an organic matrix that is subjected to a fixed, pulsed laser beam with the results collected electronically and converted from TOF measurements into the more familiar mass/charge spectra. The collection of the resulting mass patterns arising from the bacterial proteins can be used for identification at the genus and species levels [79–89]. The technique applied to bacterial identification has been comprehensively reviewed by Biswas and Rolain [90]. The one major limitation, which it shares with the sequencing techniques, is the dependence on the diagnostic database.

6.6 REAL-TIME/POINT OF CARE INFECTION DIAGNOSTICS

The early detection of infection has long been recognized as being pivotal to implementing effective management regimes, and while there are significant advances in the development of technologies to enable bacterial identification, there remains a time delay from consultation to result and the implementation of a suitable treatment. In the recent survey by Dowsett et al. [4], clinicians were found to be proactively prescribing antimicrobials for wounds that had no definitive infected diagnosis. The classic signs (used singularly or in combination) are gross indicators which cannot facilitate early treatment and, as such, there remains a substantive clinical need for technologies that can alert the patient (or healthcare professional) to the potential onset of infection and could enable more targeted diagnosis. Ideally, there is a demand for dressings that move the technology from single-shot diagnostics to systems that can remotely offer periodic monitoring of outpatients. As mentioned in Chapter 1, the Dowsett survey is illuminating in that the majority of chronic wounds are dealt within the community, and there are many more opportunities where vigilance can be compromised and infection takes hold before the clinical staff are notified [4].

There have been steady gains in the development of new diagnostic technologies targeted at detecting infection, and while they cannot offer the sophistication of the sequencing systems, they could point the way toward a simple warning system that could improve outcomes. The devices and detection rationales tend to be based around the consequence of bacterial contamination of the wound rather than directly interacting with the microbe itself. Hence, the metabolites released from the bacteria, or the immune response arising as a consequence of invading microbes, provide a host of useful biomarkers through which to raise a warning flag. The various approaches are discussed in turn in the following subsections.

6.7 MONITORING BACTERIAL METABOLITES—QUORUM SENSING

At present, bacterial infection is normally confirmed through microbial culture, but this can be far from ideal given the inherent delays between sampling and analysis. This is compounded by the possibility that the sampling can result in erroneous identification of the infective agent through the indirect culture of nonpathogenic species [91]. In response to this, a number of sensors have been developed to detect bacterial by-products—particularly quorum sensing (QS) molecules that are secreted by bacteria [92,93].

QS is a process by which bacterial cells communicate through the production, detection, and subsequent response to small molecules released within the extracellular fluid. These signaling molecules are generally termed autoinducers (AIs) and vary in structure/nature depending on the type of bacterial community involved. These AIs are pivotal elements in cell–cell communication and enable sensing of bacterial number and can enable communities to collectively alter gene expression and can involve bioluminescence, sporulation, competence, antibiotic production, biofilm formation, and virulence factor secretion [94–96].

There can be significant differences in the nature of signaling molecules and the mechanisms through which they are processed by the various bacterial communities but all function according to the following principles:

1. At low cell density, the production of AIs has little effect as diffusion within the extracellular environment mitigates against their concentration reaching the threshold for detection.
2. At high cell density however, the local concentration of the AI renders detection by neighboring bacteria inevitable [97].
3. The detection of the AIs (either by receptors in the membrane or in the cytoplasm) will activate/upregulate gene expression.
4. The detection of the AI additionally stimulates the activation of processes leading to the increased production and release of the AI and serves as a positive feedback loop [98,99].

The type of signaling system employed depends on whether the bacteria in question are gram-positive or gram-negative and four representative systems are highlighted in Fig. 6.2.

6.7.1 Gram-Positive Quorum Sensing

In the case of gram-positive bacteria, the main autoinducing systems tend to be based on small peptides (AIPs) typically ranging from 5 to 17 aminoacids which can be linear or cyclic [100–105]. When the threshold concentration of the AIP has been reached, binding to a transmembrane histidine-kinase receptor occurs and activates the kinase activity

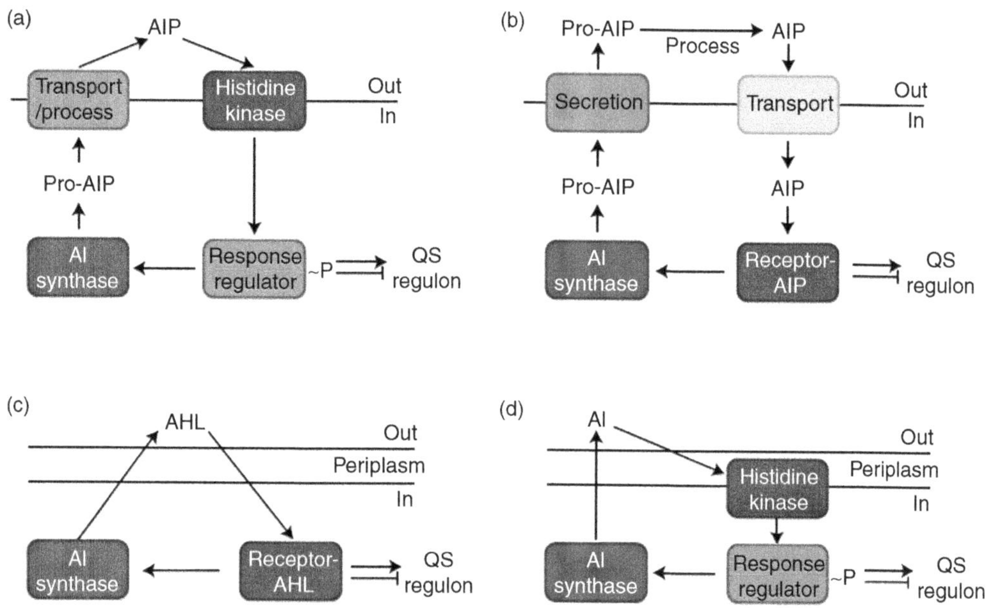

Figure 6.2 ***Quorum sensing routes for gram-positive (a and b) and gram-negative (c and d) species [100].***

which phosphorylates a "cytoplasmic response regulator" [106–108]. The latter is a key mediator not only in QS-associated gene transcription (Fig. 6.2a) but in the production of the AIP itself.

The cell membrane is generally impermeable to the peptides associated with AIPs and, therefore, the latter must be encoded as precursors (pro-AIPs) consisting of over 40 amino acid residues [100–115]. Transmembrane transporters are responsible for the secretion of the pro-AIPs and their conversion to the active AIP forms. The pro-AIP transporter, histidine kinase receptor, and response regulator are normally encoded in an operon whose expression is activated by the cytoplasmic response regulator. Thus, there is a sophisticated autoinducing positive feedback loop that effectively serves to synchronize the QS response across the bacterial community [116,117]. *S. aureus* is a typical example that follows the pathway outlined in Fig. 1a and although it is common among the human skin flora, it can be an adventitious threat where there is trauma to the epithelial barrier resulting in minor infections that can escalate to life-threatening complications [118,119]. It has been reported that *S. aureus* is presently the major cause of hospital-acquired infections and thus is a major threat to those managing chronic wounds. The extent to which it can complicate wound healing depends on the expression of an array of virulence factors which are regulated, in large part, by QS.

It has also been found that some gram-positive bacteria use an alternative AIP pathway which bypasses the histidine kinase receptor. In such cases, the AIPs are transported across the membrane from the extracellular medium to the cytoplasm (Fig. 6.2b) where they interact directly with the cytoplasmic transcription receptor which is associated with QS gene expression [120]. As with the previous case, the AIP-receptor conjugate also increases production of more pro-AIP but, in this instance, the activation of the latter is achieved through extracellular proteases. Typical examples of bacteria employing such processes are *B. subtilis* [119], *E. faecalis* [120], and Bacillus cereus group [121].

6.7.2 Gram-Negative Quorum Sensing

Gram-negative bacteria use a different class of autoinducing signaling molecules and are typically based on acyl-homoserine lactones or other molecules whose production depends on S-adenosylmethionine as a substrate [100,122]. The signaling pathways are similar in nature to those of the Gram-negative systems involving both membrane bound and cytoplasmic receptors (Figure 6.2c and d). At high cell densities, the concentration of the AI can reach the threshold level whereupon the AI binds to the histidine-kinase receptor and follows a path analogous that described for the Gram-positive system, resulting in the AI mediated gene expression (Fig. 1d). A key difference in this instance however is the ability of the AI to freely diffuse across the cell membranes and thus it is little surprise to find that the predominate pathway is through direct interaction with cytoplasmic transcription factors (Fig. 1c).

A more generic approach was taken by Ciani et al. [92] through employing impedance techniques to detect homoserine lactones (HSL) by means of a competitive binding immunoassay involving sample HSL and HSL-linked to bovine serum albumin (HSL-BSA). The presence of HSL in the sample competes with the more bulky HSL-BSA for the antibodies on gold screen-printed electrodes, whereby the greater the concentration of HSL the more HSL-BSA is displaced from binding at the electrode interface. The basic process is illustrated in Fig. 6.3. The added complexity of the sample processing necessary for the assay detracts somewhat from the clinical

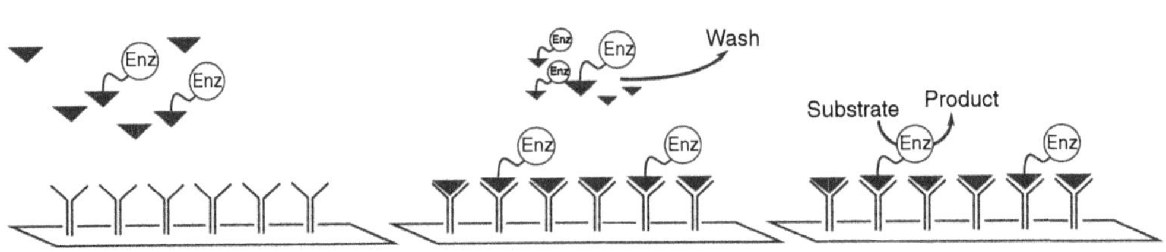

Figure 6.3 ***Idealized competitive immunoassay mechanism.***

usability of the approach, but as it represents one of the first applications of electrochemical immunoassays to wound diagnostics, it does serve as a valuable foundation for further development.

6.8 BACTERIAL TOXINS—PYOCYANIN

Pyocyanin is potent toxin secreted from *P. aeruginosa* strains and is used as weapon against both bacterial and mammalian cells. The toxicity arises in part from its redox chemistry which can be therefore used a diagnostic handle through which to detect its parent. Sharp et al. [93] demonstrated that it is possible to quantitatively measure pyocyanin at carbon fiber-based electrodes (Fig. 6.4) and validated the system against the conventional spectroscopic assay (Fig. 6.5) for a number of bacterial strains. Their approach was shown to be selective and sensitive toward the toxin. The prototype sensor is relatively simple, consisting predominately of carbon fiber modified to increase the surface activity (described in Chapter 5).

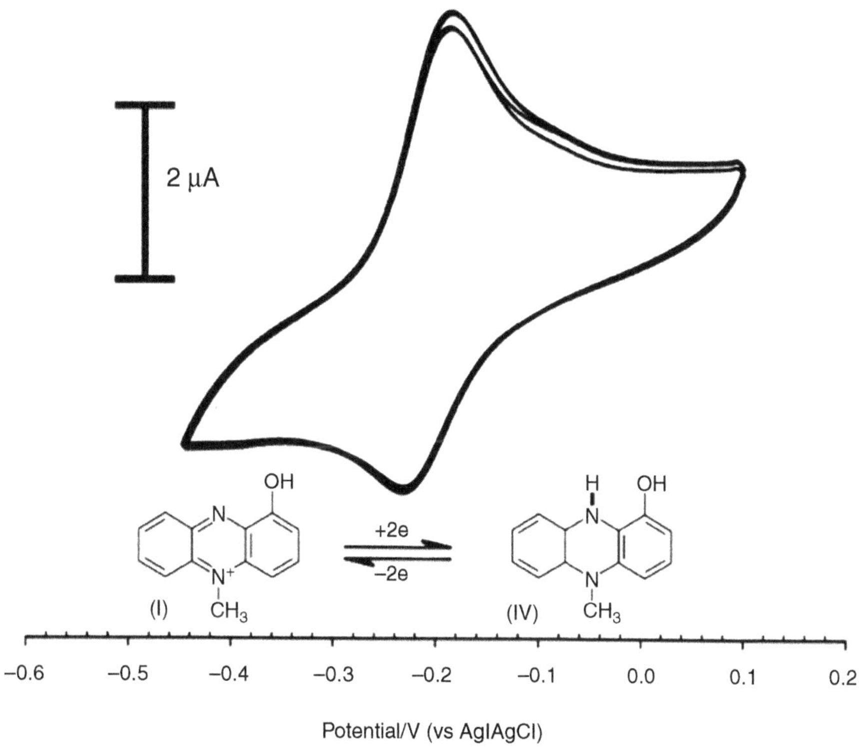

Figure 6.4 ***Cyclic voltammograms detailing the response of a carbon fiber electrode toward pyocyanin [93].***

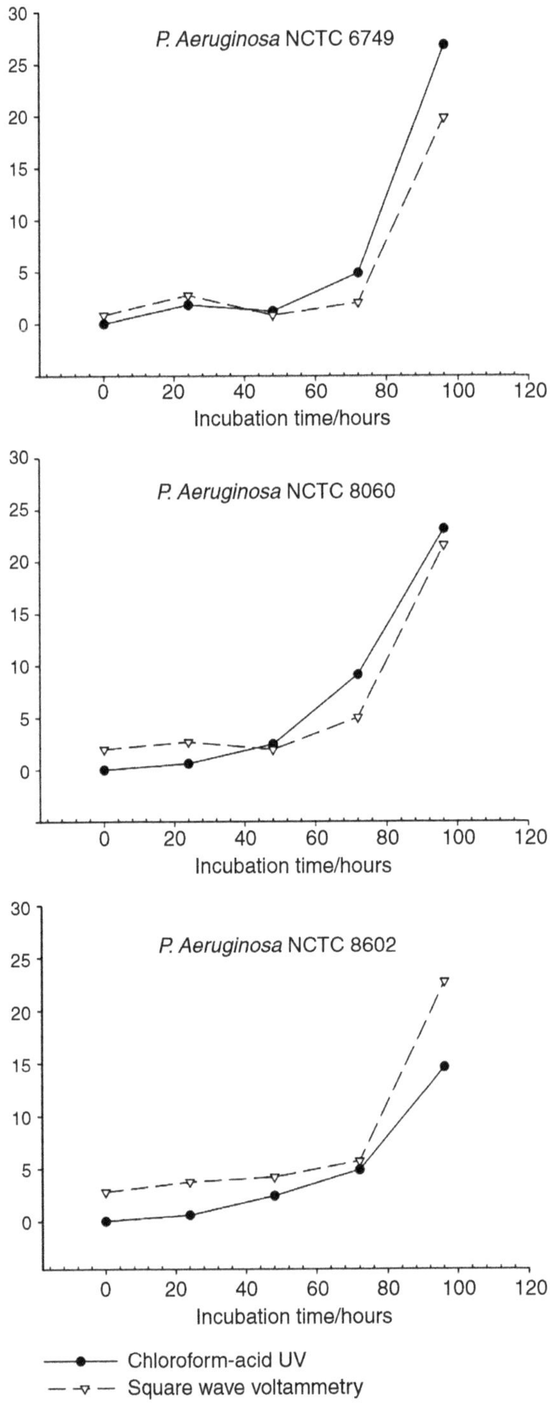

Figure 6.5 ***Comparison of electrochemical sensing and UV detection for the analysis of pyocyanin.***

A critical limitation of these approaches relates to the specificity of pyocyanin and *Pseudomonas quinolone* signal [93,100] to *P. aeruginosa* strains with the possibility of other infective agents (ie, *S. aureus*) going undetected.

6.9 BACTERIAL ENZYME EXPRESSION

The underlying rationale in this approach has been to exploit changes in the relative concentration of urate within the wound brought about through bacterial metabolism [123]. In mammalian tissue, uric acid is the final breakdown product of purine catabolism but bacteria possess uricase, an enzyme that will degrade the purine to allantoin [123]. It could be expected that in cases of low bioburden, the expression of uricase will be relatively low but the activity would increase as the bacteria begin to colonize the wound. The increased activity of uricase would therefore lead to a decrease in local urate which could be readily monitored at a carbon electrode [124]. The electrochemical detection of urate as a means of assessing pH and the severity of the wound has been mentioned in Chapter 5 and a similar methodology is employed in this instance. A schematic of the prototype smart bandage is highlighted in Fig. 6.6.

A core challenge when considering the application of sensing devices within biofluids relates to overcoming issues of nonspecific binding where macromolecular debris effectively blocks the active surfaces leading to reduced sensitivity. This was observed when the carbon fiber sensor was tested in serum samples where although

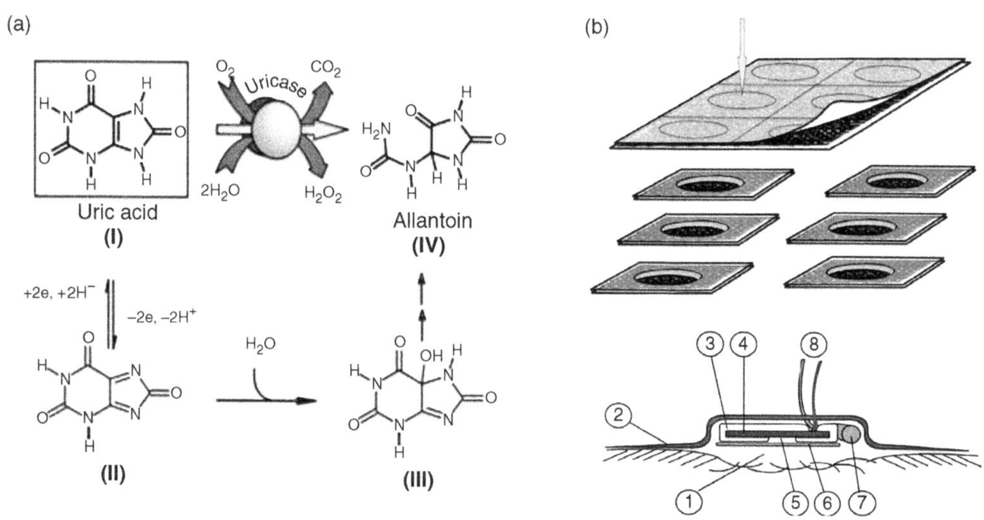

Figure 6.6 (a) Electrochemical oxidation and bacterial metabolism of urate. (b) Schematic of the lamination process and the prototype sensing assembly. (1) Wound aperture, (2) adhesive plaster backing, (3) insulating laminate, (4) carbon fiber sensor, (5) sensing window, (6) cellulose acetate barrier, (7) combined Ag/AgCl reference/counter electrode, (8) contacts to measuring device [124].

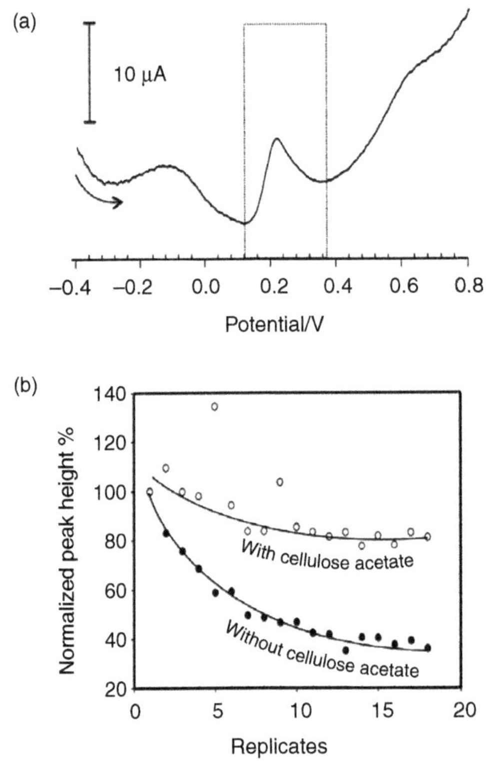

Figure 6.7 (a) Square wave voltammograms detailing the response of an anodized carbon fiber sensing assembly toward human serum. (b) Influence of cellulose acetate on the periodic response monitoring of urate in serum [124].

the urate peak is clearly resolved (Fig. 6.7a), the peak height was found to decrease on repetitive scans. The variation in peak height with increasing scan number is highlighted in Fig. 6.7b, and it is clear that the unprotected carbon sensor would be of little value for periodic measurements where there is a need to monitor the bacteria-induced removal of urate. The system can however be improved through the use of permselective barriers (ie, cellulose acetate) to filter out the large molecular weight components (Fig. 6.7b).

The efficacy of applying the sensor for assessing the bacterial metabolism of urate was trialed using *P. aeruginosa*, *S. aureus*, and *K. pneumoniae*. The electrode responses, as a function of incubation time, are highlighted in Fig. 6.8. There are considerable differences in the rate at which the different microbes metabolize the urate with *P. aeruginosa* being the more aggressive consumer. The response of the latter stands in marked contrast to the responses observed with *S. aureus* and *K. pneumoniae*. One important issue is that the latter had no effect on the urate concentration and thus can raise the issue of the susceptibility of the approach to false negatives.

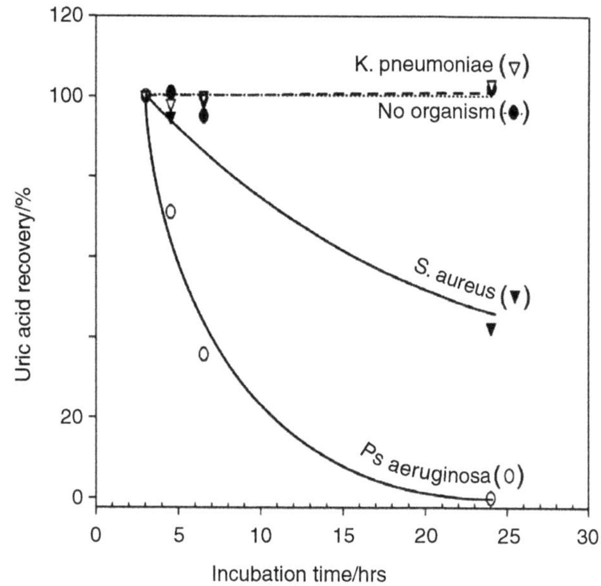

Figure 6.8 ***Influence of bacterial strain and incubation time on metabolism of exogenous urate (0.2 mM) compared with the sterile control (dotted line) [124].***

6.10 PORE-FORMING TOXINS—UNILAMELLAR VESICLES

An alternative, and electronics-free, approach has been demonstrated by Zhou et al. [125,126]. The system employs a "Trojan horse" methodology which utilizes giant unilamellar vesicles immobilized onto/within the fibers of a suitable dressing. The giant unilamellar vesicles are loaded with a fluorophore indicator that is released in the presence of bacteria that secrete pore-forming toxins (ie, α-hemolysin or phospholipase A_2). The latter are typically produced by pathogenic strains of bacteria (*S. aureus* and *P. aeruginosa*) and thus are key targets in the pursuit of simple, inexpensive dressings that can provide an early warning. The basic reaction scheme is highlighted in Fig. 6.9 and an example of a prototype dressing is illustrated in Fig. 6.10.

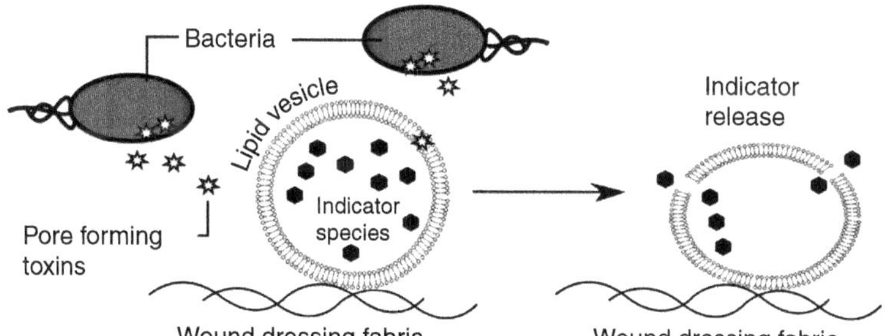

Figure 6.9 ***Schematic representation of vesicle rupture due to presence of pathogenic bacteria.*** *(Adapted from Zhou et al. [125,126]).*

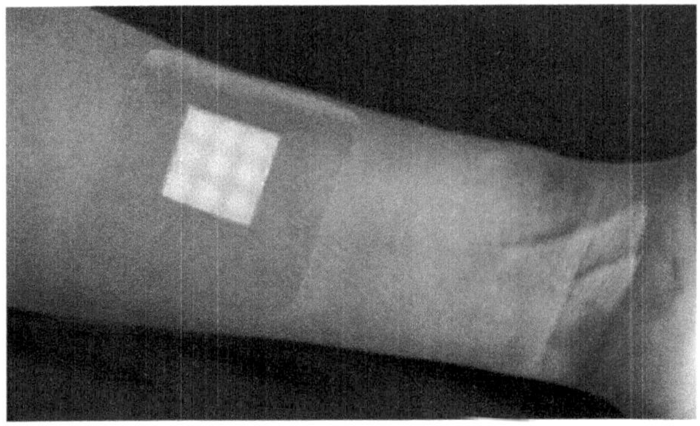

Figure 6.10 ***Proposed implementation of the smart bandage with the fluorescence of the dressing indicating the presence of pathogenic bacteria.*** *(Reproduced with permission University of Bath).*

Preliminary studies with a range of bacteria demonstrated considerable selectivity with nonpathogenic strains failing to lyse the vesicles to any significant extent and therefore it could go some way to addressing the significant clinical issue of distinguishing between harmless colonization and infection [3]. A critical advantage of the approach is that the bandage could be used to proactively target the invading bacteria with the release of an antimicrobial along with the fluorophore.

6.11 CEPHALOSPORIN-MODIFIED DRESSINGS

A similar strategy to the work conducted by Zhou and colleagues was proposed by Brocklesby and colleagues where it was postulated that the attachment of dye-modified Cephalosporin derivatives onto a dressing could be a useful visual indicator of infection [127]. The detection rationale is based on the expression beta-lactamase enzymes into the extracellular matrix which would cleave the beta-lactam functionality present within the Cephalosporin as highlighted in Fig. 6.11. The subsequent molecular rearrangement releases the drug whose diffusion cleverly reveals the word infection. There are a significant number of assumptions in this proposal and, as yet, it remains a proposition as there is no supporting to data to validate its efficacy. It does however point toward an innovative pathway which, if possible, could enable a relatively cheap means of producing dressings that can passively sense for antibiotic-resistant bacteria. The main question however will be discriminating between contamination and critical colonization.

6.12 IMMUNE RESPONSE BIOMARKERS

Once an injury has been created, neutrophil granulocytes will be among the first cell type to appear within the wound bed and are the host's primary form of decontaminating the wound. The neutrophils release a cocktail of enzymes such as human

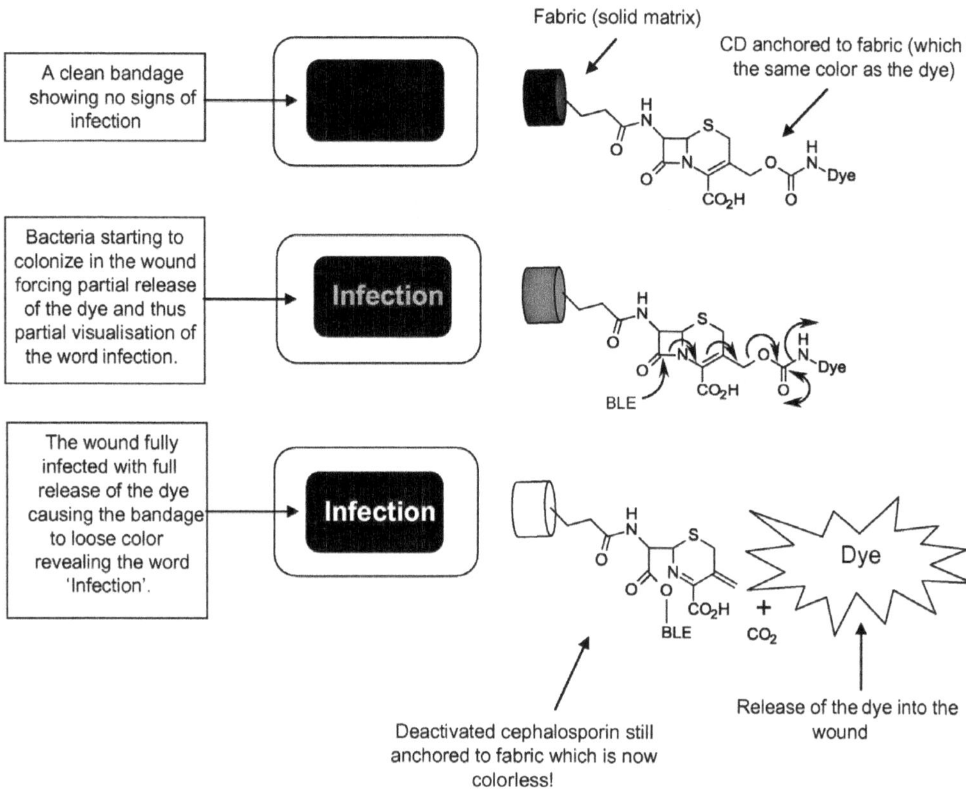

Figure 6.11 ***Proposed smart bandage based on cephalosporin-dye hybrids [127].***

neutrophil elastase (HNE), Cathepsin G (CatG), Lysozyme, Myeloperoxidase (MPO), and matrix metalloproteases (MMPs). The most sensitive detector of early infection is, in fact, the host's immune response, and therefore monitoring the changes/sudden increase in the activity of the neutrophil enzymes could provide an indication that the condition had changed from contamination to critical colonization [128–130]. There is no inherent information about the identity of the invading species—simply that there is a problem.

It must be noted that protease activity within the wound is a normal process that enables the remodeling of the extracellular matrix, connective tissues, and the removal of macromolecular debris [131]. It is recognized that the activity of the protease enzymes will be high in the early stages of the wound and can be expected to decrease the healing progress. It has already been mentioned that, in chronic wounds, protease activity can be maintained for extended periods and it is this continued activity that contributes to a failure to heal [132]. Therefore, one of the main challenges in dealing with the latter is the ability to distinguish between the different enzyme species such that a clearer picture can be obtained as to "normal elevated protease" and protease release due to infection.

Heinzle et al. [133] have demonstrated that the activities of particular proteases are elevated in response to infection when compared to wounds that are uninfected.

6.12.1 Detection of Human Neutrophil Elastase and Cathespin G

These enzymes are released from the primary (azurophil) granules of neutrophils in response to infection and have relatively broad substrate specificity. The activity of the enzymes can be determined in a conventional assay format through assessing the hydrolysis of a suitable substrate modified with a chromophore. Bopp and Goynes [134] were among the first to investigate the development of immobilized chromogenic substrates for assessing HNE activity and based their approach on the HNE promoted release of p-nitroanilide (pNA) from either Suc-AAPV-pNA and suc-AAPA-pNA. The substrates were covalently attached to an ethoxylate acrylate resin whereupon the enzyme-promoted release could be measured using a conventional colorimeter. As expected, the sterically hindered immobilized substrate exhibited slower hydrolysis rates than the freely diffusing species.

The approach was taken further by Hasmann et al. [128–130] who exploited the immobilization of N-methoxysuccinyl-AAPV-p-nitroanilide (MeOSuc-AAPVpNA) using the hydrolysable AAPV target motif. The strategy involved immobilizing the substrate on a range of polymeric materials (polyamides, polyethylene terephthalate, collagen films, and matrices of hyaluronic acid) that have traditionally been used within wound dressings (see Chapter 4). Hasmann found that when the dressing was incubated with wound fluid from "normal wounds" and those that were infected—only the latter would give rise to the color change due to the activity of the HNE enzyme [128,129]. Although the mechanism is significantly different to that developed by Zhou [125,126], the overall alert methodology is similar and outlined in Fig. 6.12.

The AAPV unit is a critical element in securing selectivity toward HNE and was further exploited as a crosslinking element linking dextran hydrogels. This detection rationale is based on a quartz crystal microbalance which, in the absence of HNE, resonates at

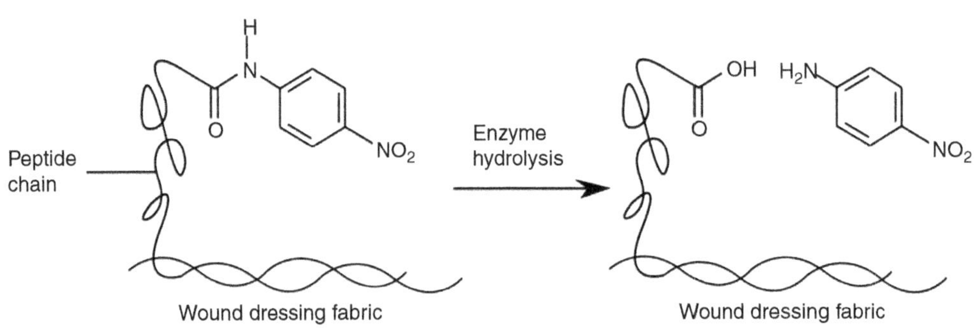

Figure 6.12 ***Protease selective dressings.***

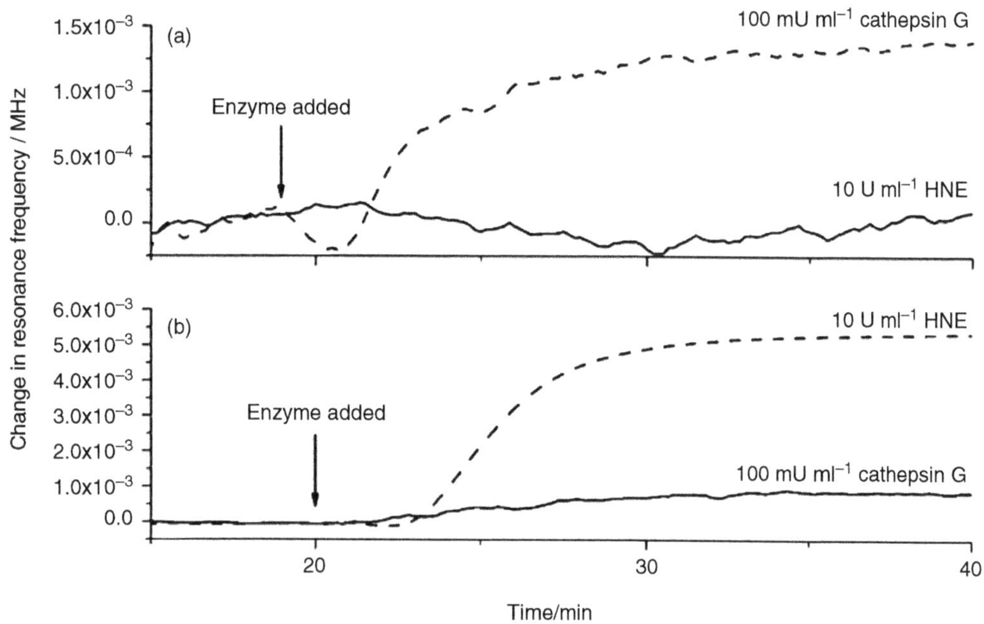

Figure 6.13 ***Effect of cross-linker sequence on activity of HNE and CatG.*** Change in resonant frequency for QCM crystals coated with hydrogels crosslinked with (a) AAPFFK and (b) AAPVAAK [135].

a set frequency [135]. Upon exposure to the HNE enzyme, hydrolysis of the AAPVAAK cross linker occurs which leads to the dissolution of the gel and a subsequent change in the frequency (Fig. 6.13). This is an innovative approach and, while its use as a diagnostic in the present context is more for curiosity value, the enzyme-promoted hydrolysis of the gel may be of use in the future where it could be envisaged that the enzyme could enable the release of an appropriate therapeutic agent.

The detection of CatG is similarly important and it acts alongside HNE in the immune response. It could be expected that as both HNE and CatG have similar roles, it would be difficult to distinguish between them; however, they have different affinities for different aminoacid motifs. Where HNE acts on the AAPV sequence, CatG targets AAPF and thus dressings containing immobilized AAPF-pNA have been shown to be selective targets for the latter. As with HNE, the color change arising from the release of the pNA chromophore was only observed when the polymer was incubated in wound fluid from infected samples [135].

6.12.2 Detection of Lysozyme

Lysozyme is categorized as a glycosidase and acts through hydrolyzing the glycosidic bonds within peptidoglycans (PG). It has considerable antimicrobial activity given the presence of the latter within bacterial cell walls. Several groups have reported the presence of elevated levels of the enzyme within infected wound fluids, and in a similar vein as HNE and CatG, its activity could be exploited as an early warning signal for impending infection. As such, there have been significant efforts to develop sensors for its detection [129,136]. The first approaches to developing a sensing system for assessing lysozyme activity were based on agarose/PG layers, whereby elevated levels of the enzyme would result in the hydrolysis of the PG layer and thereby promote a change in turbidity [129]. A more refined version was subsequently developed in which Remazol Brilliant Blue (RBB) was encapsulated with the composite framework which would ease colorimetric/visual detection. The hydrolysis of the PG upper layer was found to lead to a stained appearance in the underlying agarose hydrogel [129].

A more elaborate version of the multilayer detection system was developed by Schneider et al. [136] with the addition of laccases covalently attached to the PG layer. Laccases are copper-containing oxygen oxidoreductases and, in the presence of oxygen, are able to oxidize a variety of substrates (phenols, aromatic amines, and inorganic/organometallic complexes) [137,138]. Their role in the present instance was to oxidize (2,2-azinobis-(3-ethylbenzothiazoline-6-disulfonic acid)) (ABTS) and thereby provide a visual (or quantifiable colorimetric signal). In the absence of lysozyme, the laccase is firmly bound within the PG matrix and unable to oxidize the ABTS. In the presence of the enzyme (ie, from infected wound fluid), the PG chains are hydrolyzed, freeing the enzyme which can diffuse and oxidize the ABTS giving rise to the positive signal. The schematic of the device operation is highlighted in Fig. 6.14.

The use of aptamers, artificial single stranded nucleic acids, represents a relatively new strategy in the development of diagnostic devices and has found applications in the detection of a variety of biomedical markers such as proteins, toxins, and neurotransmitters

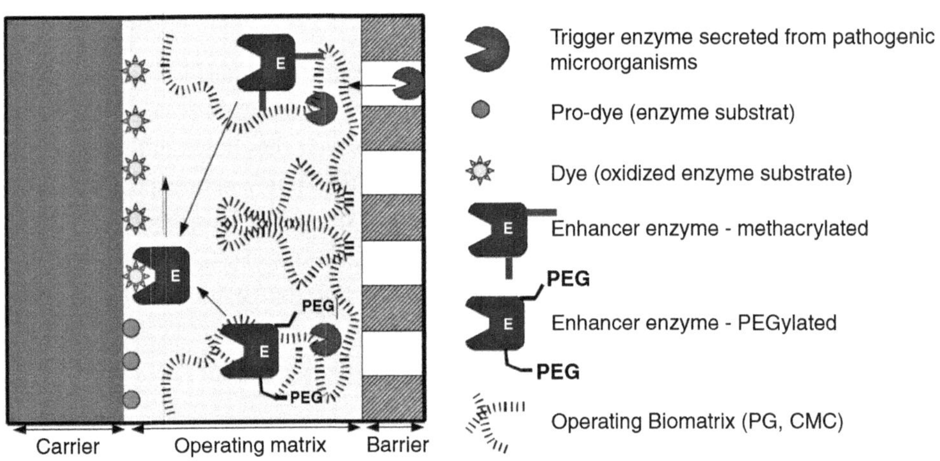

Figure 6.14 ***Format and operation of the laccase-modified sensor targeted at the detection of lysozyme activity [136].***

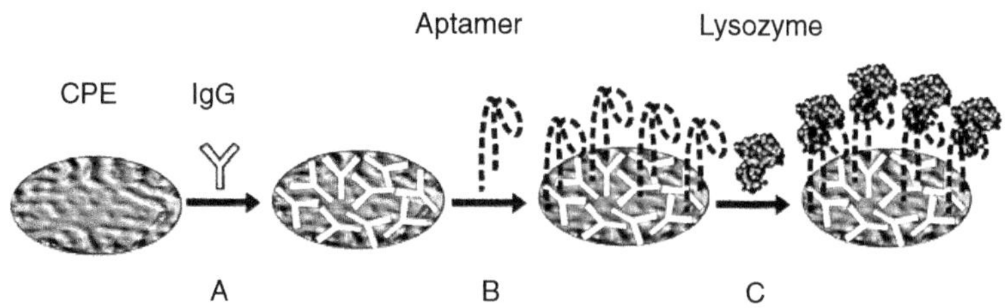

Figure 6.15 ***Electrode modification to yield aptamer functionalized surfaces selective toward lysozyme [145].***

[139–142]. Through careful design, the aptamer can exhibit tailored properties that can enable high specificity in binding target molecules and thus they have become attractive as molecular recognition elements [142]. Several aptamer sensors for the detection of lysozyme have arisen in recent years [143–147], but their application within a complex matrix such as a wound has yet to be proven. Nevertheless, the underpinning technology clearly provides some important insights when considering the design of smart bandages and their implementation could have significant advantages over conventional immunoassay-based techniques. Aptamers designed for the capture of lysozyme have employed spectroscopic [143] and electrochemical detection [144–147].

Work by Rodríguez and Rivas [145] is particularly noteworthy in that they demonstrated the ability of a carbon electrode modified with a layer of lysozyme-selective aptamer to detect the enzyme with a minimum of sample manipulation as indicated in Fig. 6.15. This "reagentless" strategy contrasts the complexity of fluorescence systems and goes some way toward a more accessible point of care device. The detection rationale centers on the electrochemical oxidation of the purine bases (adenine and guanine) within the aptamer. In the absence of the enzyme, the bases are in close proximity to the electrode and can be readily oxidized but, upon binding, there is a change in the conformation of the aptamer which reduces the electrochemical accessibility of the purine and hence a decrease in the oxidation peak is observed.

Square wave voltammograms detailing the response of the aptamer-modified electrodes toward lysozyme are highlighted in Fig. 6.16. It must also be noted that the potentials required to oxidize adenine and guanine are very large ($> +1\,V$) and thus it is inevitable that there would be substantial interference from other electroactive components within the wound fluid which would obscure the signal. Could the system be incorporated within a bandage material? The use of screen-printed or carbon composites would certainly allow the immobilization of the aptamer, but there are a number of methodological queries. The analysis is based on the oxidation of the purine bases and it is generally accepted that such electrode processes are irreversible. Thus, when oxidized, the purine is no longer able to be reoxidized. While this approach can be used for single-shot diagnostics, it would create numerous issues in terms of periodic screening.

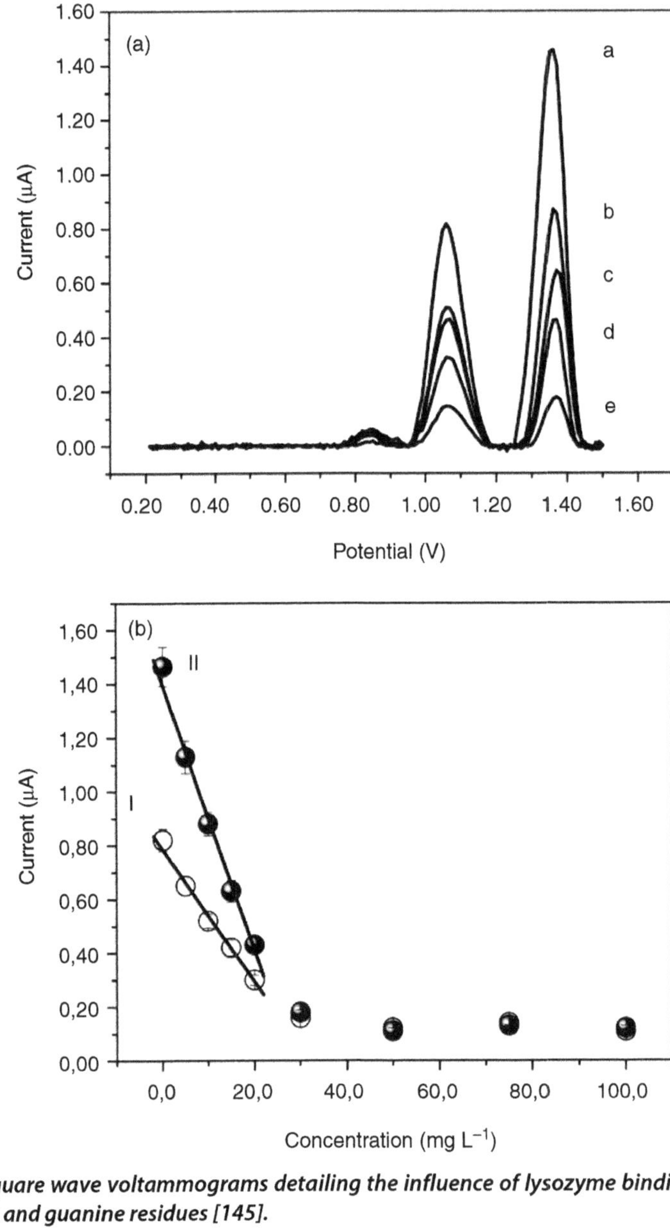

Figure 6.16 ***Square wave voltammograms detailing the influence of lysozyme binding on the oxidation of adenine and guanine residues [145].***

An alternative and potentially more appropriate approach was demonstrated by Li et al. [147]. Their method involved the immobilization of the aptamer onto gold nanoparticles but, rather than exploit the electrochemical properties of the nucleic acid strands, they employed a dual strand system with a ferrocene redox label. The latter is

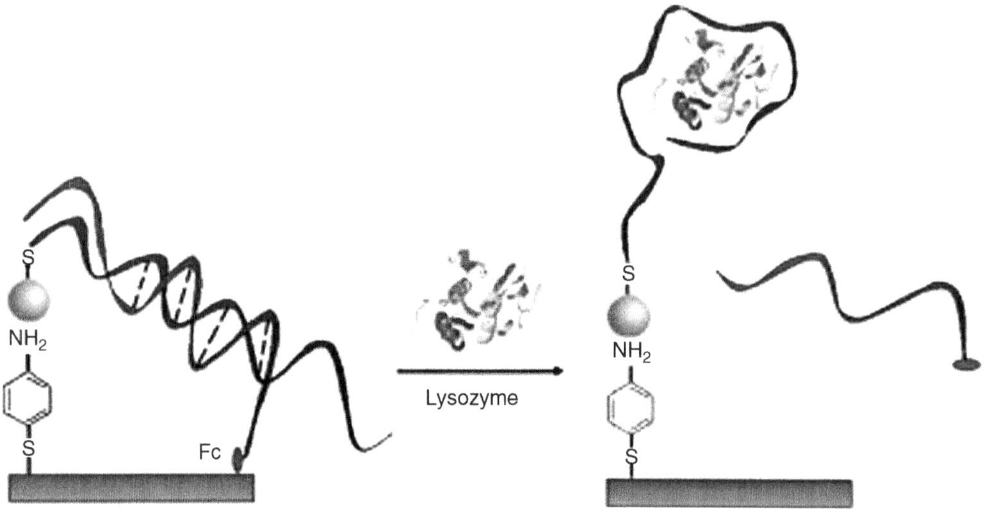

Figure 6.17 ***Change in conformation and loss of the ferrocene redox probe upon the aptamer based binding of lysozyme [147].***

a reversible redox system which could enable repeated oxidation–reduction cycles and stands in marked contrast to the irreversible purine electrochemistry described earlier. The aptamer consists of a 42-base sequence which is immobilized onto the gold nanoparticles; a second partially complementary strand bearing the ferrocene label is then added to form the double strand structure. The basic detection rationale is highlighted in Fig. 6.17. In the absence of the lysozyme target, the strand is effectively doubled over on itself which brings the terminal ferrocene group in close proximity to the electrode. The electrochemical interrogation of the latter provides an "on" signal which can be repetitively scanned. Upon the binding of lysozyme, there is a conformational change with the dismantling of the duplex structure and the release of the ferrocene chain. This has the net effect of reducing the magnitude of the ferrocene signal.

This approach is more suited to the use of periodic scanning and it is possible to envisage its adaptation to a smart dressing designed to detect lysozyme. The ferrocene label is useful in that it allows a low detection potential thereby avoiding many of the interferences liable to be present in wound fluid but, the release of the redox strand upon binding may well be an issue in terms of toxicology and biocompatibility.

Lysozyme detection has also been demonstrated through the use of fluorescence-based nanoparticle sensors and takes advantage of the glycosidic hydrolytic properties of the enzyme [148]. Carboxymethyl chitosan (CMC) modified CdTe quantum dots exhibit a high affinity for zinc ions as a consequence of the binding between the metal ion and the CMC coating. The binding of the zinc gives rise to an enhanced photoluminescence signal. In the presence of lysozyme, the CMC coating is attacked with the

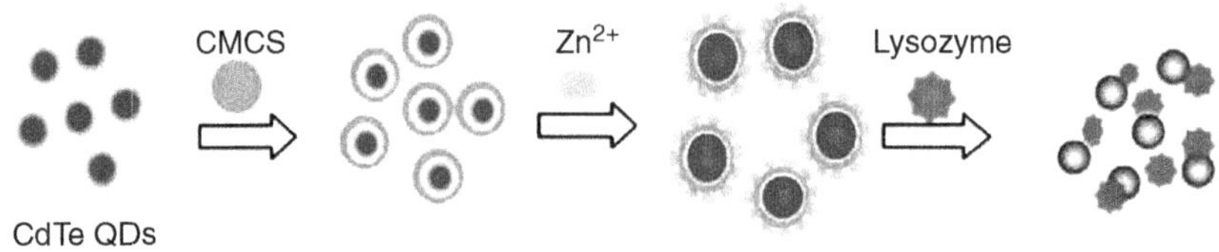

Figure 6.18 ***Fabrication of chitosan-modified quantum dots and their application toward the detection of lysozyme [148].***

subsequent hydrolysis releasing the zinc ions—diminishing the signal with the lysozyme–quantum dot complex quenching the photoluminescence. The reaction scheme is highlighted in Fig. 6.18. The quantum dot approach has been tested in a variety of biological fluids (including human sera) and found to have no significant interferences and could, in principle, prove useful as a potential technology for incorporation within a dressing.

6.12.3 Detection of Myeloperoxidase

Myeloperoxidase is a co-worker of HNE, CatG, and Lysozyme and is similarly released by neutrophils [149] but, in contrast to their hydrolytic nature, MPO functions to combine chloride and peroxide to produce hypochlorous acid. Hypochlorous acid (HOCl) is the most powerful oxidant produced by neutrophils [150] and is effectively biological bleach and will oxidize a variety of organic molecules within the wound environment. As with the other neutrophil-derived enzymes, its presence can be used as an indicator of the early signs of infection, and thus, there is considerable merit in attempting to design materials that can alert the patient/healthcare professional to its presence. Increased levels of MPO activity have been associated with increased bioburden within wound fluids [151]. There has been considerable activity in relation to the development of assays for MPO. Hasmann et al. [129] exploited its ability to oxidize phenolic compounds (guaiacol) and found significantly increased levels of MPO in infected wound fluids (92.2 + 45.0 versus 1.9 + 1.8 U/mL).

Some of the early approaches to the detection of MPO activity mirrored the approaches to HNE and CatG, whereby a suitable polymer could be loaded with a substrate that is selective to the action of MPO. While it is known that MPO can oxidize small phenolic compounds within the wound environment, it is also clear that it could similarly oxidize synthetic substrates. A number of dyes (ie, Fast Blue RR) were covalently bound to siloxane films with the development of the color arising upon oxidation by the enzyme. There are questions over the applicability within complex samples as the oxidation could be induced through a number of routes. The chlorination activity has been proffered as a more selective means of assessing MPO activity. The enzyme combines chloride ion and peroxide to form HOCl but, rather than measure HOCl

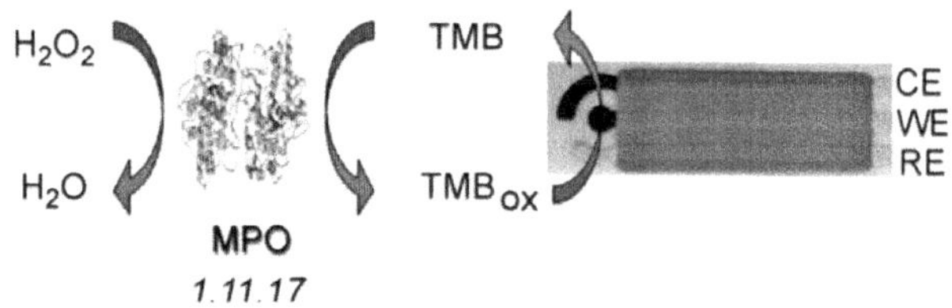

Figure 6.19 ***Mechanism for the amperometric detection of MPO at a screen-printed sensor [152].***

production, a number of authors have attempted to correlate the consumption of peroxide with MPO activity.

A screen-printed approach to measuring the depletion of peroxide was developed by Windmiller et al. [152]. The MPO has a haem redox center and, through the process of reducing the peroxide, the iron is oxidatively converted from the +2 oxidation state to +3. Windmiller employed an electron transfer mediator to shuttle electrons between the screen-printed electrode and the MPO redox center as indicated in Fig. 6.19. The electrochemical assay employs 3,3′,5,5′-tetramethylbenzidine (TMB) as a redox mediator and the analytical signal is derived from the electroreduction of the TMB which has been oxidized in the course of the enzyme reaction. In the absence of MPO, there is no catalysis and hence little response, but increased MPO will lead to an increase in reduction current as the TMB mediator begins to be oxidized. Although potentially useful as a diagnostic aid, its translation into an immobilized form could be problematic in terms of anchoring the redox mediator while still allowing it to interact with the MPO. At present, the system is based on a freely diffusing model but, within the confines of a dressing, it may be difficult for the MPO to interact with the redox mediator.

A variation in the Windmiller system was proposed by Herrasti et al. [153] who developed an immunosensor system for the detection of MPO. The detection methodology is highlighted in Fig. 6.20 where immune-functionalized magnetic microparticles

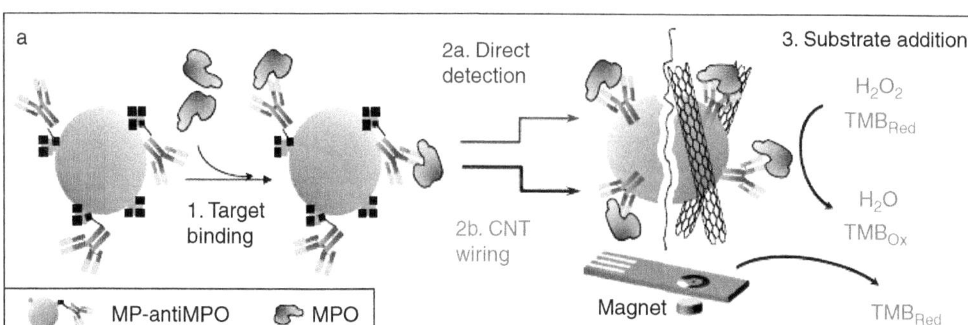

Figure 6.20 ***Steps involved in the construction of MPO-selective magnetic particles and their electroanalytical detection [153].***

were used to capture MPO at a disposable screen-printed sensor. Once captured, the introduction of the TMB mediator could enable the amperometric detection much in the same way as Windmiller et al. [152]. The principal advantage is the ability to matrix exchange (remove the interferences) and, while this is a useful addition to a point of care application, it is difficult to see how it could be implemented within an integrated dressing.

The central rationale is however supported by recent findings where there were highly significant differences in chlorination activity observed between infected and noninfected wounds [153]. In the case of a point of care test, it is possible to add standard solutions of peroxide to a given sample and then measure the difference in the concentration before and after. In attempting to translate the basic detection methodology to a smart dressing, there is an issue of the origin of the peroxide. Hajnsek et al. [151] have presented an elegant solution to this issue, whereby they have developed an in situ approach to measuring MPO peroxide consumption. The immobilization of glucose oxidase within the system enables the local generation of peroxide (through the enzymatic conversion of glucose) which can serve as the feedstock for the MPO enzyme [163]. The reaction methodology and typical signal response are highlighted in Figs. 6.21 and 6.22.

In the absence of MPO, there is a sustained production of peroxide whereas in the presence of the enzyme there is a marked decrease. The authors have used a flow system through which to characterize the sensing response but, it is unclear how the sensor would operate within a dressing. Nevertheless, it is a promising approach to MPO activity assessment.

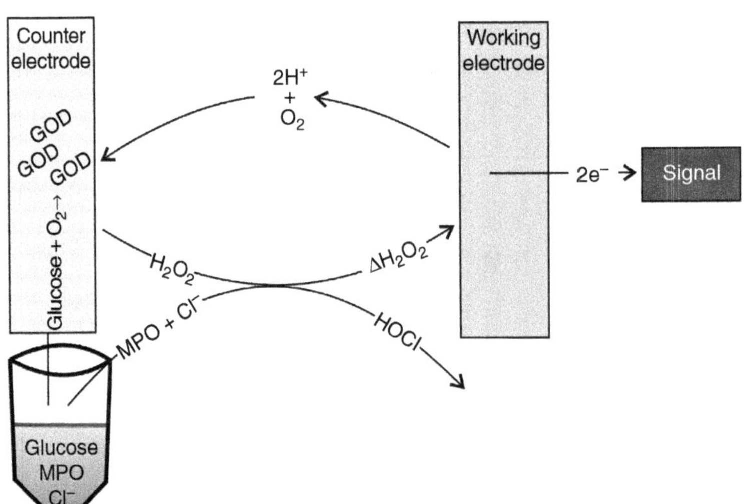

Figure 6.21 ***Reaction scheme for the electroanalytical assessment of MPO activity [151].***

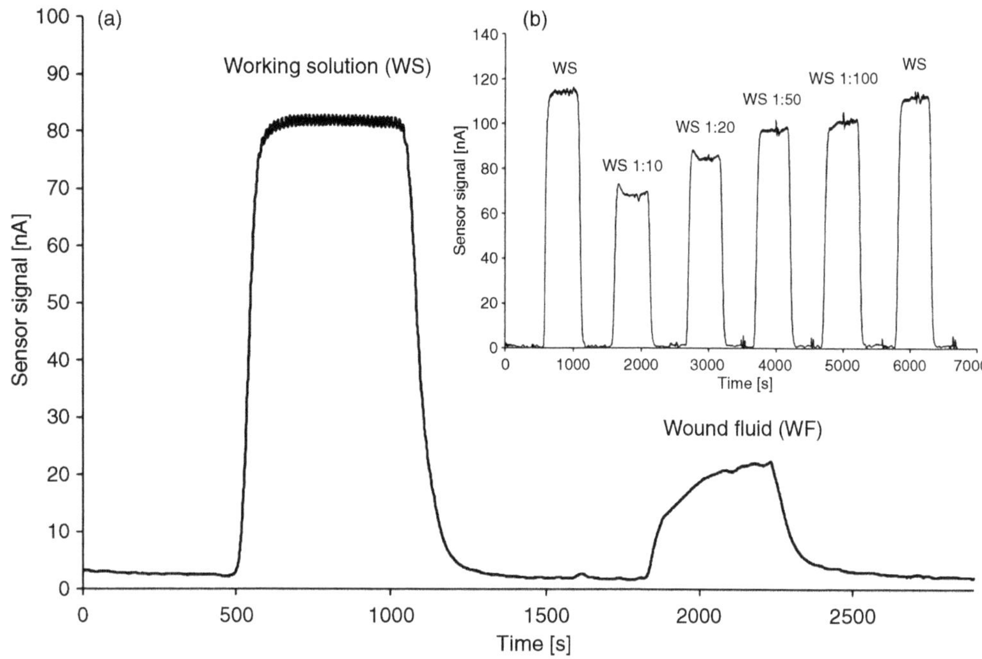

Figure 6.22 ***Flow response of the in situ generated peroxide sensing system to aliquots of a control solution and wound fluid containing MPO [151].***

6.13 SUMMARY

It has long been recognized that the early identification of infection can significantly improve patient outcome and can help prevent the development of life-threatening complications. At present, there remains considerable reliance on subjective parameters and, while there is a wealth of sophisticated detection techniques that can aid identification of individual strains, their availability for use within routine clinical practice is questionable and are, all too often, the preserve of dedicated research groups. There is little doubt that the availability of diagnostic tools that can rapidly alert the healthcare professional to the onset of infection would be a major benefit. There have been substantial advances in exploiting markers from both the invading microbe and the innate immune response of the host. It could be envisaged that these could provide an early warning to the onset of infection and could serve as the foundation of smart device.

The development of assays has traditionally been viewed from the perspective of lab-based system where sample manipulation would have been considered normal. The translation of the techniques to a format capable of serving as a smart dressing is a considerable challenge and requires a different mindset. There has been a subtle explosion in the number of articles seeking to develop smart dressings and, while many of these remain locked at the "wet end" of the sensing interface, there is a gradual shift toward systems that are reagentless and require little input from the user. This can be seen in many of the techniques presented within the chapter and it is encouraging that attention is now being trained on the particular needs of the clinician from a community treatment context.

REFERENCES

[1] World Union of Wound Healing Societies (WUWHS). Principles of best practice: Wound infection in clinical practice. An international consensus. London: MEP Ltd, 2008. Available at: www.mepltd.co.uk
[2] International Best Practice Guidelines: Wound Management in Diabetic Foot Ulcers. Wounds International, 2013. Available at: www.woundsinternational.com.
[3] Percival J. Classification of wounds and their management. Surgery 2002;20:114–7.
[4] Dowsett C, Blelby A, Searle R. Reconciling increasing wound care demands with available resources. J Wound Care 2014;23:552–62.
[5] Lavery LA, Armstrong DA, Wunderlich RP, et al. Risk factors for foot infections in individuals with diabetes. Diabetes Care 2006;29(6):1288–93.
[6] Richards JL, Lavigne JP, Got I, et al. Management of patients hospitalized for diabetic foot infection: results of the French OPIDIA study. Diabetes Metab 2011;37:208–15.
[7] Gardner SE, Frantz RA, Troia C, Eastman S, MacDonald M, Buresh K, et al. A tool to assess the clinical signs and symptoms of localized infection in chronic wounds: development and reliability. Ostomy/Wound Manage 2001;47:40–7.
[8] Gardner SE, Hillis Stephen L, Frantz RA. Clinical signs of infection in diabetic foot ulcers with high microbial load. Biol Res Nurs 2010;11:119–28.
[9] Cutting KF, Harding KG. Criteria for identifying wound infection. J Wound Care 1994;3:198–201.
[10] Gardner SE, Frantz RA, Doebbeling BN. The validity of the clinical signs and symptoms used to identify localized chronic wound infection. Wound Repair Regen 2001;9:178–86.
[11] Gardner SE, Hillis SL, Frantz RA. Clinical signs of infection in diabetic foot ulcers with high microbial load. Biol Res Nurs 2009;11:119–28.
[12] Lipsky BA, Berendt AR, Deery HG, Embil JM, Joseph WS, Karchmer AW, et al. Diagnosis and treatment of diabetic foot infections. Clin Infect Dis 2004;39:885–910.
[13] Gardner SE, Frantz RA, Saltzman CL. Diabetes and inflammation in infected chronic wounds. Wounds 2005;17:203–5.
[14] Edwards R, Harding K. Bacteria and wound healing. Curr Opin Infect Dis 2004;17:91–6.
[15] Enoch S, Harding K. Wound bed preparation: the science behind the removal of barriers to healing. Wounds 2003;15(7):213–29.
[16] Schultz G, Sibbald G, Falanga V, Ayello E, Dowsett C, Harding K, Romanelli M, Stacey MC, Teot L, Vanscheidt W. Wound bed preparation: a systematic approach to wound management. Wound Repair Regen 2003;11:S1–S28.
[17] Bowler P, Davies B. The microbiology of acute and chronic wounds. Wounds 1999;11:72–9.
[18] Dow G, Browne A, Sibbald G. Infection in chronic wounds: controversies in diagnosis and treatment. Ostomy Wound Manage 1999;45(8):23–40.
[19] Wright A, Flemming A, Colebrook L. The conditions under which the sterilization of wounds by physiologic agency can be obtained. Lancet 1918;1:831–8.
[20] Bowler P. The anaerobic and aerobic microbiology of wounds: a review. Wounds 1998;10:170–8.
[21] Haneke E. Infections in dermatological surgery. In: Harahap M, editor. Diagnosis and treatment of skin infections. Oxford: Blackwell Science; 1997. p. 416–30.
[22] Klimek J. Treatment of wound infections. Cutis 1985;15:21–4.
[23] Mayhall C. Surgical infections including burns. In: Wenzel R, editor. Prevention and control of nosocomial infections. Baltimore: Williams & Wilkins Co; 1993. p. 614–64.
[24] Nichols R, Smith J. Anaerobes from a surgical perspective. Clin Infect Dis 1994;18:S280–6.
[25] Page G, Beattie T. Infection in the accident and emergency department. In: Taylor W, editor. Infection in surgical practice. Oxford: Oxford University Press; 1992. p. 123–32.

[26] Brook I. Aerobic and anaerobic microbiology of necrotising fascitis in children. Pediatr Dermatol 1996;13:281–4.
[27] Daltrey D, Rhodes B, Chattwood J. Investigation into the microbial flora of healing and non-healing decubitus ulcers. J Clin Pathol 1981;34:701–5.
[28] Danielsen L, Balslev E, Döring G, Høiby N, Madsen S, A° gren M, Thomsen HK, Henrik H, Steen F, Westh H. Ulcer bed infection. Report of a case of enlarging venous leg ulcer colonised by Pseudomonas aeruginosa. Acta Pathol Microbiol Immunol Scand 1998;106:721–6.
[29] Gilland E, Nathwani N, Dore C, Lewis J. Bacterial colonization of leg ulcers and its effect on the success rate of skin grafting. Ann R Coll Surg Engl 1988;70:105–8.
[30] Halbert A, Stacey M, Rohr J, Jopp-McKay A. The effect of bacterial colonisation on venous healing. Australas J Dermatol 1992;33:75–80.
[31] MacFarlane D, Baum K, Serjeant G. Bacteriology of sickle cell leg ulcers. Trans R Soc Trop Med Hyg 1986;80:553–6.
[32] Madsen S, Westh H, Danielsen L, Roshahl V. Bacterial colonisation and healing of venous leg ulcers. Acta Pathol Microbiol Immunol Scand 1996;104:895–9.
[33] Schraibman I. The significance of beta-haemolytic streptococci in chronic leg ulcers. Ann R Coll Surg Med 1990;7292:123–4.
[34] Sehgal S, Arunkumar B. Microbial flora and its significance in pathology of sickle cell disease in leg ulcers. Infection 1992;20:86–8.
[35] Twum-Danso K, Grant C, Al-Suleiman A, Abdel- Khaders S, Al-Awami M, Al-Breiki H, Taha S. Microbiology of postoperative wound infection: a prospective study of 1770 wounds. J Hosp Infect 1992;21:29–37. 34.
[36] Bowler P, Duerden I, Armstrong G. Wound microbiology and associated approaches to wound management. Clin Microbiol Rev 2001;14:244–69.
[37] Washinton J. The role of the microbiology laboratory in antimicrobial susceptibility testing. Infect Med 1999;16:531–2.
[38] Dow G. Bacterial swabs and the chronic wound: when, how, and what do they mean. Ostomy Wound Manage 2003;49:8–13.
[39] Gardner S, Frantz R, Bradley N, Dobbeling M. The validity of the clinical signs and symptoms used to identify localized chronic wound infection. Wound Repair Regen 2001;9:178–86.
[40] Kingsley A. The wound infection continuum and its application to clinical practice. Ostomy Wound Manage 2003;49:1–7.
[41] Robson M. A failure of wound healing caused by an imbalance of bacteria. Surg Clin North Am 1997;77:637–50.
[42] Robson M, Heggers J. Bacterial quantification of open wounds. Military Med 1969;134:19–24.
[43] Rudensky B, Lipschits M, Isaacsohn M, Sonnenblick M. Infected pressure sores: comparison of methods for bacterial identification. South Med J 1992;85:901–3.
[44] Stotts N. Determination of bacterial burden in wounds. Adv Wound Care 1995;8:28–46.
[45] Thompson P, Smith D. What is infection? Am J Surg 1994;167:S7.
[46] Fleck C. Identifying infection in chronic wounds. Adv Skin Wound Care 2006;19:20–1.
[47] Kelly F. Infection control: validity and reliability in wound swabbing. Br J Nurs 2003;12:959–64.
[48] Cooper R, Lawrence J. The isolation and identification of bacteria from wounds. J Wound Care 1996;5:335–40.
[49] Donovan S. Wound infection and wound swabbing. Prof Nurs 1998;13:757–9.
[50] Kingsley A. Audit of wound swab sampling: why protocols could improve practice. Prof Nurs 2003;18:338–43.
[51] Walker JT, Verran J, Boyle B, Percival SL. Microscopy methods to investigate the structure of potable water biofilms. Methods Enzymol 2002;337:243–55.
[52] Walker JT, Percival SL. Control of biofouling in drinking water systems. In: Walker JT, Surman S, Jess J, editors. Industrial biofouling: detection, prevention and control, vol. 1. Chichester, UK: John Wiley and Sons; 2001. p. 103–21.
[53] Percival SL, Thomas JG, Williams DW. The world of microbiology and biofilmology. In: Percival SL, Cutting K, editors. Microbiology of wounds. London, UK: CRC Press; 2010. p. 1–58.
[54] Percival SL, Rogers AA. The significance and role of biofilms in chronic wounds. In: McBain A, Allison D, Pratten J, Spratt D, Upton M, Verran J, editors. Biofilms, persistence and ubiquity. Bioline: Cardiff; 2005. p. 171–80.

[55] Percival SL, Kite P, Stickler D. The use of urinary catheters and control of biofilms using TEDTA. Urol Res 2009;37:205–9.
[56] Percival SL, Walker JT. Biofilms and public health significance. Biofouling 1999;14:99–115.
[57] Percival SL, Kite P, Donlan RM. Assessing the effectiveness of tetrasodium ethylene diaminetetraacetic acid as a novel central venous catheter (CVC) lock solution against biofilms using a laboratory model system. Infect Control Hosp Epidemiol 2005;26:515–9.
[58] Kite P, Eastwood K, Sugden S, Percival SL. Use of in-vivo generated biofilms from haemodialysis catheters to test the efficacy of a novel antimicrobial catheter lock for biofilm eradication in-vitro. J Clin Microbiol 2004;42:3073–6.
[59] Donlan RM, Costerton JW. Biofilms: survival mechanisms of clinically relevant microorganisms. Clin Microbiol Rev 2002;15:167–93.
[60] Sauer K, Camper AK, Ehrlich GD, Costerton JW, Davies DG. Pseudomonas aeruginosa displays multiple phenotypes during development as a biofilm. J Bacteriol 2002;184:1140–54.
[61] Wysocki A. Evaluating and managing open skin wounds: colonization versus infection. Am Assoc Crit Care Nurs Clin Issues 2002;13:382–97.
[62] Sibbald R, Orsted H, Schultz G, Coutts P, Keast D. Preparing the wound bed 2003: focus on infection and inflammation. Ostomy Wound Manage 2003;49:24–51.
[63] Enoch S, Harding K. Wound bed preparation: the science behind the removal of barriers to healing. Wounds 2003;15:213–29.
[64] Association for the Advancement of Wound Care. A. Advancing your practice: understanding the role of biofilms. USA: Malvern PA; 2008.
[65] Percival S, Cutting K. Biofilms: possible strategies for suppression in chronic wounds. Nurs Standard 2009;23:64–72.
[66] Costerton J, Stewart P, Greenberg E. Bacterial biofilms: a common cause of persistent infections. Science 1999;284:1318–22.
[67] Kolter R, Losick R. One for all and all for one. Science 1998;280:226–7.
[68] Potera C. Forging a link between biofilms and disease. Science 1999;283:1837–9.
[69] Wolcott RD. Economic aspects of biofilm-based wound care in diabetic foot ulcers. J Wound Care 2015;24:189–94.
[70] Price LB, Liu CM, Melendez JH, Frankel YM, Engelthaler D, Aziz M, Bowers J, Rattray R, Ravel J, Kingsley C, Keim PS, Lazarus GS, Zenilman JM. Community analysis of chronic wound bacteria using 16S rRNA gene-based pyrosequencing: impact of diabetes and antibiotics on chronic wound microbiota. PLoS One 2009;4:e6462.
[71] Sibley CD, Peirano G, Church DL. Molecular methods for pathogen and microbial community detection and characterization: current and potential application in diagnostic microbiology. Infect Genet Evol 2012;12:505–21.
[72] Stotts N, Whitney J. Identifying and evaluating wound infection. Home Healthcare Nurs 1999;17:159–65.
[73] Wolcott RD, Dowd SE. A rapid method for characterising bacterial bioburden in chronic wounds. J Wound Care 2008;17:513–6.
[74] Carbonnelle E, Beretti JL, Cottyn S, Quesne G, Berche P, Nassif X, Ferroni A. Rapid identification of Staphylococci isolated in clinical microbiology laboratories by matrix-assisted laser desorption ionization-time of flight mass spectrometry. J Clin Microbiol 2007;45:2156–61.
[75] Carbonnelle E, Beretti JL, Cottyn S, Quesne G, Berche P, Nassif X, Ferroni A. Rapid identification of Staphylococci isolated in clinical microbiology laboratories by matrix-assisted laser desorption ionization-time of flight mass spectrometry. J Clin Microbiol 2007;45:2156–61.
[76] Croxatto A, Prod'hom G, Greub G. Applications of MALDI-TOF mass spectrometry in clinical diagnostic microbiology. FEMS Microbiol Rev 2012;36:380–407.
[77] Seng P, Drancourt M, Gouriet F, La Scola B, Fournier PE, Rolain JM, Raoult D. Ongoing revolution in bacteriology: routine identification of bacteria by matrix-assisted laser desorption ionization time-of-flight mass spectrometry. Clin Infect Dis 2009;49:543–51.
[78] Welham KJ, Domin MA, Scannell DE, Cohen E, Ashton DS. The characterization of micro-organisms by matrix assisted laser desorption/ionization time-of flight mass spectrometry. Rapid Commun Mass Spectrom 1998;12:176–80.

[79] Wunschel SC, Jarman KH, Petersen CE, Valentine NB, Wahl KL, Schauki D, Jackman J, Nelson CP, White E. Bacterial analysis by MALDI-TOF mass spectrometry: an inter-laboratory comparison. J Am Soc Mass Spectrom 2005;16:456–62.
[80] Arnold RJ, Reilly JP. Fingerprint matching of E. coli strains with MALDI-TOF MS of whole cells using a modified correlation approach. Rapid Commun Mass Spectrom 1998;12:630–6.
[81] Bundy J, Fenselau C. Lectin based affinity capture for MALDI-MS analysis of bacteria. Anal Chem 1999;71:1460–3.
[82] Domon B, Aebersoldm R. Mass spectrometry and protein analysis. Science 2006;312:212–7.
[83] Freiwald A, Sauer S. Phylogenetic classification and identification of bacteria by mass spectrometry. Nat Protoc 2009;4:732–42.
[84] Graham R, Graham C, McMullan G. Microbial proteomics: a mass spectrometry primer for biologists. Microb Cell Fact 2007;6:26.
[85] Haag AM, Taylor SN, Johnston KH, Cole RB. Rapid identification of Haemophilus bacteria by matrix assisted laser desorption ionization time of flight mass spectrometry. J Mass Spectrom 1998;33:750–6.
[86] Platt JA, Uy OM, Heller DN, Cotter RJ, Fenselau C. Computer-based linear regression analysis of desorption mass spectra of microorganisms. Anal Chem 1988;60:1415–9.
[87] Russell SC. Microorganism characterization by single particle mass spectrometry. Mass Spectrom Rev 2009;28:376–87.
[88] Sauer S, Kliem M. Mass spectrometry tools for the classification and identification of bacteria. Nat Rev Microbiol 2010;8:74–82.
[89] Wall DB, Lubman DB, Flynn SJ. Rapid profiling of induced proteins in bacteria using MALDI-TOF mass spectrometric detection of nonporous RP HPLC-separated whole cell lysates. Anal Chem 1999;71:3894–900.
[90] Biswas S, Rolain JM. Use of MALDI-TOF mass spectrometry for identification of bacteria that are difficult to culture. J Microbiol Methods 2013;92:14–24.
[91] Angel DE, Lloyd P, Carville K, Santamaria N. The clinical efficacy of two semi-quantitative wound-swabbing techniques in identifying the causative organism(s) in infected cutaneous wounds. Int Wound J 2011;8:176–85.
[92] Ciani I, Schulze H, Corrigan DK, Henihan G, Giraud G, Terry JG, Walton AJ, Pethig R, Ghazal P, Crain J, Campbell CJ, Bachmann TT, Mount AR. Development of immunosensors for direct detection of three wound infection biomarkers at point of care using electrochemical impedance spectroscopy. Biosens Bioelectron 2012;31:413–8.
[93] Sharp D, Gladstone P, Smith RB, Forsythe S, Davis J. Approaching intelligent infection diagnostics: carbon fibre sensor for electrochemical pyocyanin detection. Bioelectrochemistry 2010;77:114–9.
[94] Novick RP, Geisinger E. Quorum sensing in staphylococci. Annu Rev Genet 2008;42:541–64.
[95] Ng WL, Bassler BL. Bacterial quorum-sensing network architectures. Annu Rev Genet 2009;43:197–222.
[96] Williams P, Camara M. Quorum sensing and environmental adaptation in Pseudomonas aeruginosa: a tale of regulatory networks and multifunctional signal molecules. Curr Opin Microbiol 2009;12:182–91.
[97] Kaplan HB, Greenberg EP. Diffusion of autoinducer is involved in regulation of the Vibrio fischeri luminescence system. J Bacteriol 1985;163:1210–4.
[98] Novick RP, Projan SJ, Kornblum J, Ross HF, Ji G, Kreiswirth B, Vandenesch F, Moghazeh S. The agr P2 operon: an autocatalytic sensory transduction system in Staphylococcus aureus. Mol Gen Genet 1995;248:446–58.
[99] Seed PC, Passador L, Iglewski BH. Activation of the Pseudomonas aeruginosa lasI gene by LasR and the Pseudomonas autoinducer PAI: an autoinduction regulatory hierarchy. J Bacteriol 1995;177:654–9.
[100] Rutherford ST, Bassler BL. Bacterial quorum sensing: its role in virulence and possibilities for its control. Cold Spring Harb Perspect Med 2012;2:a012427.
[101] Magnuson R, Solomon J, Grossman AD. Biochemical and genetic characterization of a competence pheromone from B. subtilis. Cell 1994;77:207–16.
[102] Havarstein LS, Coomaraswamy G, Morrison DA. An unmodified heptadecapeptide pheromone induces competence for genetic transformation in Streptococcus pneumoniae. Proc Natl Acad Sci 1995;92:11140–4.

[103] Mayville P, Ji G, Beavis R, Yang H, Goger M, Novick RP, Muir TW. Structure-activity analysis of synthetic autoinducing thiolactone peptides from Staphylococcus aureus responsible for virulence. Proc Natl Acad Sci 1999;96:1218–23.
[104] Okada M, Sato I, Cho SJ, Iwata H, Nishio T, Dubnau D, Sakagami Y. Structure of the Bacillus subtilis quorum-sensing peptide pheromone ComX. Nat Chem Biol 2005;1:23–4.
[105] Bouillaut L, Perchat S, Arold S, Zorrilla S, Slamti L, Henry C, Gohar M, Declerck N, Lereclus D. Molecular basis for group-specific activation of the virulence regulator PlcR by PapR heptapeptides. Nucleic Acids Res 2008;36:3791–801.
[106] Hoch JA, Silhavy TJ. Two-component signal transduction. Washington, DC: ASM Press; 1995.
[107] Inouye M, Dutta R. Histidine kinases in signal transduction. London: Academic; 2003.
[108] Simon MI, Crane BR, Crane A. Two-component signalling systems. San Diego, CA: Academic; 2007.
[109] Otto M, Sussmuth R, Jung G, Gotz F. Structure of the pheromone peptide of the Staphylococcus epidermidis agr system. FEBS Lett 1998;424:89–94.
[110] Lazazzera BA. The intracellular function of extracellular signaling peptides. Peptides 2001;22:1519–27.
[111] Nakayama J, Cao Y, Horii T, Sakuda S, Akkermans AD, de Vos WM, Nagasawa H. Gelatinase biosynthesis-activating pheromone: a peptide lactone that mediates a quorum sensing in Enterococcus faecalis. Mol Microbiol 2001;41:145–54.
[112] Kalkum M, Lyon GJ, Chait BT. Detection of secreted peptides by using hypothesis-driven multistage mass spectrometry. Proc Natl Acad Sci 2003;100:2795–800.
[113] Okada M, Sato I, Cho SJ, Iwata H, Nishio T, Dubnau D, Sakagami Y. Structure of the Bacillus subtilis quorum-sensing peptide pheromone ComX. Nat Chem Biol 2005;1:23–4.
[114] Thoendel M, Kavanaugh JS, Flack CE, Horswill AR. Peptide signaling in the staphylococci. Chem Rev 2011;111:117–51.
[115] Ji G, Beavis RC, Novick RP. Cell density control of staphylococcal virulence mediated by an octapeptide pheromone. Proc Natl Acad Sci 1995;92:12055–9.
[116] Peterson KM, Mekalanos JJ. Characterization of the Vibrio cholerae ToxR regulon: identification of novel genes involved in intestinal colonization. Infect Immun 1988;56:2822–9.
[117] Lowy FD. Staphylococcus aureus infections. N Engl J Med 1998;339:520–32.
[118] Massey RC, Horsburgh MJ, Lina G, Hook M, Recker M. The evolution and maintenance of virulence in Staphylococcus aureus: a role for host-to-host transmission? Nat Rev Microbiol 2006;4:953–8.
[119] Pottathil M, Lazazzera BA. The extracellular Phr peptide-Rap phosphatase signaling circuit of Bacillus subtilis. Front Biosci 2003;8:d32–45.
[120] Dunny GM. The peptide pheromone-inducible conjugation system of Enterococcus faecalis plasmid pCF10: cell-cell signalling, gene transfer, complexity and evolution. Philos Trans R Soc Lond B Biol Sci 2007;362:1185–93.
[121] Slamti L, Lereclus D. A cell–cell signaling peptide activates the PlcR virulence regulon in bacteria of the Bacillus cereus group. EMBO J 2002;21:4550–9.
[122] Wei Y, Ng WL, Cong J, Bassler BL. Ligand and antagonist driven regulation of the Vibrio cholerae quorum sensing receptor CqsS. Mol Microbiol 2012;83:1095–108.
[123] Dutt JSN, Cardosi MF, Livingstone C, Davis J. Diagnostic implications of uric acid in electroanalytical measurements. Electroanalysis 2005;17:1233–43.
[124] Sharp D, Davis J. Integrated urate sensors for detecting wound infection. Electrochem Commun 2008;10:709–13.
[125] Zhou J, Loftus AL, Mulley G, Jenkins ATA. A thin film detection/ response system for pathogenic bacteria. J Am Chem Soc 2010;132:6566–70.
[126] Zhou J, Tun TN, Hong S, Mercer-Chalmers JD, Laabei M, Young AER, Jenkins ATA. Development of a prototype wound dressing technology which can detect and report colonization by pathogenic bacteria. Biosens Bioelectron 2011;30:67–72.
[127] Brocklesby KL, Johns SC, Jones AE, Sharp D, Smith RB. Smart bandages—a colourful approach to early stage infection detection and control in wound care. Med Hypotheses 2013;80:237–40.
[128] Hasmann A, Gewessler U, Hulla E, Schneider KP, Binder B, Francesko A, Tzanov T, Schintler M, Van der Palen J, Guebitz GM, Wehrschuetz-Sigl E. Sensor materials for the detection of human neutrophil elastase and cathepsin G activity in wound fluid. Exp Dermatol 2011;20:508–13.
[129] Hasmann A, Wehrschuetz-Sigl E, Kanzler G, Gewessler U, Hulla E, Schneider KP, Binder B, Schintler M, Guebitz GM. Novel peptidoglycan-based diagnostic devices for detection of wound infection. Diagn Microbiol Infect Dis 2011;71:12–23.

[130] Hasmann A, Wehrschuetz-Sigl E, Marold A, Wiesbauer H, Schoeftner R, Gewessler U, Kandelbauer A, Schiffer D, Schneider KP, Binder B, Schintler M, Guebitz GM. Analysis of myeloperoxidase activity in wound fluids as a marker of infection. Ann Clin Biochem 2013;50:245–54.
[131] Ågren MS, Mirastschijski U, Karlsmark T, Saarialho-Kere UK. Topical synthetic inhibitor of matrix metalloproteinases delays epidermal regeneration of human wounds. Exp Dermatol 2001;10:337–48.
[132] Moore WGI, Bodden MK, Windsor LJ, Decarlo A, Engler JA. Matrix metalloproteinases: a review. Crit Rev Oral Biol Med 1993;4:197–250.
[133] Heinzle A, Papen-Botterhuis NE, Schiffer D, Schneider KP, Binder B, Schintler M, Haaksman IK, Lenting HB, Gübitz GM, Sigl E. Novel protease-based diagnostic devices for detection of wound infection. Wound Repair Regen 2013;21:482–9.
[134] Bopp AF, Goynes W. Detection of human neutrophil elastase with ethoxylate acrylate resin analogs. J Pept Res 2005;66:160–8.
[135] Schiffer D, Verient V, Luschnig D, Blokhuis-Arkes MHE, Palen JVD, Gamerith C, Burnet M, Sigl E, Heinzle A, Guebitz GM. Lysozyme-responsive polymer systems for detection of infection. Eng Life Sci 2015;.
[136] Schneider KP, Gewessler U, Flock T, Heinzle A, Schenk V, Kaufmann F, Sigl E, Guebitz GM. Signal enhancement in polysaccharide based sensors for infections by incorporation of chemically modified laccase. N Biotechnol 2012;29:502–9.
[137] Nyanhongo GS, et al. Biodegradation of 2,4,6-trinitrotoluene (TNT): an enzymatic perspective. Biocatal. Biotransfor. 2005;23:53–69.
[138] Riva S. Laccases: blue enzymes for green chemistry. Trends Biotechnol 2006;24:219–26.
[139] Tombelli S, Minunni M, Mascini M. Analytical applications of aptamers. Biosens Bioelectron 2005;20:2424–34.
[140] Zayats M, Huang Y, Gill R, Ma CA, Willner IJ. Label-free reagentless aptamer based sensors for small molecules. J Am Chem Soc 2006;128:13666–7.
[141] Willner I, Zayats M. Electronic aptamer-based sensors. Angew Chem Int Ed 2007;46:6408–18.
[142] Yoshida W, Abe K, Ikebukuro K. Emerging techniques employed in aptamer-based diagnostic tests. Expert Rev Mol Diagn 2014;14:143–51.
[143] Chen C, Zhao J, Jiang J, Yu R. A novel exonuclease III-aided amplification assay for lysozyme based on graphene oxide platform. Talanta 2012;101:357–61.
[144] Erdem A, Eksin E, Muti M. Chitosan-graphene oxide based aptasensor for the impedimetric detection of lysozyme. Colloids Surf B Biointerfaces 2014;115:205–11.
[145] Rodríguez MC, Rivas GA. Label-free electrochemical aptasensor for the detection of lysozyme. Talanta 2009;78:212–6.
[146] Lian Y, He F, Mi X, Tong F, Shi X. Lysozyme aptamer biosensor based on electron transfer from SWCNTs to SPQC-IDE. Sens Actuators B Chem 2014;199:377–83.
[147] Li L-D, Chen Z-B, Zhao H-T, Guo L, Mu X. An aptamer-based biosensor for the detection of lysozyme with gold nanoparticles amplification. Sens Actuators B Chem 2010;149:110–5.
[148] Song Y, Li Y, Liu Z, Liu L, Wang X, Su X, Ma Q. A novel ultrasensitive carboxymethyl chitosan-quantum dot-based fluorescence "turn on-off" nanosensor for lysozyme detection. Biosens Bioelectron 2014;61:9–13.
[149] Hansson M, Olsson I, Nauseef WM. Biosynthesis, processing, and sorting of human myeloperoxidase. Arch Biochem Biophys 2006;445:214–24.
[150] Dale DC, Boxer L, Liles WC. The phagocytes: neutrophils and monocytes. Blood 2008;112:935–45.
[151] Hajnsek M, Schiffer D, Harrich D, Koller D, Verient V, Palen JVD, Heinzle A, Binder B, Sigl E, Sinner F, Guebitz GM. An electrochemical sensor for fast detection of wound infection based on myeloperoxidase activity. Sens Actuators B Chem 2015;209:265–74.
[152] Windmiller JR, Chinnapareddy S, Santhosh P, Halámek J, Chuang MC, Bocharova V, Tseng TF, Chou TY, Katz E, Wang J. Strip based amperometric detection of myeloperoxidase. Biosens Bioelectron 2010;26:886–9.
[153] Herrasti Z, Martínez F, Baldrich E. Carbon nanotube wiring for signal amplification of electrochemical magneto immunosensors: application to myeloperoxidase detection. Anal Bioanal Chem 2014;406:5487–93.

CHAPTER SEVEN

Connected Health Approaches to Wound Monitoring

D. Finlay
School of Engineering, Ulster University, Jordanstown, Northern Ireland, United Kingdom

7.1 INTRODUCTION

It is clear from the previous chapters that there are still many challenges to the development of robust wound-monitoring solutions. While much of the technology underpinning the biochemical recognition elements with the sensor is relatively mature, the extraction and reporting of the signal is often overlooked in the literature, yet it will be a critical component of the eventual device. The current application concept is for these systems to function in what is effectively a standalone mode. By this, we mean they require the observer, or person who will act upon the outcome of the monitoring process, to be in close proximity to the device. It is envisaged that the next generation of these devices will incorporate connectivity to allow a more integrated use with the "connected health" context [1].

7.2 THE EVOLUTION OF CONNECTED HEALTH

Connected Health has recently emerged as a domain that considers the full exploitation of electronic devices, connectivity, and people as being fundamental to promoting health. The notion of devices and technology supporting healthcare and well-being is of course not new, and the healthcare domain has seen much benefit from the use of technology over the years [2]. A number of key terms and nomenclature that have shaped the definition of what, is today, known as "connected heath" are explored in the following sections. We explore this material to build a foundation for the discussion of technologies and approaches that will ultimately provide advanced and "connected" solutions for wound monitoring.

7.2.1 Telemedicine, Telehealth, and Telecare

The term telemedicine was one of the first terms to become popular in the reference to the combination of medicine and technology [3]. Fundamentally, the term "telemedicine" referred to the execution of medical practice remotely. Although the term has really only been recognized in the past few decades, and usually relies on the use of telecommunications technology, its definition would indicate that any exchange of information (eg, a letter between two physicians a century ago) could be considered telemedicine. Early telemedicine systems were usually based on video conferencing. This could be used, for example, by two medical professionals at opposite sides of the world, to discuss some rare case of a disease. It could also enable a specialist to conduct a remote assessment of a patient who has no means of transport to the specialist's clinic. Although video conferencing has played a large part in this domain, new techniques are being introduced. One such new example of telemedicine is the use of robots to conduct surgery remotely [4].

Telehealth is a term which is often used interchangeably with telemedicine but, in fact, refers to a much broader collection of services and activities [5]. For example, telemedicine generally refers only to the provision of clinical services whereas telehealth can refer to both clinical and nonclinical aspects. Services which are examples of telehealth but are not considered examples of telemedicine include administration (record keeping) and education (training of medical experts). This comparison with telemedicine is analogous to comparing medicine within the broader domain of healthcare where wellness is also considered.

The term telecare is a further term that describes a service distinct from those mentioned above. Telecare, while referring to the technology used, also encompasses the data transferred and the response to the transmission of this data. The term telecare is most widely used in the description of services that relate to providing technology-enhanced care for those who need support to remain at home [6], for example, systems that are used to promote elderly support and independent living (living at home without needing continual care).

7.2.2 eHealth and mHealth

eHealth is a term that has emerged over this past decade and has been described as the practise of healthcare using electronic means. More specifically, the term ehealth usually applies to scenarios where the Internet is used as the communication technology [7]. This definition therefore excludes applications that use telecommunications technologies that do not rely on Internet technologies, for example, older video conferencing systems used in telemedicine that do not rely on Internet communications protocols for operation. Although we distinguish e-health systems as being those that rely on Internet protocols, there is an increasing convergence of this approach. For example, more and more systems now rely on some form of Internet protocol for transmission of data.

mHealth is a more recent addition to the collection of terminology and can be considered to be a subgroup of eHealth. The term mHealth appears mostly in applications where some form of conventional mobile device is utilized such as a smartphone or tablet PC [8]. There are of course more specific situations where bespoke-monitoring devices provide a mobile form of intervention in the absence of a smartphone or tablet computer. While the latter is effectively mobile health, the term mHealth is less often used. For the purposes of our discussion in the later sections, we will focus on the use of smartphone technology and therefore consider our proposed approaches to wound monitoring as being a form of mHealth system.

7.3 WOUND-MONITORING TECHNOLOGY COMPONENTS

The other chapters in this text provide the rationale and background for wound monitoring and also introduce the type of sensors that can be used to measure wound condition. In this section, our attention is focused on how such sensors must be integrated to provide a true connected health solution. Our discussion in the following paragraphs is based on consideration of the high-level component diagram illustrated in Fig. 7.1. In this diagram we have identified the various relevant stages required in the handling of signals in wound-monitoring solutions.

Almost all connected health-monitoring systems are concerned with measuring quantities that are continuous and vary over time. By continuous we mean that the quantity in question will always have a value at any instant in time. An example of this is the electrocardiogram, which is a measure of voltage on the surface of the body [9]. There will always be a voltage as long as the person's heart is beating. Signals with this continuous property are said to be "analogue." Classically, such signals were recorded and analyzed using "analogue" electronic circuitry. In this approach any analysis or processing of the signal would rely on analogue electronic circuit components (eg, resistors, capacitors). Processing of such signals would involve, for example, circuit components physically arranged and connected in a certain order to filter the signal to reduce unwanted electrical noise.

In more recent years, the trend has been to move away from the use of analogue circuitry for such applications. Instead, nowadays, signals are usually handled digitally. In this approach analogue signals are "sampled" and then processed digitally [10]. The

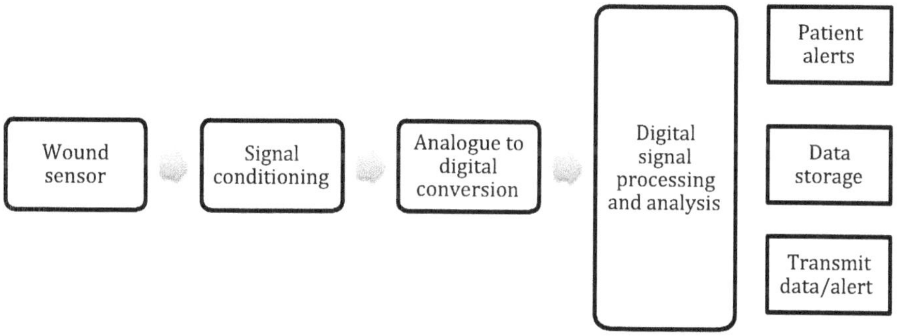

Figure 7.1 ***Main components in wound-monitoring system.***

sampling process involves using an analogue-to-digital converter (ADC) to periodically observe the analogue time varying quantity and store a number that corresponds to the measurement of the data.

In this text, we will only consider the handling of digital signals as analogue systems for handling connected health data are now uncommon. While our attention is focussed on digital handling of these signals, we must not neglect that these signals are fundamentally analogue at their source/origin. With this in mind, our description in the following paragraphs will pay particular attention to how digitization of analogue signals must be performed in a fashion that preserves enough information to reflect the underlying source.

7.3.1 Analogue-to-Digital Conversion

Fundamental to handling analogue signals digitally is the ADC. The ADC is not the first stage of the overall process as highlighted in Fig. 7.1; however, it is where we begin our discussion. Sampling, as discussed earlier, involves periodically observing a time varying quantity and somehow storing its value. There are two important aspects of this process that must be considered when an ADC is being chosen for a particular application. The first relates to how often the analogue signal is observed/measured. We will refer to this from now on as sample frequency. Sample frequency is a particularly important consideration in situations where the signals value is changing quickly over time. This is perhaps less problematic in wound-monitoring situations where measurements are not likely to change considerably over the course of a few seconds. In other applications such as ECG recording sample frequencies in the region of 500 Hz (500 samples per second) are employed. It is possible to select a minimum value of sampling frequency for any application. This choice is based on a sampling theory introduced by Nyquist [11]. Nyquist's rule states that the sampling frequency (f_s) must be greater than twice the highest frequency content (f_h) of the signal:

$$f_s >> 2f_h \tag{7.1}$$

Clearly, this rule relies on some insight into what the highest frequency content of the raw signal is. This must be determined using other methods that are beyond the scope of the current text. For the sake of wound-monitoring applications, we are assuming that the changes in the signal are of low frequency so a value of less than 1 for f_s is likely to be sufficient.

The second consideration in the sampling process is how the resulting sampled number is stored. We refer to this consideration as "quantization." At a very low hardware level all sampled numbers are stored in a binary format. Binary numbers are used inside digital hardware to represent decimal numbers, which humans are more familiar with, as a sequence of bits. Bits are set as either ones or zeros and the combination of the ones and zeros dictates which decimal number is being stored. Quantization is an important consideration as binary numbers made up of a greater number of bits are capable of representing larger decimal numbers. For example, 8 bits can represent a decimal number between 0 and 255 whereas 10 bits can represent numbers between 0 and 1,023. In the context of quantization this means that if we are measuring analogue values between a range of 0 and 5 V we will have 255 discrete values in steps of 19.5 mV steps when using an 8 bit ADC. Or, if we were measuring the same voltage range using 1,023 discrete values, possibly using a 10 bit ADC, we would be capable of measuring in 4.9 mV steps. The latter will obviously provide a better representation of the original signal.

These are important theoretical underpinnings that should underline the choice of ADC for an application. The question of why this is important is worth addressing. Generally, ADCs of high specification (supporting a high sampling rate and a large number of bits) are more complex and more expensive than those of lower specification. Therefore, it is important that the characteristics of the signal are well understood and the correct choice of ADC hardware is made.

7.3.2 Signal Conditioning Stage

While the ADC convertor is fundamental in converting any time varying analogue quantity to discrete values, ADCs are usually not designed for connecting directly to the acquisition sensor on their own. In this section, we discuss the components that typically exist between the sensor and the ADC. This stage will typically consist of amplification circuitry, patient isolation, and possibly presample filtering among other things. In the majority of cases the signal amplitudes produced by medical sensors are very small, often of the order of millivolts or smaller. Signals of these amplitudes are not usually compatible for direct connection to an ADC, which will likely have a maximum input range of the order of volts. By way of example, we want to consider the range of voltages that are typical of that produced by a pH-based wound sensor. In this application a voltage range of approximately 2 V is typically observed. In this application a voltage range of approximately 2 V is typically observed. The ADC specification employs 8 bits in the input and a supply range between 0 and 5 V. This number of bits will give us 19.6 mV step sizes as described above. To effectively measure smaller changes in the signal we amplify the signal prior to its digitization. To do this we use amplifier circuitry. The main purpose of the amplifier is to take a small input signal and increase its amplitude by a predetermined factor referred to as the "gain." The gain of the amplifier should be consistent across the range input voltages. Using the above example, if we scaled our input voltage by a gain of 2.5 then we would use the entire range of the ADC (ie, 0–5 V) and we could then assume that the 19.6 mV step size actually represented value changes of 19.6/2.5 = 7.8 mV. Clearly, the combination of input voltage range, amplifier gain, and number of ADC bits influence the resolution of signal change that we can measure.

In medical applications the kind of amplifier employed is usually what is known as an "instrumentation amplifier." Instrumentation amplifiers are especially designed for applications where certain qualities of the measured system are unknown. Specifically, they are designed for applications where there is likely to be a mismatch in impedance between the measured system and the amplifier itself. Instrumentation amplifier circuitry used in medical applications is usually referred to as "medical instrumentation." Medical instrumentation is an extensive area of engineering and readers are directed to more specialized texts such as those by Webster [12] for further reading on this subject.

While detailed discussion of medical instrumentation is somewhat beyond the scope of the current text, there are several other tasks that do merit a mention in consideration of the signal conditioning stage. First, this stage may also provide some rudimentary filtering of the signal. The instrumentation amplifier will itself likely be designed to reject some firms of noise or unwanted signal; however, further filtering may also be employed to remove unwanted parts of the signal. Second, the signal conditioning stage may also provide some form of electrical isolation. This is an extremely important aspect of medical instrumentation and ensures electrical isolation of the patient from the device. This ultimately protects the patient from leakage current from the recording hardware. This can be achieved in circuitry which seamlessly converts the electrical signal to a light-based signal and then immediately uses this light signal to drive a receiver that converts the light back to an electrical signal. This process is referred to as opto-isolation. The reader should be aware that there are several ways in which electrical isolation can be implemented and opto-isolation is just one approach.

7.3.3 Digital Signal Processing Stage

In this text we have focused on the scenario where any signal sampled from the sensor is almost immediately digitized. We should stress that this is not always the case as some approaches may rely on more analogue processing of the signal downstream. In our approach we are assuming that all significant processing of the signal will take place on the digital signal subsequent to sampling. This does represent a trend in most commercial and medical electronic systems. For example, although many systems which we use everyday deal with analogue quantities (eg, mobile telephone conversations, listening to music) the underlying systems handle signals digitally. Digital signal processing (DSP) itself offers many advantages over analogue signal processing. The main advantages include the fact that:

- DSP system parameters are usually determined via software that can be easily reprogrammed even when a system or device is in use (via a software/firmware update). Analogue systems will usually require the alteration of hardware components to make changes to processing requirements.

- DSP systems are much less susceptible to environmental variations (eg, changes in temperature). Discrete analogue components are much more susceptible to such variations.
- DSP systems allow processing tasks that are simply not possible with conventional electronic components, for example, substantial numeric calculations, etc.

While the advantages of digital signal processing-based systems stand up in their own right digitization of signals in smart wound monitoring is particularly applicable. This is because most connected health applications will rely on transmission of the recorded data in some way. In later sections, we will introduce a number of technologies that can provide a modular approach to digital data communication.

DSP systems can either be implemented in bespoke DSP hardware or they can be implemented in more generic microcontrollers. The former are often used when there are few other computational tasks and where very high sample rates are required. The latter microcontroller-based approach is perhaps more appropriate to smart wound-monitoring connected health applications where the microcontroller will also provide communication functionality over and above DSP tasks. DSP tasks will likely include the initial conditioning of the signal and any further processing that is required prior to transmission or handling of the signal. Signal conditioning will include filtering of the signal. Filtering of the signal will remove unwanted parts of the signal by eliminating parts of the signal that change at a certain unwanted frequency. This means that unwanted fluctuations in the signal are smoothed out. While the design and implementation of digital filters is a complex area of DSP, the basic concept is easy to envisage. A very basic example of a digital filter is the moving average filter. In a moving average filter a sampled signal value is modified to make it an average of itself and a predetermined number of previous samples. The new value is stored as the filter output. This has the obvious effect of removing any unwanted jitter that may emerge during the recording process. In this approach, we are effectively taking an average of a number of observations of our signal to get a reliable measurement. While this is a very basic type of filter, much more complex filter implementations are possible, for example, a filter to eliminate electromagnetic noise in a signal that comes about from power line interference.

After DSP tasks related to basic signal condition are complete, the next stage is to perform some basic analysis on the cleaned signals. For wound-monitoring applications where pH levels relate directly to the sensed voltage, the basic task will be to identify if a predetermined threshed in pH level has been attained. Slightly more elaborate analysis may involve conducting trending-type analysis on the incoming data. This form of analysis could be used to intelligently predict the onset of undesirable wound conditions prior to their occurrence. Many types of machine-learning approach are now available which offer the ability to easily perform signal analysis in a way that an unobvious trend could be identified [13].

7.4 POSTPROCESSING STAGE

After data has been processed and analysis has been conducted, the next stage is to act upon and events that are highlighted during the thresholding or trending stage. There a number of ways in which action can be taken. We split these into three distinct approaches. The first is concerned mostly to alerting the individual who is wearing the smart bandage. The second relates to storage of the recorded data or alerts for future analysis. The third relates to alerting someone who is responsible for the patient's care. There is no reason why a wound-monitoring system may not consider all three of these aspects. We devote more attention to these as follows.

7.4.1 Patient Alerts

The most obvious way for the smart bandage to raise an alert with the patient is to provide an audible or visual alert from the bandage itself. This is entirely feasible and requires no transmission of information from the bandage unit. This does however require the integration of components into the bandage unit that are capable of providing this type of patient interface. While this does require additional components, these components could be as simple and inexpensive, for example, a light-emitting diode (LED) which would be illuminated once an event is raised. More advanced approaches could include incorporating LCD displays into the bandage. At the time of writing there is much interest in the development of "flexible" display technology that could be suitable for this type of application.

7.4.2 Data Storage

Data storage options are a possible requirement for clinical use of wound-monitoring systems. This would allow review of wound status during clinical follow-up. For wound-monitoring systems used in the research setting this is likely to be a more definitive requirement as retrospective analysis of data on wound status is likely to be an important part of any retrospective analysis. Data storage could include the storage of all data values obtained from the sensor or just the storage of alert information (with time stamp). In either case some sort of nonvolatile (memory that is not erased once power is removed) is required. Today, such memory is relatively inexpensive; however, the circuitry required to write to and manage this memory is not trivial and its integration in a bandage will greatly include the complexity of the system. New approaches to connected health that are discussed in the coming section may however provide solutions that still permit the storage of the data but do not require the integration of this functionality in the bandage itself.

7.4.3 Transmission of Data/Alerts

The possibility of the transmission of data and alerts from the bandage opens up a range of possibilities that take a big step in the direction of making wound-monitoring solutions a truly connected health concern. We briefly discuss the transmission of data and alerts in this section but have devoted a much more extensive discussion of connectivity in wound monitoring in the following sections. In short transmission of data/alerts will require the implementation of communications functionality in the bandage unit. An advantage of this approach is that the patient interface and data storage functionality outlined above can easily be migrated to another supplementary device that the bandage simply communicates with. The supplementary device could be a bespoke unit that could reside in the person's home. Development of a bespoke unit for this purpose is, of course, resource intensive; however, there is a compelling argument for considering technology that most patients (certainly patients of the future) are already likely to have in their pocket. The technology we are referring to is the now somewhat ubiquitous smartphone. Smartphones are already widely equipped to perform many of the tasks required. In the following paragraphs, we take a much more detailed look at the relevant technology and how this can be exploited to envisage a "connected" model for wound monitoring.

7.5 ARCHITECTURES FOR CONNECT HEALTH APPROACHES TO WOUND MONITORING

Connected health solutions inevitably rely on the use of technology to connect individuals and devices. Today, many medical devices and systems still rely on wired connections between recording sensors and acquisition hardware. Furthermore, many medical devices are connected to computer networks and hospital information systems using wired connections. Wireless solutions, which effectively replace cable connections, have however become more common. Almost all modern wireless solutions rely on the use of radio technology. While the term "wireless" is largely synonymous with radio technology, it should be appreciated that the term can refer to the use of other communication mediums (eg, infrared light, ultrasound); however, these are used very infrequently nowadays. Due to the dominance of radio technologies for wireless communications, these other, less commonly used, technologies receive no further attention here.

Radio communications rely on the oscillation of electrical signals at certain frequencies (radio frequency (RF)) that in turn allow them to propagate through the air as electromagnetic waves. The development of RF technology is a complex discipline that includes advanced electronic engineering topics such as complex circuit design, signaling, and antenna design.

Over this past two decades, several well-known standards have emerged that allowed us to now take a much more modular approach to RF-based wireless adoption in connected health applications. In this approach, a wireless module can be incorporated into our connected health devices and this module will take care of all aspects of radio communication (electronic circuits, power management, antennas, etc). In the following section, we discuss several of the communications technologies that are seeing widespread use in connected health applications.

7.5.1 Bluetooth

The Bluetooth standard emerged as a result of developments relating to mobile device technology in the mid to late 1990s. The rationale for the development of the Bluetooth standard was driven by the desire to replace wired communication between mobile devices, for example, communication between mobile phone and a headset or between mobile phone and a personal computer. The intention was to develop a standard that would provide a modular low-powered cable replacement technology that was compatible between different manufactures. The standard includes specification of parameters such as communication frequency, data format, link control, management, etc.

While Bluetooth was intended to be a low-power solution the power consumption of Bluetooth-enabled devices remains relatively high. Bluetooth communications links usually facilitate wireless transmission of data over distances between 10 and 100 m. Bluetooth is based around transmission of signals at 2.4 GHz. Most current smartphones, tablet computers, and notebook computers are Bluetooth enabled. The development of Bluetooth is overseen by the Bluetooth Special Interests Group [14].

7.5.2 Wi-Fi

Wi-Fi came about through the desire to facilitate wireless computer networks. The Wi-Fi standard is based on IEEE standard 802.11 and its development is overseen by the Wi-Fi Alliance [15]. The standard differs from Bluetooth in that it was more so intended to allow portable devices to gain access to the Internet—a connection that was traditionally achieved using cable. In this mode, the portable device establishes connection with a wireless access point that is in turn connected to the Internet. Wi-Fi can be used to create what are known as ad-hoc networks that allow two devices to communicate directly with each other without the need for a wireless hot spot. This ad-hoc mode is used less frequently. The communication range of Wi-Fi is comparable to Bluetooth (of the order of tens of meters); however, it typically offers greater bandwidth, that is, faster data transfer. The cost of Wi-Wi technology is typically more than Bluetooth technology. Wi-Fi uses a number of frequencies which include 2.4 gigahertz and 5 gigahertz. Wi-FI is widely supported and implemented in most notebook computers, smartphone, and tablet computers.

7.5.3 Bluetooth Low Energy

There are several variations and versions of the Bluetooth standard as introduced previously. As the name suggests Bluetooth Low Energy (BLE), also referred to as Bluetooth Smart, is touted as a variant of the Bluetooth standard that is designed to provide lower power consumption [16]. As a result, BLE has the potential to offer significant improvements in battery life and can operate for weeks on a standard coin-cell-sized battery. This is a significant improvement over standard Bluetooth technology that causes noticeable battery drain when enabled, in devices whose normal battery life does not extend much beyond 1 day (eg, current-generation smartphones). BLE does, however, offer reduced bandwidth but does have specific operating modes, known as "profiles" which are especially designed to be suited to healthcare applications. This, in turn, allows better compatibility between devices. At the time of writing BLE remains a relatively new technology; however, it is seeing growing support in many consumer devices such as tablets and smartphones.

7.6 WOUND-MONITORING COMMUNICATION ARCHITECTURES

The above section introduces well-known technologies that are suitable for supporting wireless communication in connected health applications. This is just a modest subset of the range of technologies/standards that can be used for this application. An extensive list is beyond the scope of the current text; however, the reader should be aware that other technologies are available. The above paragraphs also relate to standards that are largely concerned with short-range cable replacement technologies. We have intentionally refrained from discussing long-range wireless communication technologies such as 3G and 4G wireless technologies. These are the technologies that provide fast wireless connections to the Internet on our smartphones. These technologies rely on a connection to a mobile phone network. Our reason for neglecting these technologies is that we envisage that such technology is less likely to see direct incorporation in wound-monitoring devices. Instead, it is more likely that the wound-monitoring device will follow the trend in other wearable electronics applications where short-range radio links are typically used to connect the body worn part of the system to another device that will itself have fast Internet access.

With this in mind, we want to introduce an overall architecture that is common in many emerging medical and current lifestyle device applications [17]. By lifestyle device applications we are referring to systems such as those that measure parameters such as heart rate during activities or exercise but are not generally used for healthcare assessment. We believe this is an appropriate model to also meet the needs of wound-monitoring applications. This approach relies on the notion of creating a small network in the vicinity of the patient that allows the wound-monitoring device to communicate directly with other devices. Indeed, the notion of such a network is already recognized in the general telecommunications domain. As a result, two specific forms of network have become recognized.

7.6.1 Personal Area Networks

A personal area network is a network concerned with the exchange of information in the vicinity of a person. Typically, these systems are wireless and involve the transmission of data between devices such as smartphones, personal computers, tablet computers, etc. The purpose of such a network is usually to allow either transmission of data or information between such devices or to server as the network that allows further up link to the Internet. Developments in the area of Personal Area Networks (PANs) are largely overseen by the IEEE 802.15 working group [18].

7.6.2 Body Area Network

A body area network is distinct from a PAN in that it is concerned with a network of devices that are in much closer proximity to the person. Typically, these devices will be attached to or located on the person's body. In some cases devices may even be implanted. Clearly, this is very applicable to medical applications [19,20]. A Body Area Network (BAN) may use a PAN to transmit data over longer distances. As with most systems BANs rely on RF-based communications. At the time of writing the latest standard for BANs is IEEE802.15.6 [21].

Our model for wound-monitoring connectivity incorporates aspects of both the PAN and BAN models. More importantly, this approach ultimately allows us to exploit existing technology that many patients already have in their possession. Specifically, we envisage the smartphone as a hub or gateway device for our PAN/BAN architecture suitable for wound monitoring. To fully appreciate the benefits that this model brings, we must consider what features and functionality a connected wound-monitoring solution would have.

Wound-monitoring wish list:

1. Ability to interpret and analyze data acquired from a wound sensor.
2. Ability to display this information to a patient or a caregiver.
3. Ability to record/store data for future analysis.
4. Communications functionality to allow this information to be transmitted to a remote carer.

While it is reasonable to assume that the solution here could lie in a custom device incorporating all of the above functionalities, developing a bespoke device with this level of functionality would require significant development effort and hence cost. As alluded to in the previous sections, the production of a device with components such as displays, data storage functionality is also costly. Fortuitously, smartphone technology offers much of the above functionality. If we consider the following key features of modern smartphones, there is obvious mapping to all of the above wish list:

Key smartphone features:

- Powerful microprocessor for signal analysis.
- High-resolution display.
- Short-range (eg, Bluetooth and Wi-Fi) and long-range (4G) network connectivity options.
- Significant storage capability usually of the order of Gigabytes.

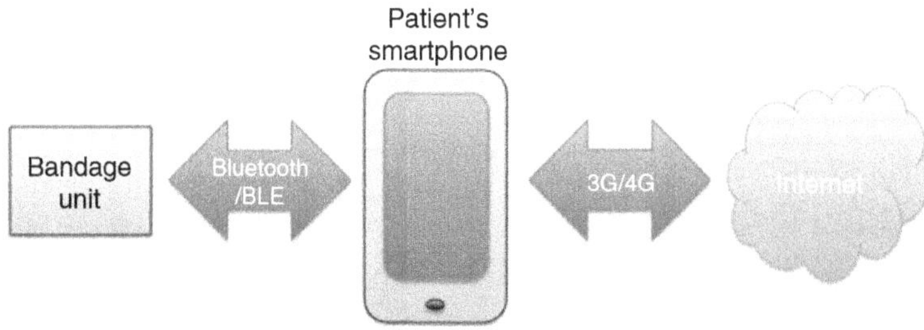

Figure 7.2 ***mHealth architecture for wound monitoring.***

This mapping leads us to envisage that a suitable model for a connected health approach to wound monitoring be one where the smartphone forms the gateway in a PAN/BAN architecture and the wound-monitoring device, which is attached to the patient, has limited functionality that merely allows acquisition of wound status. The key aspect of this approach is allowing a very basic wound-monitoring device to communicate with the smartphone. The smartphone is then programmed to provide all of the required functionality. Communication between the wound monitor and the smartphone device can be achieved by incorporating either a Bluetooth or a BLE module into the wound-monitoring device. At the time of writing, such a module can be purchased for just a few dollars and these modules are highly discrete in that they offer all the functionality including antenna in one easily integrated package.

In Fig. 7.2 the basic architecture is outlined. We briefly discuss the basic components of this diagram as follows.

7.6.3 Patient Unit/Bandage Electronics

In this approach basic electronics are located in a unit attached to the bandage itself. This unit will include the actual sensor and the associated electronics that will allow signal acquisition, digitization, and transmission of our data. We know from our previous discussion that acquisition will involve amplification and analogue-to-digital conversion of the sensor signals. If we think back to Fig. 7.1, we can map everything up to the analogue-to-digital conversion into this bandage unit. After that we envisage that data will be transmitted top the smartphone where further digital signal processing will take place. Aside from the signal amplification hardware this unit is likely to include some form of modest microcontroller (small computer). This microcontroller is required to control all data acquisition and will be connected to a communication module as described above (likely Bluetooth or BLE). Some microcontrollers also have in-built ADC functionality and are relatively low cost. In recent years, several initiatives have been introduced to allow easy access to microcontroller for experimental project [arduino]. These systems are definitely suitable for prototype and proof of concept applications; however, more advanced microcontroller systems are likely to be used in any commercial/medical device grade system. All electronics in the bandage unit will require some sort of power source.

7.6.4 Smartphone Component

As we have noted previously, the smartphone serves as the gateway in our PAN/BAN topology. The advantage of this model is that we can exploit the advanced features that the smartphone has to offer. To utilize these features, a software application, more commonly referred to as an "app," must be developed. This app will be responsible for establishing communication with the patient unit and receiving data sent from this unit. The app can then be developed to process, store, display, or transmit this data to the Internet. The app development process is dependant on the type of smartphone technology used. The two dominant smartphone platforms at the time of writing are Apple iOS and Android. In either case, the most challenging part of the app development process is communication with the patient unit. This is less so with the Android platform due to its less proprietary nature.

As stated, the app will be developed to intercept data that is sent from the bandage unit. We envisage that most of the processing of this data and any trending analysis, described in the previous sections, would be carried out on the smartphone app as opposed to on the microcontroller embedded in the bandage unit. The motivation for migrating as much of this functionality to the smartphone is two-fold. First, smartphones currently possess processing power which is easily on a par or in some cases well in excess of that available on an embedded microcontroller. Second, smartphone app software can be easily updated or upgraded. We see this frequently as smartphone apps are updated online in a process that is relatively seamless to the user.

The app will also have the ability to present information to the screen of the user in an appropriate format and to store this information in the phones memory in turn allowing later retrieval of the data. Finally, the app can be developed to utilize a smartphones fast 3G/4G Internet connection with a remote system via the Internet. This is further described later.

7.6.5 Internet Aspect

This aspect of our architecture receives just modest discussion here. The key thing is that data is transferred from the smartphone device (if required) via the Internet. This can be to facilitate storage of data in the "cloud" or it can be to allow the data and any associated alerts to be passed onto a relevant carer for example. The specific actions on the data or any alerts are more a feature of the healthcare system relevant to the patient rather than technical constraints. The flow of information is also dependant on the use case. For example, we already noted that the ideal would be to migrate processing functionality away from the embedded microcontroller to the smartphone application. If necessary, this functionality could even be migrated to the Internet "cloud" if desired.

7.6.6 Constraints

We should point out that other architectures, using very similar technology or, using a different arrangement of the same technology, are possible. These all can be configured to offer the same functionality as above. One model that is perhaps close to that above is where the smartphone component is bypassed and the communication from the patient unit is directly to the cloud. A possible technical solution in this case is to integrate Wi-Fi technology to the patient unit and have some from of Wi-Fi access point that in turn links the patient unit to the cloud. This could be achieved in the mobile setting by configuring the patient smartphone as the Wi-Fi "hotspot." This is distinct from the model described in Fig. 7.2 as, in this approach, the data would not normally be intercepted on the device. The device will merely serve as a proxy for Internet access.

7.7 SUMMARY

There are several limitations to the above discussion, which should also be acknowledged. The model we propose here is, for the moment, somewhat theoretical and faces certain barriers. From a technical perspective, there is no reason why such a system cannot be realized at low cost. The technology is all accessible and the costs of such technology continue to reduce. The first main issue is that regulation of such technology from a medical device perspective is not well defined. Specifically, medical device regulators, at the time of writing, are still adjusting their processes for the consideration of some of the above technology. A particular aspect that has received much coverage of late relates to how medical apps are regulated [22]. A further issue is how such a system would integrate with the current process. Technology developers have faced this issue in many aspects of healthcare technology development as, in many cases, it requires a change of practice for clinicians and, sometimes that change is met with some reluctance.

Our text in this chapter should come with some form of disclaimer. The description of devices and technology is extremely high level and serves in no way as an in-depth primer to support the technical development of such systems. There are, for example, several important issues that are omitted from the discussion. The first is the discussion of power sources—we have made very little reference to how the bandage unit receives its power and how this is impacted upon with power-demanding processes such as communication. Second, our description of the bandage electronics is extremely limited and any developments must pay particular attention to issues around patient safety, ensuring that patients are adequately protected from any unintentional malfunction of the device.

REFERENCES

[1] Caulfield BM, Donnelly SC. What is connected health and why will it change your practice? QJM 2013;106(8):703–7.
[2] Faulkner A. Medical technology into healthcare and society. Palgrave Macmillan, Basingstoke; 2008.
[3] Perednia DA, Allen A. Telemedicine technology and clinical applications. JAMA 1995;273(6):483–8.
[4] Ghodoussi M, Wang Y. Robotic surgery—the transatlantic case. In: Proc. 2002 IEEE international conference on robotics and automation ICRA'02 (Vol. 2, 1882–1888).
[5] Koch S. Home telehealth—current state and future trends. Int J Med Inform 2006;75(8):565–76.
[6] Celler BG, Lovell NH, Chan DK. The potential impact of home telecare on clinical practice. Med J Australia 1999;171(10):518–21.
[7] Kreps GL, Neuhauser L. New directions in eHealth communication: opportunities and challenges. Patient Educ Counseling 2010;78(3):329–36.
[8] Istepanian R, Laxminarayan S, Pattichis CS. M-health. Berlin: Springer Science+ Business Media, Incorporated; 2006.
[9] McFarlane PW, Lawrie TD, eds. Comprehensive electrocardiology. New York: Pergamon Press; 1989.
[10] McClellan JH, Schafer RW, Yoder MA. Signal processing first. Pearson/Prentice Hall, New Jersey; 2003.
[11] Nyquist H. Certain topics in telegraph transmission theory. Trans Am Inst Electr Engineers 1928;47(2):617–44.
[12] Webster JG. Medical instrumentation—application and design. J Clin Eng 1978;3(3):306.
[13] Finlay DD, Nugent CD, Wang H, Donnelly MP, McCullagh PJ. Mining, knowledge and decision support. Technol Health Care 2010;18(6):429–41.
[14] Bluetooth Special interest Group [Internet]. 2015 [cited 15 December 2015]. Available at: www.bluetooth.org.
[15] Wi-Fi Alliance [Internet]. 2015 [cited 18 December 2015]. Available at: http://www.wi-fi.org/.
[16] Bluetooth Smart [Internet]. 2015 [cited 10 December 2015]. Available at: https://www.bluetooth.com/what-is-bluetooth-technology/bluetooth-technology-basics/low-energy.
[17] Burns W, Nugent C, McCullagh P, Finlay D, Cleland I, McClean S, Scotney B, McCann J. A smart garment for older walkers. Impact analysis of solutions for chronic disease prevention and management. Berlin Heidelberg: Springer; 2012. pp. 258–261.
[18] IEEE 802.15 Working Group for WPAN [Internet]. 2015 [cited 18 December 2015]. Available at: http://www.ieee802.org/15/.
[19] Li HB, Takizawa K, Kohno R. Trends and standardization of body area network (BAN) for medical healthcare. In: IEEE European conference on wireless technology. EuWiT 2008. Oct 27, 2008 (pp. 1–4).
[20] Kohno R, Hamaguchi K, Li HB, Takizawa K. R&D and standardization of body area network (BAN) for medical healthcare. In: IEEE international conference on ultra-wideband. ICUWB 2008. Sep 10, 2008 (Vol. 3, pp. 5–8).
[21] 802.15.6-2012—IEEE Standard for Local and metropolitan area networks—Part 15.6: Wireless Body Area Networks [Internet]. 2016 [cited January 11, 2016]. Available at: https://standards.ieee.org/findstds/standard/802.15.6-2012.html.
[22] Hamel MB, Cortez NG, Cohen IG. FDA regulation of mobile health technologies. New Engl J Med 2014;371(4):372–9.

GLOSSARY

Acyl-homoserine lactones (AHLs) A class of small molecules used in signaling between bacteria.

Analog digital converter (ADC) Device typically used to acquire a measurement signal from a sensing device allowing it to be interpreted by appropriate software.

Analyte A substance or chemical constituent that is of interest in an analytical procedure.

Anodization Typically an electrolytic passivation process used to increase the thickness of the natural oxide layer on the surface of metal parts. In this case, it involves the fracturing of carbon particles to increase surface area and incorporate oxygen functionalities.

Antigenicity Capacity of a chemical structure to bind specifically with a certain product that has adaptive immunity

Autoinducing peptides (AIPs) A class of small molecules used in signaling between bacteria.

Bandage A strip of woven material used to bind up a wound or to protect an injured part of the body.

Bioactive A chemical species or material that has an effect upon a living organism, tissue, or cell.

Bioburden The number of bacteria living on a surface that has not been sterilized.

Biocompatibility The ability of a material to perform with an appropriate host response in a given application.

Biofilm A thin, usually resistant, layer of microorganisms that form on and coat various surfaces.

Biomaterial A natural or synthetic material that is suitable for introduction into living tissue, especially as part of a medical device.

Cell degranulation A cellular process that releases antimicrobial cytotoxic or other molecules from secretory vesicles called granules found inside some cells.

Chronic venous insufficiency (CVI) Occurs when the venous wall muscles and/or valves in the leg veins fail to work effectively. The net result is that return of blood to the heart is compromised.

Comorbid condition The presence of one or more additional disorders or disease co-occurring with a primary disease or disorder.

Cyclic voltammetry One of the most widely used techniques for qualitative analysis relating to electrochemical reactions such as redox processes, heterogeneous electron-transfer reactions, and adsorption processes. The method employs a triangular waveform in which the potential of a stationary working electrode is scanned linearly over a defined range and the current measured. The nature of the resulting profile can be used to extract diagnostic information on the species present within the sample.

Cytotoxic A material or chemical species that is toxic to living cells.

Deacetylation Removal of acetate groups from polymers such as Chitosan.

Diabetic foot ulcer (DFU) Typically a patch of broken skin usually on the lower leg or feet. Nerve damage and peripheral vascular disease are among the main contributors and without adequate blood flow, healing is compromised and the wounds can become chronic.

Dressing A piece of material used to cover and protect a wound.

eHealth The transfer of health resources and health care by electronic means.

Electroblowing Process of blowing air in conjunction with electrospinning in order to increase the flow rate and alter the dimensions of the spun fibers. Net effect is the drawing the solution from the nozzle while generating a strong initial stretching force.

Electrospinning A method of producing small diameter fibers typically in the low micron to nanometer range. An electric force is employed to draw charged threads of polymer solutions or polymer melts up into the requisite fiber structure.

Enzyme-linked immunosorbant assay (ELISA) Antibody-based diagnostic procedure in which an immobilized antibody is used to capture the target analyte (typically a protein). A second antibody is then introduced which binds to the captured protein. This second antibody is bound to an enzyme which when provided with the appropriate substrate generates a measurable signal that enables quantification of the target protein.

Etiology The investigation or attribution of the cause or reason for a disease or condition.

Extracellular matrix (ECM) A diverse collection of molecules and polymeric components secreted by cells with the aim of providing a physical framework and biochemical environment to support neighboring cells.

Extracellular polymeric substances (EPS) Material that is typically deposited by bacteria prior to establishing a biofilm.

Exudate A mass of cells and fluid that seeps out of blood vessels or an organ, especially in inflammation.

Film dressing Thin polymeric layer—typically transparent and semipermeable to oxygen and water vapor while being impermeable to bacteria. They can be applied directly onto the wound or as an addition to other dressings to improve the fluid barrier properties.

Foam dressing Film consisting of a porous polymeric network and typically used for moderate/high draining wounds. Their ability to absorb wound fluid is dependent on the foam thickness and the polymeric material.

Gauze A loosely woven surgical dressing, usually made of cotton.

Hemocompatibility Compatibility of a substance with blood.

Hydrocolloid A moist wound dressing with a backing material such as a semipermeable film, foam, or nonwoven polyesters fibers.

Hydrogel Dressings composed of a single or mixed hydrated polymer that can retain at least 20% of their weigh in water.

Hydrophilic Materials that possesses the tendency to mix with, dissolve in, or be wetted by water.

Hydroxyl groups An oxygen containing group based on an alcohol or OH group.

Hyperglycemia The presence of excess glucose in the bloodstream.

Hypoxia The deficiency of the amount of oxygen reaching tissues.

Immunoassay Diagnostic technique in which target proteins (the antigen) are captured by the appropriate antibody. There is a wide spectrum of approaches but most involve sandwich based assays (ELISA) or lateral flow to provide a quantitative measure.

In vivo Process performed or taking place in a living organism.

Isoelectric Two or more molecular entities that have the same number of valence electrons and the structure.

Lateral flow immunoassay A disposable strip based on a modified ELISA methodology.

Maceration The softening and breaking down of skin as a result of prolonged exposure to moisture.

Matrix metalloproteinases (MMPs) Class of protein which, when present at elevated levels, can prolong inflammation and delay wound healing.

mHealth Abbreviation for mobile health, a term used for the practice of medicine and public health supported by mobile devices.

Negative pressure wound therapy (NPWT) Wound management technique in which the wound is subject to negative pressure in an attempt to remove excess exudate from wound.

Nernst equation Relates the reduction potential of a half cell at any point in time to the standard electrode potential, temperature, activity, and reaction quotient of the underlying reactions and species used.

Neuroischemia The combined effect of diabetic neuropathy and ischemia, whereby macrovascular disease and, in some instances, microvascular dysfunction impair perfusion in a diabetic foot.

Nitric oxide (NO) Versatile molecule that has an antibacterial action but is also used for intercell signaling.

Nyquist's theorem Also known as the sampling theorem, it is used in the digitization of analog signals. For analog-to-digital conversion (ADC) to result in a faithful reproduction of the signal, samples of the analog waveform must be taken frequently.

Osmolarity The total concentration of a solution expressed as the total number of solute particles per liter.

Oxidation A chemical reaction in which an atom or ion loses an electron, and therefore undergoes an increase in valence.

Pathophysiology The disorder physiological processes associated with disease or injury.

pH A figure relating to the acidity or alkalinity of a solution on a logarithmic scale. The pH is equal to $\log_{10}c$, where c is the hydrogen ion concentration in moles per liter.

Plaster Colloquial term for an adhesive strip of material for covering cuts and wounds.

Point of care testing (POCT) Medical diagnostic testing performed outside the clinical laboratory and in a location close to where the patient is receiving care—either by the bedside or in the home.

Polycatonic A molecule or chemical complex having positive charges at several sites.

Potentiometry A method used in electroanalytical chemistry, usually to find the concentration of a solute in solution. In poteniometric measurements, the potential between two electrodes is measured using a high impedance voltmeter.

Quorum sensing A process through which bacteria (Gram positive or negative) sense one another through cell-to-cell interactions transmitted by signaling molecules (AHLs or AIPs). This enables gene expression to be regulated according to the density of bacterial population and modulates the behavior of the community.

Radiofrequency identification (RFID) Small antenna that can be used to wirelessly relay information to and from a device.

Reactive oxygen species (ROS) Chemical species such as superoxide, peroxide, and hydroxyl radical, which are released by the host's immune defenses.

Redox The process of both oxidation and reduction reactions considered together as complimentary processes

Reduction A half reaction in which a chemical species decreases its oxidation number, usually by gaining electrons

Screen printed electrode Development of electrochemical sensor arrays through a print technique that would normally be applied to art and fabric designs. Rather than deposit pigments, the printing processes use conductive (typically carbon based) inks.

Selectivity The extent to which particular analyte(s) in a complex mixture can be determined without interference from other components in the mixture

Square wave voltammetry (SQWV) A sensitive differential technique in which a waveform of a symmetrical square wave (with one pulse in the forward direction and one in the reverse), superimposed on a base staircase potential, is applied to the working electrode. The current is sampled during each square wave cycle, once at the end of the forward pulse and once at the end of the reverse pulse. The difference between the two measurements is plotted versus the base staircase potential. The resulting peak shaped voltammogram is symmetrical about the half wave potential and the peak current is proportional to the concentration.

Telecare Remote care for the elderly and the physically less able people, providing the care and reassurance needed to allow them to remain living in their homes

Telehealth The collection of means or methods for enhancing health care, public health, and health education delivery, and support using telecommunications

Telemedicine The remote diagnosis and treatment of patients by means of telecommunications technology

Tissue inhibitors of metalloproteinase (TIMPs) Chemical species—natural and synthetic that can, when incorporated within a dressing, aid attenuation of the activity of metalloproteinase activity.

Ulcer The loss of full skin thickness with exposure of dermal, potentially, subdermal tissue. Ulcers are associated with a loss of normal tissue viability

Venous leg ulcer (VLU) Estimated to be the predominant source of chronic wounds, VLU are thought to result from the improper/inefficient operation of the venous valves. See also CVI.

Viscosity The state of being thick, sticky, and semifluid in consistency, due to internal friction.

Voltammetry An electroanalytical method used in analytical chemistry to determine the chemical make-up of a sample substance by measuring the current as the potential is varied.

Wound The disruption of the anatomic structure and its function in any body part.

X-ray photoelectron spectroscopy (XPS) Surface characterization technique in which the chemical composition and functionality can be determined.

SUBJECT INDEX

E

F

G

H

X

Edwards Brothers Malloy
Ann Arbor MI. USA
July 25, 2016